Cardiovascular Pathophysiology

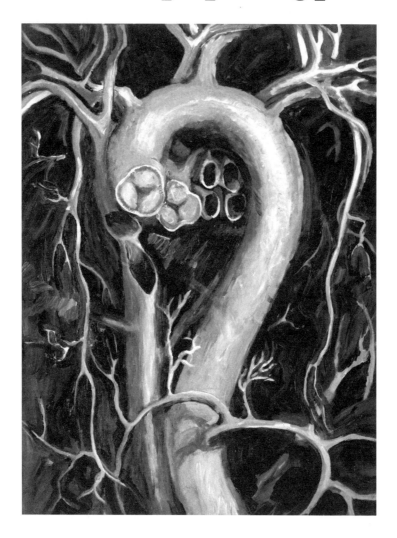

Cardiovascular Pathophysiology

Fred M. Kusumoto, M.D.

Assistant Clinical Professor
Department of Medicine
Division of Cardiology
University of New Mexico School of Medicine
Director, Electrophysiology and Pacing Service
Lovelace Medical Center
Albuquerque, New Mexico

Fence Creek
Publishing

Madison,
Connecticut

Typesetter: Pagesetters, Brattleboro, VT
Printer: Port City Press, Baltimore, MD
Illustrations by Visible Productions, Fort Collins, CO
Distributors:

United States and Canada
Blackwell Science, Inc.
Commerce Place
350 Main Street
Malden, MA 02148
Telephone orders: 800-215-1000 or 781-388-8250
Fax orders: 781-388-8270

Australia
Blackwell Science, PTY LTD.
54 University Street
Carlton, Victoria 3053
Telephone orders: 61-39-347-0300
Fax orders: 61-39-347-5001

Outside North America and Australia
Blackwell Science, LTD.
c/o Marston Book Service, LTD.
P.O. Box 269
Abingdon Oxon, OX 14 4XN England
Telephone orders: 44-1-235-465500
Fax orders: 44-1-235-465555

1 2 3 4 5 6 7 8 9 10

TABLE OF CONTENTS

CONTRIBUTORS

Phoebe Ashley, M.D.
Cardiology Fellow
Department of Medicine
Division of Cardiology
University of New Mexico School of Medicine
Albuquerque, New Mexico

Andrew U. Chai, M.D.
Clinical Instructor
Department of Medicine
Division of Cardiology
University of New Mexico School of Medicine
Albuquerque, New Mexico

James C. Fields, M.D.
Medical Center Physicians
Nampa, Idaho

Sreenivas Gudimetla, M.D.
Senior Cardiology Fellow
Department of Medicine
Division of Cardiology
University of New Mexico School of Medicine
Albuquerque, New Mexico

Fred M. Kusumoto, M.D.
Assistant Clinical Professor
Department of Medicine
Division of Cardiology
University of New Mexico School of Medicine
Director, Electrophysiology and Pacing Service
Lovelace Medical Center
Albuquerque, New Mexico

The heart has always occupied an important spiritual and medical position for humanity. The number of people affected by heart disease has rapidly expanded over the past 50 years; it is now estimated that approximately 20 million people in the United States alone have some form of heart disease. In the United States, cardiovascular disease is responsible for more than 70% of the deaths in people over 70 years of age. Fortunately, medical knowledge about the cardiovascular system has undergone a dramatic expansion, which is, in part, responsible for a 49% reduction in the death rate due to cardiovascular causes and the emergence of the subspecialty of cardiology. In particular, exciting discoveries of the pathophysiologic basis of cardiovascular diseases have provided the impetus for the development of new treatment strategies and technologies.

Cardiovascular Pathophysiology has been designed for anyone interested in a comprehensive introduction to the pathophysiology of cardiovascular diseases. The book is divided along anatomic lines: heart muscle, the specialized conduction system, coronary arteries, valves, pericardium, congenital abnormalities, and great vessels are sequentially discussed. In each chapter, relevant anatomy and physiology are reviewed before an extended discussion of pathophysiologic processes. I hope that this chapter structure will facilitate the application of basic science concepts to the disease process. An intended consequence of this chapter structure is that some concepts are discussed separately in several chapters. For example, pressure–volume loops, which are important for understanding the effects of different loading conditions on the heart, are discussed extensively in both the cardiomyopathies and valvular abnormalities chapters. I believe this repetition is important since it allows each chapter to be read separately and also implicitly stresses the interrelated nature of cardiovascular pathophysiology. Two appendices review the patho-physiologic mechanisms of physical examination findings and introduce the reader to some of the diagnostic tests available to the cardiologist. These appendices are not intended as exhaustive discussions of these two broad topics but rather provide a means by which the student can integrate pathophysiologic concepts from different chapters.

Many new discoveries at the molecular level have fundamentally changed our clinical understanding of heart disease. I have attempted to incorporate some of these important findings into *Cardiovascular Pathophysiology* to help students form sequential bridges from molecular biology to organ pathophysiology and finally to the bedside of the patient. Each chapter begins with a clinical case, and as the chapter proceeds, relevant pathophysiology is applied to the case until the clinical case's final resolution at the end of the chapter. This chapter format has been chosen to illustrate the importance of the scientific foundation of medicine and the application of pathophysiology to disease processes.

The book has been specifically designed for second- and third-year medical students. However, I hope that college students interested in cardiovascular pathophysiology and fourth-year medical students preparing for their board certification, and physicians interested in a basic guide to the new pathophysiologic basis of cardiology will find this book useful. However, this book is not intended to provide a guide for the management of patients with heart disease. Discussion of treatment is limited to only specific situations that illuminate the practical applications of pathophysiology.

I hope that you find this text interesting and rewarding. I welcome your comments and suggestions.

Fred M. Kusumoto, M.D.

ACKNOWLEDGMENTS

The production of any book requires the concerted input from a number of people. I would like to thank Matt Harris for his understanding over repeated missed deadlines. His patience and thoughtful recommendations were always appreciated. Thank you to Jane Edwards for her fine editing. It has been a special privilege for me to work with my coauthors who took large amounts of time during particularly busy periods in their lives to contribute to *Cardiovascular Pathophysiology*.

I would like to acknowledge Betty Wise, Beth Mooney, Carleen Kimber, Kim D'Lao, and Bert Danielson who provided superb secretarial support for this project. Ratana Gross, Donna Rollinson, Sharon Walker, Carolyn Johns, Joe Jaramillo, Ginny Sigler, Conni Brooks, Gail West, Cindy Boyson, Julia Stone, Judy Ridgon, Jamie Rivet, Esther Hattler, Barbara Dillard, and Cheri Miller were particularly invaluable for helping me keep my clinical responsibilities in relative order during this project. I would like to thank Steven Mickelsen, Murali Bathina, and Chamisa MacIndoe for technical support and their feedback on several of the chapters.

A very special thank you to Haruo and Sumiko Kusumoto for teaching me the importance of being constantly inquisitive (and putting up with far more than the usual 434 questions a 5-year-old asks a day). Finally, as I write these last words amidst the barking of a Labrador retriever, the building of a Duplo house, and the smell of fresh foccacio, I thank Hana, Miya, and Laura for their constant understanding, personal support, and encouragement, which make tasks like this possible.

To Hana, Miya, and Laura for their heartfelt support and love.

INTRODUCTION

Cardiovascular Pathophysiology is one of six titles in the *Pathophysiology Series* from Fence Creek Publishing. These books have been designed as course supplements and aids for board review for second- and third-year medical students who are studying the pathophysiology of individual organ systems. Each book in the series is an overview of a major organ system with an emphasis on pathophysiology. Diagnosis, treatment, and management of specific diseases are also covered at a level appropriate for preclinical study. Each chapter has one or more clinical cases integrated throughout the text; the resolution of these cases requires mastery of the pathophysiologic concepts presented in the chapter.

Each book in the *Pathophysiology Series* shares common features and formats. Difficult concepts are presented in a brief and focused format to provide a pedagogical aid that facilitates both knowledge acquisition and review. Extensive use of margin notes, figures, tables, and board-review questions illuminates the basic science principles of pathophysiology.

Given the long gestation period necessary to publish a book, it is often impossible for publishers to keep pace with the rapid changes and advances. However, the authors and the publisher recognize the need to have access to the most current information and are committed to keeping *Cardiovascular Pathophysiology* as up-to-date as possible between editions. As the field of cardiovascular pathophysiology evolves, updates to this text may be posted on our web site periodically at http://www.fencecreek.com.

We hope that the student finds the format and the text material relevant, interesting, and challenging. The Fence Creek staff and the author welcome your comments and suggestions for use in future editions.

Chapter 1

CARDIOMYOPATHIES

James C. Fields, M.D., and Fred M. Kusumoto, M.D.

Case Study: Introduction	Mr. Kurt Buecheler was a 59-year-old man with a history of high blood pressure since his early 30s. He had been poorly compliant with medicines but had no significant sequelae to his hypertension. However, over the previous several weeks Mr. Buecheler noted shortness of breath with exertion. In addition, during this period, he woke up at night and felt as though he was "gasping for air."
	On examination in the physician's office Mr. Buecheler was noted to have a blood pressure of 208/106 mm Hg. On auscultation of his lungs he was noted to have fine crackles at both bases on inspiration. Auscultation of his heart revealed a loud fourth heart sound (S_4). What are the possible pathophysiologic processes that were occurring in Mr. Buecheler?

▌ INTRODUCTION

Systole: Greek for contraction.
Diastole: From the Greek *diastellein*, which means ''to expand.''

While philosopher-scientists have identified and described the heart since the Middle Ages, it was not until William Harvey's seminal treatise *De motu cordis et sanguinis*, published in 1628, that cardiovascular anatomy and physiology were first described accurately. The principal function of the heart is to provide an adequate supply of blood to the tissues of the body. When the heart does not perform this basic function, heart failure is present.

Heart failure is a condition that produces a characteristic constellation of symptoms (e.g., fatigue, shortness of breath). Heart failure can arise from several mechanisms: abnormalities of the heart muscle, abnormal valvular function, abnormal heart rhythms, and congenital structural abnormalities. This chapter focuses on heart failure caused by

Mechanisms of Heart Failure Caused by Abnormal Cardiac Myocytes
Poor contractile function (systolic dysfunction)
Abnormal filling (diastolic dysfunction)
Hypertrophy associated with obstruction

abnormalities of the heart muscle (*cardiomyopathies*). Valvular abnormalities, arrhythmias, and congenital abnormalities are discussed in later chapters.

Abnormalities of heart muscle can cause heart failure by three mechanisms: poor contractile function (*systolic dysfunction*), abnormal filling of the ventricle (*diastolic dysfunction*), and hypertrophy that is associated with *obstruction to flow*. This chapter is divided into two sections: first, normal cellular physiology of the cardiac myocyte, normal cardiac anatomy, and normal cardiac organ physiology are sequentially reviewed; second, the pathophysiology of different types of heart failure is discussed. In general, our discussion of heart failure focuses on the left ventricle; however, in the last section we discuss the effects of right ventricular failure.

■ NORMAL CARDIAC PHYSIOLOGY

NORMAL CELLULAR PHYSIOLOGY

Cellular Architecture. The heart has four chambers whose walls are composed of muscular tissue. Individual cardiac myocytes are large cells (approximately 100 μm in length) with a similar architecture to skeletal muscle. Within the cardiac myocyte are longitudinally arranged myofibrils that are composed of serially connected contractile units called sarcomeres (Fig. 1-1).

FIG. 1-1
CELLULAR ARCHITECTURE FOR TWO ADJACENT MYOCYTES. Each myocyte has a number of myofibrils that are composed of longitudinally arranged sarcomeres. The cell membrane of the myocytes, or sarcolemma, has deep invaginations known as T tubules that allow rapid spread of membrane depolarization to all regions of the myocyte. Around the myofibrils is a densely branching system of tubules called the sarcoplasmic reticulum. The sarcoplasmic reticulum is important for the storage of intracellular calcium.

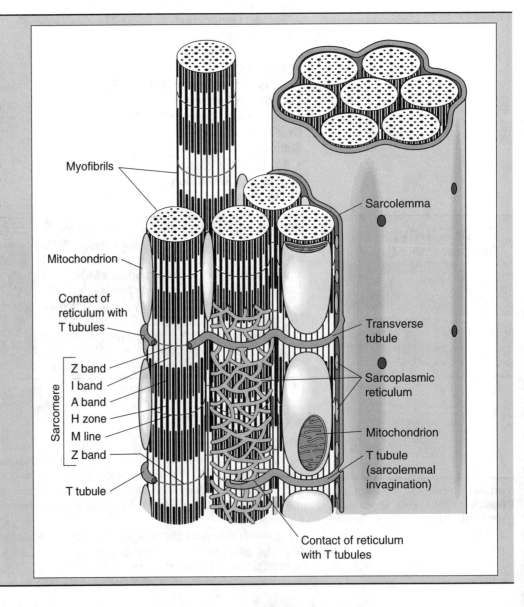

Each sarcomere is composed of specialized protein molecules that can interact with one another and cause shortening of the sarcomere, which in turn causes myocyte contraction. The proteins of the sarcomere are arranged in thick and thin filaments (Fig. 1-2). The thick filaments are composed of *myosin*, and the thin filaments are composed of *actin*, as well as the regulatory proteins *troponin* and *tropomyosin*. The thick filaments are anchored at the M line, and the thin filaments are anchored at the Z line. The thick and thin filaments are interleaved at their free ends. The overlapping of the thick and thin filaments results in a dark band between the Z lines called the A band.

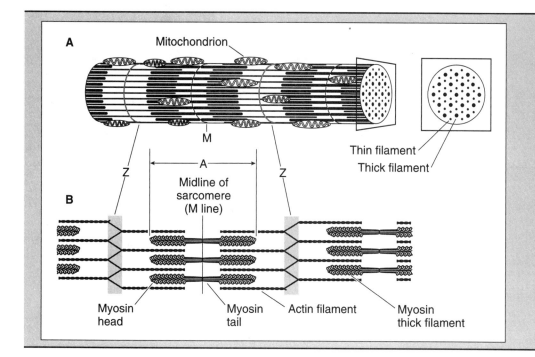

FIG. 1-2
SARCOMERE ARCHITECTURE.
(A) A drawing of a sarcomere is shown. Notice that each thick filament is surrounded by six thin filaments. (B) A closer view of the molecules making up the thick and thin filaments is shown. The thick filament is made up of bunches of 300–400 myosin molecules. The thin filament is composed, in part, by two actin molecules twisted in a helical arrangement.

Thick Filaments. The myosin molecule is a dimer of two myosin heavy chains (MHCs), each with a globular head and a filamentous, intertwined tail. Thick filaments are formed when 300–400 myosin molecules are packed together in a parallel fashion, with their tails attached to the M line. Each pair of MHCs is associated with two pairs of smaller proteins called myosin light chains (MLCs) [each with a molecular weight of 16,000 to 20,000 D]. The light chains are located on the globular head of the myosin molecule (see Chap. 3, Fig. 3-5). In addition, the myosin head contains adenosine triphosphatase (ATPase) and an actin-binding site.

Approximately 10–15 distinct *MHC* genes have been identified. In cardiac myocytes, two types of *MHC* genes, which produce proteins with different ATPase activity (α-MHC and β-MHC), are located adjacent to each other on chromosome 14. The α-MHC has greater ATPase activity than the β-MHC. In the fetus, equal amounts of α- and β-MHCs are observed in the heart. However, shortly after birth and through adulthood, the β-MHC becomes predominant (90%–95%).

Thin Filaments. A double helix polymer of actin molecules arranged on a backbone of filamentous tropomyosin dimers forms the thin filament (Fig. 1-3). At 400 Angström (Å) intervals, each tropomyosin molecule is associated with a troponin complex, which functions as the regulatory subunit of the actin–myosin complex. The filamentous actin polymer is approximately 42,000 D and combines with another actin polymer to form a helical dimer. Six different actin proteins with a significant amount of amino acid homology have been identified. In addition to being an important component of the thin filament of myocytes, actin is an ubiquitous molecule that forms the cytoskeleton in nearly all cells.

FIG. 1-3
THIN FILAMENT STRUCTURE.
The thin filament is formed from a double helix of actin. The ends of the thin filaments intertwine with the ends of thin filaments from an adjacent sarcomere to form the Z line. Within the groove formed by the actin helix are two strands of tropomyosin. At 400 Å intervals, a troponin complex (made up of T, I, and C polypeptides) is present. The troponin complex "covers" the myosin-binding site in the absence of calcium ions.

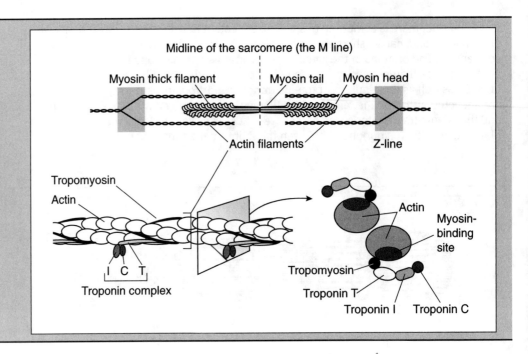

Thick filaments are "bunches" of myosin molecules; **thin filaments** include actin, tropomyosin, and the troponin complex (T, I, and C).

Tropomyosin is also formed as an α-helical dimer from polypeptides approximately 280 amino acids long. Tropomyosin filaments are embedded into the groove formed by the twisted actin filaments. Associated with each tropomyosin molecule is a complex of three troponin peptides (troponin-T, troponin-I, and troponin-C), which provide important regulatory functions for contraction. Troponin-T (so named because it binds tropomyosin) serves to link tropomyosin to troponin-I and troponin-C. Troponin-I (inhibitory subunit) interacts with tropomyosin to allow only weak binding between the myosin globular heads and actin and inhibits the myosin ATPase. Troponin-C (calcium ion [Ca^{2+}]–binding subunit), which has considerable homology to calmodulin, when bound to Ca^{2+} removes the inhibitory effect of troponin-I, which allows a strong interaction between myosin and actin and allows activation of the myosin ATPase.

Thick Filament–Thin Filament Orientation. The thick filaments extend in both directions from their anchor at the M line. In a similar fashion, the thin filaments extend in both directions from their anchor at the Z line. The thick and thin filaments are interleaved in such a way that the myosin globular heads are in proximity to the helix of actin molecules along the length of the filaments. Each thick filament is surrounded by six thin filaments, and each thin filament is surrounded by three thick filaments (see Fig. 1-2).

Thick Filament and Thin Filament Interaction (Contraction and Relaxation). Interaction between the thick and thin filaments is responsible for both cardiac myocyte contraction and relaxation. The sliding filament hypothesis was originally proposed by Huxley and Hanson in 1954 and has gained widespread acceptance as the mechanism of contraction for all types of muscle. Cytosolic Ca^{2+} concentrations play a central role in the regulation of thick and thin filament interaction.

Contraction. The process of contraction is produced by a cycle of cross-linking between the globular head of the myosin molecule and a myosin-binding site on the actin molecule (Fig. 1-4). Repeated conformational changes in the myosin molecule with each cycle of cross-linking slides the thin filament relative to the thick filament. Since the thin and thick filaments are anchored at the Z lines and M lines, respectively, the movement of the filaments relative to one another causes shortening of the sarcomere. This is seen histologically as shortening of the distance between the Z lines and widening of the A band.

The current molecular model for contraction is illustrated in Fig. 1-4. In the relaxed state, the troponin complex blocks the myosin-binding site of the actin molecule. The binding of Ca^{2+} to the troponin complex causes tropomyosin to become more deeply

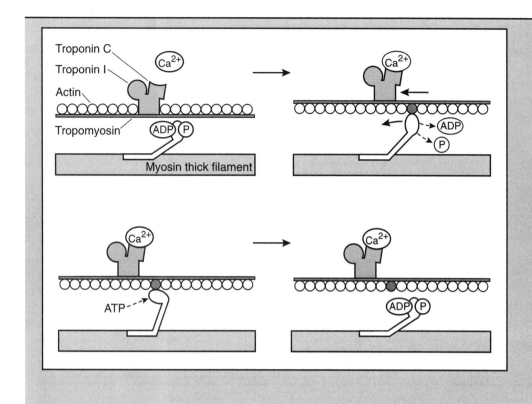

FIG. 1-4
PROPOSED CELLULAR MECHANISM OF CONTRACTION. During diastole, tropomyosin keeps the head of the myosin molecule from strongly interacting with actin. With contraction, intracellular calcium ions (Ca^{2+}) released from the sarcoplasmic reticulum diffuse to the sarcomere. Ca^{2+} binding to troponin-C causes the tropomyosin molecule to move deeper into the thin filament groove, which uncovers actin-binding sites. The myosin head and actin form a strong attachment, and the myosin head flexes with the removal of adenosine diphosphate (ADP) and phosphate (P). An adenosine triphosphate (ATP) molecule attaches to the myosin head and is hydrolyzed to ADP and P, causing separation of the myosin head and actin. The cycle continues to repeat until Ca^{2+} concentrations drop as a result of resequestration of Ca^{2+} in the sarcoplasmic reticulum, which initiates diastole.

embedded in the thin filament groove, which exposes actin-binding sites that allow a strong interaction between actin and myosin. This interaction leads to the release of bound adenosine diphosphate (ADP) and bound phosphate (P) and flexion of the myosin head, and since the actin and myosin filaments are tightly bound, causes the actin filament to slide relative to the myosin filament. Once the "stroke" is completed, ADP is released, and adenosine triphosphate (ATP) becomes bound to the myosin head, which causes "release" of actin from the myosin head and returns the myosin head to its original 90-degree orientation. The strong binding between actin and myosin increases the myosin ATPase activity by 200-fold. The cycle is then repeated with the myosin head attaching to a new actin-binding site farther along the actin filament. Thus, the chemical energy of ATP is converted to the mechanical energy of contraction.

The percentage of troponin-binding sites occupied by Ca^{2+} determines the number of filaments recruited during contraction. Thus, the magnitude of contractile force generated is to some degree dependent on the cytosolic Ca^{2+} concentration achieved.

Relaxation. Relaxation is initiated by removal of Ca^{2+} from the cytosol. At low Ca^{2+} concentrations, the troponin complex blocks the myosin-binding sites on actin. The thick and thin filaments are allowed to slide past one another. The sarcomere lengthens passively to a neutral position. This neutral position is defined by forces extrinsic to the sarcomere. As outlined below, Ca^{2+} efflux from the cytosol is mediated by ATP, and therefore, in part, relaxation is an energy-requiring process. The efficiency of relaxation depends on the degree to which actin–myosin cross-linking is inhibited. The extrinsic forces that stretch the sarcomere to its length just prior to contraction, taken together, are termed *preload*.

Regulation of Intracellular Ca^{2+} Concentrations.

Since the classic experiments by Ringer in 1882, it has been known that contraction of the heart depends on the presence of Ca^{2+}. Control of intracellular Ca^{2+} concentrations is critical in controlling the cycle of contraction and relaxation. There are two mechanisms by which intracellular Ca^{2+} is increased: *entry of extracellular Ca^{2+}* and the *release of intracellular stored Ca^{2+}* (Fig. 1-5).

FIG. 1-5

CALCIUM ION (CA^{2+}) MOVE-MENT IN THE CARDIAC MYO-CYTE DURING THE CARDIAC CYCLE. (A) Initially, cytosolic Ca^{2+} concentrations are very low (10^{-7} mol/L), although there is a large amount stored in the sarcoplasmic reticulum. (B) The membrane is depolarized, which causes a relatively small amount of Ca^{2+} to flow into the cell from the extracellular space. The small increase in intracellu-lar Ca^{2+} stimulates the release of a large amount of the Ca^{2+} stored in the sarcoplasmic re-ticulum via the Ca^{2+}-release channels. (C) The increased in-tracellular Ca^{2+} diffuses to the sarcomere and leads to contrac-tion (systole). (D) Ca^{2+} is then re-sequestered into the sarcoplas-mic reticulum by Ca^{2+}–aden-osine triphosphatase (Ca^{2+}-ATPase).

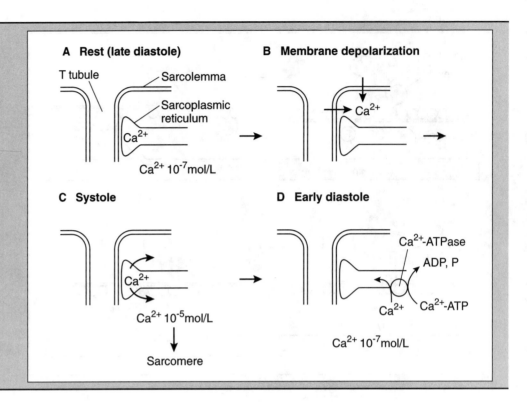

Sarco is from the Greek word *sarkos*, which means "flesh."

Ca^{2+}-release channels are also known as ryanodine recep-tors, because they bind to ryan-odine, a plant alkaloid.

Steps in Cardiac Myocyte Contraction:
1. Depolarization of the surface membrane causes a small in-crease in intracellular Ca^{2+}.
2. The small increase in intra-cellular Ca^{2+} leads to release of a large amount of Ca^{2+} from the sarcoplasmic retic-ulum.
3. Increased intracellular Ca^{2+} diffuses to the sarcomere and binds to troponin, and the sar-comere contracts.

Ca^{2+} is also removed from the intracellular space by two pro-teins in the sarcolemma. The Ca^{2+}-ATPase protein is also lo-cated in the sarcolemma. In addi-tion the Na$^+$–Ca^{2+}-exchanger removes Ca^{2+} from the cyto-plasm (see Chap. 2).

Cardiac myocyte contraction is initiated by cell membrane depolarization. When the cell membrane of the cardiac myocyte is depolarized, extracellular sodium ions (Na$^+$) and Ca^{2+} flow into the cell via voltage-sensitive ion channels (see Chap. 2). The surface membrane of the cardiac myocyte (sarcolemma) has deep invaginations called *trans-verse tubules* (or *T tubules*) that allow rapid spread of the depolarizing wave throughout all regions of the cell (see Fig. 1-1). This cell architecture leads to a widespread but small increase in intracellular Ca^{2+} concentrations. However, the amount of Ca^{2+} that enters the cell from the extracellular space is not sufficient for contraction. Extracellular Ca^{2+} influx triggers the release of intracellular Ca^{2+}, which is stored an organelle called the *sarcoplasmic reticulum*. The sarcoplasmic reticulum is composed of a widespread branching system of tubules floating within the intracellular space (sarcoplasm). The actual mechanism by which the small amount of Ca^{2+} influx from the extracellular space causes release of large stores of sarcoplasmic reticulum Ca^{2+} is not known. It is, however, known that the Ca^{2+} is released from the cisternae of the sarcoplasmic retic-ulum via specialized channels (Ca^{2+}-release channels). (The sarcoplasmic reticulum is well developed in mammalian hearts; however, in the frog heart, cardiac myocytes have a much less extensive sarcoplasmic reticulum, which suggests that Ca^{2+} fluxes across the sarcolemma have a greater role.) Release of intracellular stores of Ca^{2+} causes a 100-fold increase in intracellular Ca^{2+} (from 10^{-7} mol/L to 10^{-5} mol/L). Ca^{2+} diffuses throughout the sarcomere and binds to troponin, which allows strong binding between thick and thin filaments and thus contraction.

After the sarcomere contracts, its relaxation is observed. Relaxation (diastole) is mediated by decreasing intracellular concentrations of Ca^{2+}. The actual triggering mechanisms are unknown, but it appears that Ca^{2+} is resequestered into the sar-coplasmic reticulum by Ca^{2+}-ATPase. Ca^{2+}-ATPase has a large "head" that protrudes into the cytoplasm and contains the ATP-binding site and a series of 10 α-helical transmembrane segments that are important for Ca^{2+} binding (Fig. 1-6). The activity of the Ca^{2+}-ATPase is regulated by a 22 kD protein embedded in the wall of the sarco-plasmic reticulum, *phospholamban*.

Since both systole and diastole are mediated by cytosolic Ca^{2+} concentrations, both systole and diastole can be regulated by processes that control intracellular Ca^{2+} con-centrations. For example, catecholamines activate a cyclic adenosine monophosphate

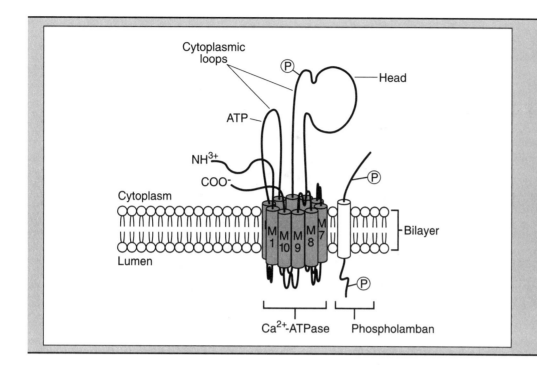

FIG. 1-6
STRUCTURE OF THE CALCIUM PUMP (CA^{2+}-ATPASE). Ca^{2+}-ATPase has a complex structure with ten transmembrane α-helical segments that form a Ca^{2+} channel (M$_1$–M$_{10}$). The adenosine triphosphate (ATP)–binding site is located in the cytoplasmic portion of the protein. The Ca^{2+}-ATPase is associated with a smaller protein called phospholamban, which has important regulatory effects. Phosphorylation sites on the Ca^{2+}-ATPase and phospholamban are designated by P.

(cAMP) second messenger system via cell membrane β-adrenergic receptors, which leads to the phosphorylation of various proteins involved in the regulation of cytosolic Ca^{2+} concentrations. The phosphorylation of cell membrane Ca^{2+} channels increases the influx of Ca^{2+} and enhances systole. The phosphorylation of phospholamban activates Ca^{2+}-ATPase, which causes increased sequestration of Ca^{2+} in the sarcoplasmic reticulum and thus enhances relaxation. Therefore, the activation of β-adrenergic receptors enhances both systole and diastole.

ANATOMY

The heart is composed of four chambers: the left and right atria and the left and right ventricles. The ventricles are muscular, pumping chambers, and the atria are thin-walled chambers that act as "priming pumps" for the ventricles and are responsible for the final 20%–30% of ventricular filling.

The course of blood is summarized in Figs. 1-7 and 1-8. Unoxygenated blood from the inferior vena cava and superior vena cava enter the right atrium. From the right atrium blood flows through the tricuspid valve into the right ventricle.

The right ventricle, the most anterior structure of the heart, is made up of the free wall, the intraventricular septum, and the right ventricular outflow tract. The endocardial surface of the right ventricle is heavily trabeculated. The right ventricle pumps blood into the low-resistance vessels of the lungs and therefore has relatively thin walls compared to the left ventricle. The right ventricle's semilunar shape is defined by the circular shape of the intraventricular septum, which conforms to the shape of the left ventricular chamber (Fig. 1-9).

From the right ventricle blood flows through the pulmonic valve to the lungs. In the lungs blood becomes oxygenated and returns to the left atrium via the pulmonary veins. Blood flows through the mitral valve and into the left ventricle (see Fig. 1-8).

The left ventricle is the muscular pumping chamber of the heart and accounts for the majority of the cardiac mass. It is a cylindrical, or "bullet-shaped," chamber made up of the anterior, lateral, inferior, septal, and apical walls, as well as the left ventricular outflow tract. The endocardial surface is less trabeculated than that of the right ventricle. The anterior and posterior papillary muscles of the mitral valve extend from the anterolateral and posteriomedial endocardial surfaces, respectively, and attach to the mitral valve leaflets via the chordae tendineae (Fig. 1-9; see Fig. 1-8).

FIG. 1-7
RIGHT-SIDED CHAMBERS OF THE HEART. Blood returns to the right atria via the inferior and superior venae cavae. Blood flows into the right ventricle via the tricuspid valve. Right ventricular contraction causes blood to be ejected into the pulmonary arteries via the pulmonic valve.

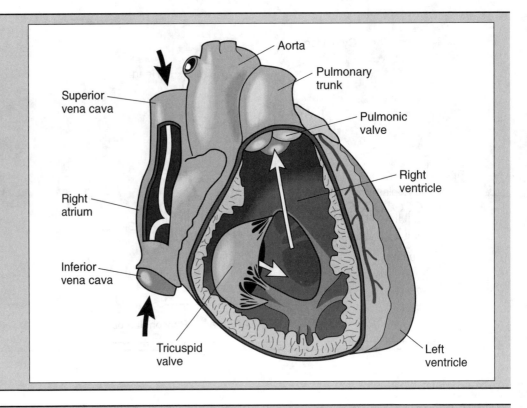

FIG. 1-8
LEFT-SIDED CHAMBERS OF THE HEART. Heart with the anterior portions of the right ventricle and left ventricle removed. Oxygenated blood returns to the left atrium via the four pulmonary veins. Blood flows into the left ventricle via the mitral valve. Left ventricular contraction causes blood to be ejected through the aortic valve into the aorta and out to the body.

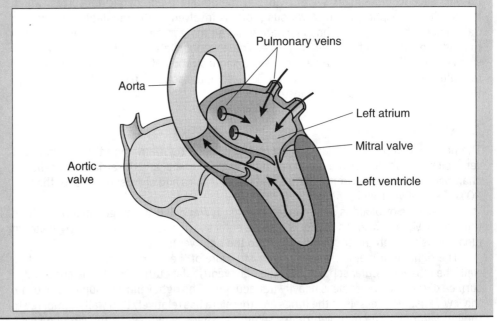

The heart lies freely in the pericardial sac and is attached to the mediastinum only at the great vessels. The valve plane of the heart is referred to as the *base* of the heart, and the tip of the left ventricle is called the *apex*. The heart is oriented with the base in the mediastinum and the apex extending inferiorly, laterally, and anteriorly. Since the apex is relatively close to the chest wall, the motion of the apex (called the apical impulse) can be felt by placing the palm over the chest wall.

ORGAN PHYSIOLOGY

Cardiac Cycle (Pressure–Time Analysis). The cardiac cycle is normally considered *temporally* by dividing the heartbeat into systole and diastole. During diastole, blood flows from the peripheral circulation into the right atrium and from the

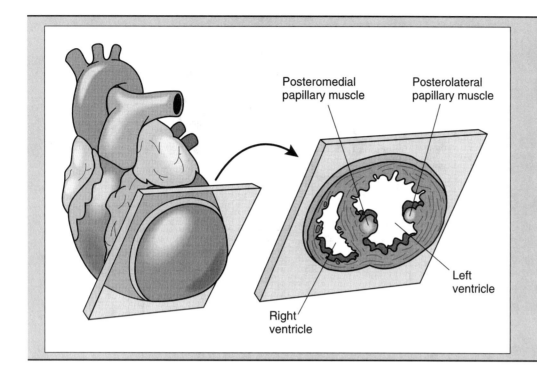

FIG. 1-9
CROSS-SECTION OF THE VEN-TRICLES. The right ventricle is anterior and has a crescent shape. The left ventricle is a thick-walled, doughnut-shaped structure. Both of the ventricles are efficient for the types of loads they handle.

Posteromedial papillary muscle

Posterolateral papillary muscle

Left ventricle

Right ventricle

pulmonary circulation into the left atrium (Fig. 1-10). There is free communication between the atrial and ventricular chambers through the open tricuspid and mitral valves, so that during early diastole, blood flows freely from the venous circulation into the atria and through the tricuspid and mitral valves, and fills both the left and right ventricles. Early diastolic filling normally accounts for most ventricular filling.

The contraction of the atrial chambers (atrial systole) occurs at the end of ventricular diastole. The contraction of the atrial chambers moves additional blood into the ventricular chambers and accounts for the final 20%–30% of ventricular filling.

After atrial contraction, the period of systole begins (see Fig. 1-10). During systole, the right and left ventricles contract. As the ventricles contract, the intraventricular cavitary pressures increase, and when ventricular pressure rises above atrial pressure the mitral and tricuspid valves are forced closed. As ventricular contraction continues, there is a brief period of time when all four valves of the heart are closed. This occurs because the pressure in the ventricular chambers is high enough to close the mitral and tricuspid valves but is not high enough to force open the aortic and pulmonic valves. Since all of the cardiac valves are closed and blood is not entering or leaving the ventricular chambers, the ventricular volumes are constant. This short period of time in early systole is called *isovolumic contraction*.

When the pressure in the ventricular chambers exceeds the pressures in the aorta and pulmonary artery, the aortic and pulmonic valves open, and the blood in the ventricular chambers is ejected. As systole ends, the pressures in the ventricular chambers fall. When the pressure falls below the pulmonary artery and aortic pressures, the pulmonic and aortic valves close. During early diastole there is another short period when all four cardiac valves are closed. Blood neither enters nor leaves the ventricular chambers, and the ventricular volumes are constant. This early diastolic period is called *isovolumic relaxation*.

There are actually three identifiable phases of ventricular filling during diastole. First, there is a *rapid filling phase* (also referred to as the early filling phase) resulting from sudden opening of the mitral and tricuspid valves and flow of blood from the left and right atria that has accumulated during systole. After this period of rapid filling, filling of the ventricles slows as the atria act as a conduit for blood return from the venous system (*diastasis*). The final phase of ventricular filling is *atrial contraction* (atrial systole), as discussed above.

In conditions associated with thickening of the left ventricle, left atrial contraction can be responsible for up to 40% of ventricular filling.

Systole (Ventricular Contraction)
  Isovolumic contraction
  Ejection phase
Diastole (Ventricular Relaxation)
  Isovolumic relaxation
  Rapid filling phase
  Diastasis
  Atrial contraction

FIG. 1-10
CARDIAC CYCLE. Schematics and pressures are shown for the left ventricle only. At the beginning of diastole, just after aortic valve closure (AC), the ventricle is relaxing; ventricular pressure being less than aortic pressure but greater than atrial pressure, both the aortic and mitral valves are closed. This short period with no ventricular volume change is called the *isovolumic relaxation period.* With continued ventricular relaxation, ventricular pressure drops below atrial pressure, which causes the mitral valve to open (MO), and blood accumulated in the atrium flows into the ventricle (*ventricular filling*). Ventricular filling has three recognizable periods: early (rapid) filling phase, diastasis and atrial contraction. At *atrial contraction*, the ventricle is filled to its end-diastolic volume. During atrial contraction, blood flows backward at the pulmonary vein orifices (since there are no valves). Contraction of the ventricle increases ventricular pressure. The mitral valve closes (MC). Again, there is a short period when ventricular pressure has an intermediate value between atrial and aortic pressure and both the mitral and aortic valves are closed (*isovolumic contraction*). When ventricular pressure exceeds aortic pressure, the aortic valve opens (AO), and the *ejection phase* begins.

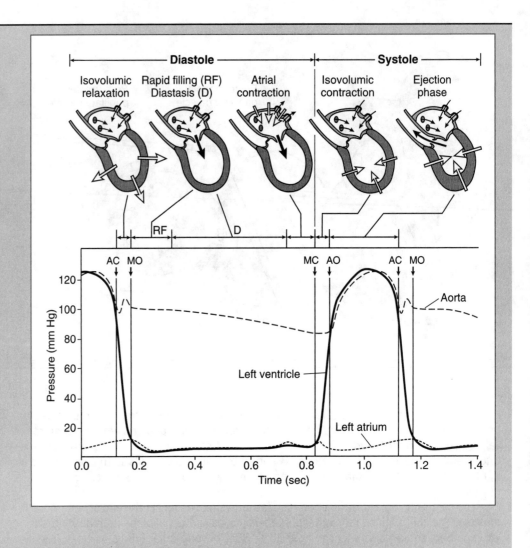

Right heart (right atrium, right ventricle) = highly compliant, low-pressure system.
Left heart (left atrium, left ventricle) = less compliant, high-pressure system.

Differences between Right and Left Heart Physiology. While the cardiac cycles of the right and left heart are perfectly analogous, the physiology of the two systems is somewhat different. The circulation through the right heart (the right atrium and ventricle) and the pulmonary circulation is a low-pressure, high-compliance system.

Compliance is a measure of the relationship between pressure (P) and volume (V) in a closed hemodynamic system (compliance = $\Delta V/\Delta P$). A highly compliant system has very little increase in pressure with the addition of volume. A system with low compliance has a marked increase in pressure with small additions of volume.

The highly compliant venous systems undergo large fluctuations in volume over the range of normal physiologic conditions without significant increases in pressure. Similarly, the highly compliant vascular pulmonary arterial circulation accepts the entire blood volume at a relatively low pressure. As shown in Fig. 1-11, normal systolic pulmonary pressures range from 25 to 30 mm Hg, which is approximately one-quarter to one-fifth of normal systemic arterial pressures (100–140 mm Hg). The thin-walled right ventricle is well suited for the task of pumping large volumes of blood at low pressure.

In contrast to the right heart and pulmonary circulation, the left heart and systemic circulation is a less compliant, high-pressure system. The systemic arteries are muscular, thick-walled conduits. Normal systolic arterial pressures range from 100 to 140

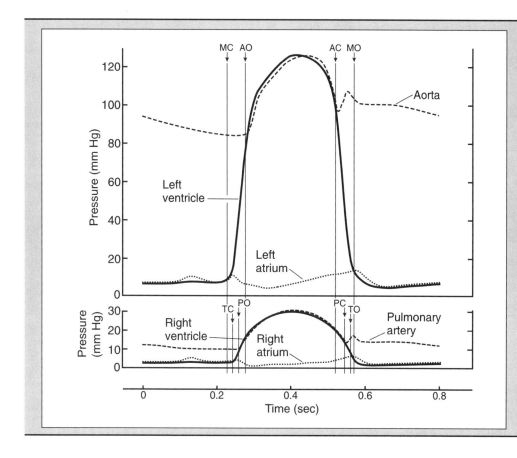

FIG. 1-11
COMPARISON OF PRESSURES IN THE RIGHT VENTRICLE AND PULMONARY ARTERY AND THE LEFT VENTRICLE AND AORTA. AC = aortic valve closing; AO = aortic valve opening; MC = mitral valve closing; MO = mitral valve opening; PC = pulmonic valve closing; PO = pulmonic valve opening; TC = tricuspid valve closing; TO = tricuspid valve opening. (*Source:* Reprinted with permission from Mountcastle VB: *Medical Physiology*, 14th ed. St. Louis, MO: C. V. Mosby, 1980, Fig. 37-10.)

mm Hg. The left heart structures serve this function well. The left ventricle is thicker and more massive than the right. The aortic and mitral valve leaflets are thicker and stronger than the pulmonic and tricuspid valves.

Measurement of Pressures and Resistances in the Circulatory Systems.
Basic hemodynamic properties govern blood flow in the human circulation. The flow of a fluid through a chamber or conduit is determined by the pressure of the fluid and the resistance of the conduit. The flow through an orifice demonstrates these basic principles and can be used as a starting point in the understanding of the hemodynamics of the human circulation. The pressure of the fluid upstream of the orifice produces flow across the orifice. The energy expended in generating the flow results in a drop in pressure across the orifice. The magnitude of the drop in pressure is proportional to the resistance of the orifice. Therefore, the flow across an orifice is directly proportional to the pressure difference (ΔP) across the orifice and inversely proportional to the resistance of the orifice (flow = ΔP/resistance). This is analogous to Ohm's law, which describes the relationship of resistance (R), current (I), and voltage (V) in an electronic circuit (I = V/R).

These principles can be applied directly to the human circulation. For example, left ventricular systole produces pressure in the aorta and other large arteries, which drives the flow of blood from the systemic arterial circulation to the systemic venous circulation. The resistance of the capillary system results in a drop in pressure from the arteries to the veins (Fig. 1-12). Pressures and flows can be directly measured by various instruments (a blood pressure cuff can indirectly measure systemic arterial pressure, a small catheter placed within the lumen of a vessel or chamber can directly measure pressure and flows), and the resistance of the system can be calculated.

These parameters are used to characterize the physiologic state of the cardiovascular system. For example, the *cardiac output*, which is the measure of blood flow from the heart, is directly proportional to the difference in pressure from the arterial to the venous circulation and inversely proportional to the resistance of the peripheral circulation. The resistance of the peripheral circulation is termed the *systemic vascular resistance* (*SVR*).

FIG. 1-12
MEASUREMENT OF THE SYSTEMIC VASCULAR RESISTANCE (SVR). The mean pressure in the arterial system (MAP) is 85 mm Hg, and the pressure in the inferior vena cava (IVC) or right atrium (RA) is 3 mm Hg. (Normally, pressures in the RA and the IVC are very similar.) Cardiac output (CO) is 5 L/min, or 83.3 mL/sec. The ratio of the pressure difference and the CO must be multiplied by a conversion factor of 1132 to express the answer in dynes-sec/cm^5. In this example, the systemic vascular resistance is 1114 dynes-sec/cm^5, which is within the normal range (see Table 1-1).

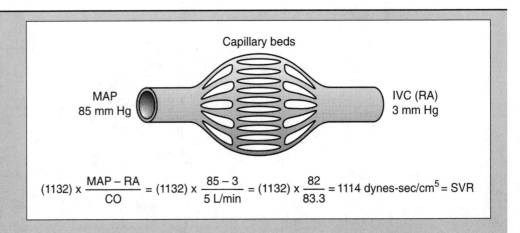

Capillary beds

MAP 85 mm Hg

IVC (RA) 3 mm Hg

$$(1132) \times \frac{MAP - RA}{CO} = (1132) \times \frac{85 - 3}{5 \text{ L/min}} = (1132) \times \frac{82}{83.3} = 1114 \text{ dynes-sec/cm}^5 = SVR$$

The SVR can be calculated by measuring the cardiac output (CO), the arterial pressure, and the venous pressure. The arterial pressure is usually measured as the mean arterial pressure (MAP), and the venous pressure can be taken as the mean right atrial pressure (MRA). Using the formula resistance = ΔP/flow, SVR = (MAP − MRA)/CO. Similarly, the pressure across the pulmonary circulation, termed the *pulmonary vascular resistance* (*PVR*), is equal to the difference in pressure across the pulmonary circulation (difference between pulmonary artery and pulmonary venous pressure) divided by the CO. Normal ranges for CO, SVR, PVR, MAP, and MRA are given in Table 1-1.

Mean arterial pressure (MAP):

$$MAP = DBP + \frac{SBP - DBP}{3}$$

SBP = systolic blood pressure
DBP = diastolic blood pressure

Table 1-1
Normal Cardiac Values in Humans

PARAMETER	NORMAL VALUES
Mean arterial pressure	70–105 mm Hg
Mean right atrial pressure	0–8 mm Hg
Mean pulmonary artery pressure	9–16 mm Hg
Mean left atrial pressure	1–10 mm Hg
Cardiac output	2.5–3.6 L/min/m^2
Systemic vascular resistance	1170 ± 270 dynes-sec/cm^5
Pulmonary vascular resistance	67 ± 30 dynes-sec/cm^5

Activation of α-adrenergic receptors causes vasoconstriction of arteries and veins. Drugs such as prazosin that block α-adrenergic receptors and reduce SVR are sometimes used for treatment of hypertension. Conversely, dopamine, which activates α-adrenergic receptors at high concentrations, is used for treatment of sepsis.

There are direct clinical applications of these relationships. For example, high systemic arterial pressure (commonly referred to as high blood pressure) can be caused by increased SVR or CO, since MAP is the product of CO and SVR. Several types of high blood pressure medication cause arterial vasodilation, which reduces SVR. Another clinical application of this relationship occurs in the setting of severe systemic infections (*sepsis*). Endotoxins produced by bacteria can cause dramatic reductions in SVR, which result in low blood pressures and high COs. To maintain blood pressure, vasoconstrictors are given to increase the SVR. Understanding the relationships between resistance, pressures, and CO creates the basis for understanding the behavior of the cardiovascular system in normal as well as pathologic states.

Cardiac Output. CO, as stated above, is the measure of blood flow from the heart and is a basic measure of cardiac performance. CO is the volume of blood pumped over time and is usually expressed in liters per minute corrected for body surface area (to allow comparisons between different-sized individuals). Normal values for CO can be quite varied but, interestingly, for large animals (e.g., dog, cow, horse, human) the CO is linearly related to body weight. *Stroke volume* (*SV*) is the volume of blood ejected during a single cycle of contraction. Therefore, the CO is equal to the SV times the number of contractions per minute, or heart rate (HR) [CO = SV × HR].

There is a direct relationship between HR and CO; as HR increases, CO increases. The increase in CO achieved through tachycardia is dependent on ability to maintain cardiac filling. As HR increases, the time required for systole being relatively constant, the relative proportion of time that the heart is in diastole decreases. Therefore, maintaining cardiac filling during tachycardia requires more efficient diastolic filling. In the normal exercising heart, which is beating at less than approximately 170 beats/min, filling is not compromised by the shortening of diastole. In the normal heart, as HR increases, cardiac relaxation becomes more rapid, and complete cardiac filling can be achieved during the short diastolic filling periods. As discussed above, this effect is partly mediated through the stimulation of β-receptors by catecholamines, which enhance relaxation by increasing removal of intracellular Ca^{2+}. At HRs above approximately 170 beats/min, complete relaxation can no longer occur, cardiac filling begins to be compromised, and further increases in CO cannot be achieved.

Stroke Volume. There are three parameters that determine SV, the other determinant of CO: *preload*, *afterload*, and *inotropic state*. These three concepts are important determinants of function both in an isolated muscle fiber and in the intact ventricle.

Isolated Muscle Fiber. The concepts of preload, afterload, and inotropic state can be understood by studying a model developed by A. P. Hill in the late 1930s, which has been used by numerous investigators to evaluate the functions of skeletal, smooth, and cardiac muscle. In this model a muscle fiber is stretched to varying lengths (Fig. 1-13). Preload is the load or tension required to stretch the myocardial fiber to its initial length. If the myocardial fiber is now allowed to contract, afterload is the load against which the fiber contracts, and inotropic state is a measure of the contractile strength of the fiber.

Myocyte contraction in the ventricles generates the force of systole. This force is generated at the biochemical level by the coordinated action of individual sarcomeres. The force generated by the sarcomere depends on the degree of overlapping of the thin and thick filaments.

Cardiac output is the product of heart rate and stroke volume. Stroke volume is determined by preload, afterload, and inotropic state.

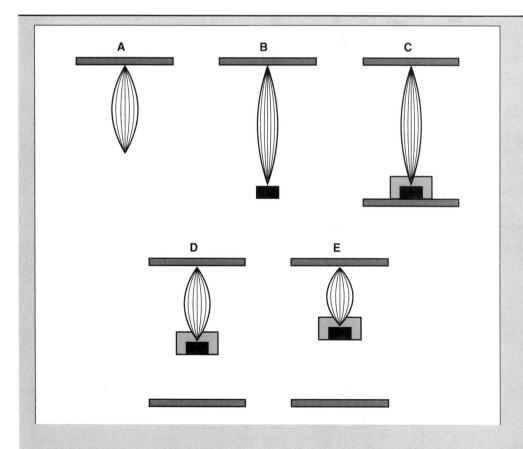

FIG. 1-13
SCHEMATIC SHOWING THE RELATIONSHIPS AMONG PRELOAD, AFTERLOAD, AND INOTROPIC STATE FOR AN ISOLATED MYOCYTE. (A) The first panel shows a myocyte at rest. (B) In the second panel, the myocyte is stretched by placing a small weight on the end of the muscle fiber. This initial weight is the *preload* for the muscle fiber. (C) In the third panel, the weight is supported to keep the muscle fiber at its stretched length. An additional, larger weight is placed on the end of the muscle fiber. The total load the myocyte must now overcome before it can lift the weight off the support is called the *afterload*. (D) In the fourth panel, the tension produced by myocyte contraction surpasses the afterload, and the myocyte shortens. (E) The myocyte in the fifth panel is bathed in a solution with an increased Ca^{2+} concentration and thus has a greater inotropic state and shortens to a greater extent for a given preload and afterload.

The sarcomere length at the initiation of contraction determines the degree of thin and thick filament overlap. As the initial length of the sarcomere increases, the degree of overlapping increases and more cross-bridge interactions can occur. This results in greater contractile force. Beyond a certain point, further increases in sarcomere length do not increase the overlapping of the thin and thick filaments, and the force no longer increases.

This relationship can be graphically illustrated using our experimental model of an isolated myocardial fiber. The initial fiber length is preset to different fixed lengths (by increasing the preload), and contraction is stimulated, but *the fiber is not allowed to shorten*. The tension produced by myocyte activation is measured. Since the fiber length is fixed, this type of "contraction" is called *isometric* contraction, and the relationship between initial myocyte length and tension is illustrated in Fig. 1-14. The length of the myocardial fiber at the beginning of the contraction is a function of the preload. As the fiber length is increased, the tension generated during an isometric contraction increases. However, as the fiber length is increased beyond a threshold value, the resultant force plateaus and begins to decrease. This information can be combined graphically as a length–tension diagram (Fig. 1-15). As a myocyte is passively stretched to different lengths and the muscle is stimulated but not allowed to contract, the measured tension increases, plateaus, and then decreases.

The second determinant of SV is *inotropic state*, which is a measure of the force generated by the fiber at a fixed preload and afterload. At a given length, a fiber generates

FIG. 1-14
RELATIONSHIP BETWEEN PRE-LOAD AND GENERATED MYO-CYTE TENSION. An isolated myocyte is stretched to increasing lengths by increasing the preload (A–D). The myocyte is stimulated but not allowed to contract (isometric contraction). The generated muscle tension at each of the four preloads is shown on the right. As preload is increased from A to C, generated tension increases. However, at preload D, the overlap of thick and thin filaments begins to decrease, and the generated tension during an isometric contraction falls.

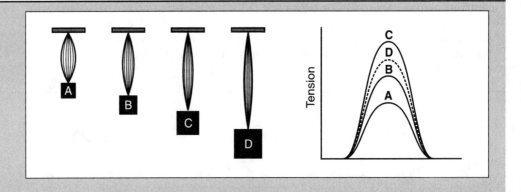

FIG. 1-15
LENGTH–TENSION DIAGRAM FOR THE EXAMPLES IN FIG. 1-14. A myocyte is stretched to different lengths (A through D) and excited but not allowed to contract. The developed tension increases with increasing myocyte length until preload D, in which developed tension falls.

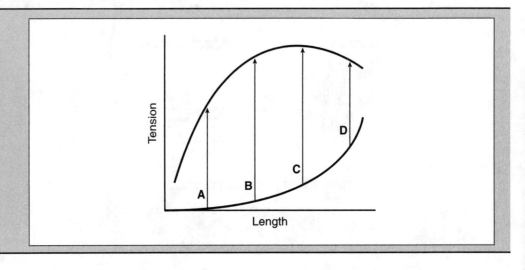

more or less force depending on the conditions of the fiber. For example, in the presence of norepinephrine a fiber generates more force. A fatigued fiber generates less force. The state of the fiber relative to its strength is termed the *inotropic* state, also called the *contractile* state. If the muscle tissue is exposed to high concentrations of Ca^{2+}, the developed tension in response to stimulation becomes higher. As already noted, increased intracellular Ca^{2+} favors increased interaction between the thin and thick filaments. In the length–tension diagram, for a given initial preload, during isometric contraction the generated tension is higher for an increased inotropic state (Fig. 1-16).

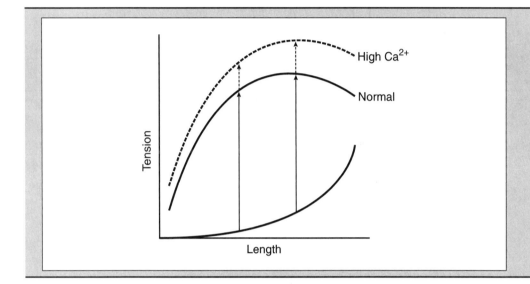

FIG. 1-16
LENGTH–TENSION DIAGRAM FOR TWO DIFFERENT INOTROPIC STATES. If the myocyte is perfused with a high-Ca^{2+} solution (increased inotropic state), for a given preload the myocyte generates a higher tension during isometric contraction.

An alternative setup to the isometric contraction experiments we have discussed to this point is to measure *isotonic* contraction, in which the myocyte is *allowed to shorten* against a preset force or load (Fig. 1-17). The change in fiber length, or fiber shortening, with contraction is measured. The initial force that the fiber must overcome before it can shorten is termed the *afterload*. The length–tension diagram for changes in afterload is shown in Fig. 1-18.

It is thus apparent that the function of an isolated myocyte is determined by preload, inotropic state, and afterload.

Intact Ventricle. The length–tension relationships that we have discussed for the isolated muscle fiber can now be applied to the pressure–volume relationships of the intact ventricle. Although the same principles can be applied to any cardiac chamber, for the

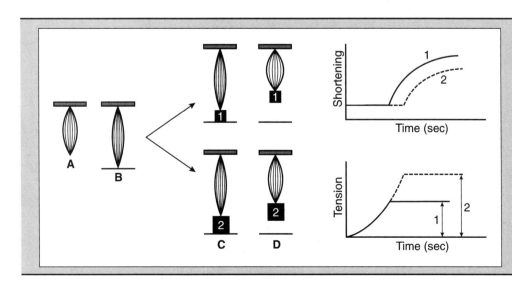

FIG. 1-17
SEQUENCE OF EVENTS FOR A GIVEN CONTRACTION AGAINST DIFFERENT AFTERLOADS. (A) First, the myocyte is stretched to a given preload (B). (C) The myocyte is then allowed to contract against different weights 1 and 2. (D) The amount of developed tension required before the muscle can shorten is called the afterload. For the higher afterload (2), the necessary tension before shortening can occur is higher, and the absolute amount of shortening is smaller.

16   **CARDIOVASCULAR PATHOPHYSIOLOGY**

FIG. 1-18
LENGTH–TENSION DIAGRAM FOR THE EXAMPLES GIVEN IN FIG. 1-17. A myocyte is stretched to a given preload and allowed to contract. Once tension 1 or 2 is reached (the afterload), the myocyte begins to shorten. The amount of shortening is greater when the myocyte is faced with a lower afterload (1).

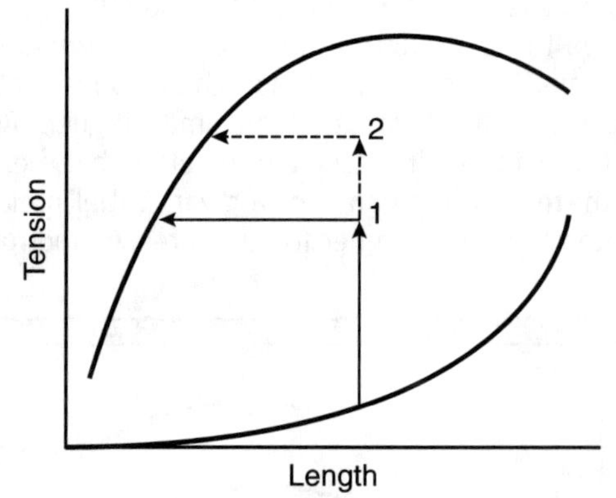

purposes of this discussion we focus on the left ventricle since this chamber is responsible for pumping blood to the systemic circulation. For the intact ventricle, the analogue to preload is the amount of filling of the left ventricle (causing stretching of the myocytes); the analogue to inotropic state is the intrinsic contractility of the heart (independent of preload and afterload); and the analogue to afterload is the pressure the heart must overcome to eject blood.

In the late 1800s several investigators (Frank, Wiggers, and Starling) independently described the fact that increased ventricular filling (end-diastolic volume) [preload] would lead to increased generated force and increased CO. This property of the heart is commonly referred to as the *Frank-Starling law of the heart*.

Frank-Starling law. For a given contraction, blood ejected by the ventricle (SV) is a function of ventricular filling (end-diastolic volume).

If the left ventricle is filled to varying amounts and allowed to contract but kept at a constant volume, the isovolumic systolic pressure curve can be derived (Fig. 1-19). This curve is analogous to the length–tension curve for isometric contraction described for the isolated muscle cell in Fig. 1-15. Within limits, as the ventricle is filled to increasing amounts, the generated intracavitary pressure produced by ventricular contraction becomes higher.

The position of the isovolumic systolic pressure curve is related to the contractile state of the ventricles (inotropic state). If the ventricle is stimulated by adrenergic agents, β-adrenergic receptors are stimulated, which increases intracellular Ca^{2+} concentrations. Increased intracellular Ca^{2+} leads to increased contractility. The isovolumic systolic pressure curve is shifted upward (greater generated pressure for a given amount of ventricular filling) [see Fig. 1-19].

The load that the intact ventricle must contract against (*afterload*) is the pressure

FIG. 1-19
If the intact left ventricle is filled to varying amounts (A, B, and C), the intracavitary pressure increases slowly since the ventricle is relatively compliant. At a given fixed volume the ventricle is allowed to contract (but not allowed to eject blood), and the intracavitary pressure is measured. The generated pressure falls on the isovolumic systolic pressure curve. If the inotropic state for the ventricle is increased, the isovolumic systolic pressure curve is shifted upward (*dashed line*).

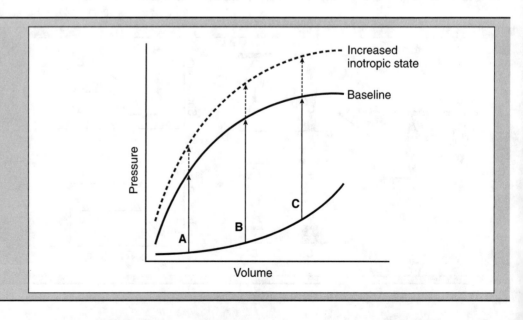

within the aorta. As the left ventricle contracts, when left ventricular pressure rises above aortic pressure, the aortic valve opens, and blood is expelled from the left ventricle. If aortic pressure is increased, the force generated by the ventricle must be greater (increased afterload) to produce intracavitary left ventricular pressures high enough to open the aortic valve and allow blood flow to the systemic circulation.

Mr. Buecheler's systolic arterial pressure was extremely high (208 mm Hg; normal systolic pressures are 100–140 mm Hg). What abnormal force was his heart being exposed to?

Case Study:
Continued

Pressure–Volume Curves. The concepts of preload, inotropic state, and afterload are combined into a useful graphical relationship, the pressure–volume curve, in which the events of the cardiac cycle are summarized by the relationship between pressure and volume.

When the mitral valve opens, the left ventricle begins filling with blood (Fig. 1-20). The pressure–volume relationship of the left ventricle follows the diastolic pressure curve, which is a function of the compliance of the left ventricle. Normally, the left ventricular volume increases without much increase in pressure because the left ventricle is generally fairly compliant (although less compliant than the right ventricle). The slope of the diastolic pressure curve is a measure of left ventricular diastolic stiffness. Stiffness ($\Delta P/\Delta V$) is the inverse of compliance. For example, a stiff and thick-walled ventricle is noncompliant and has a higher intracavitary pressure for a given volume.

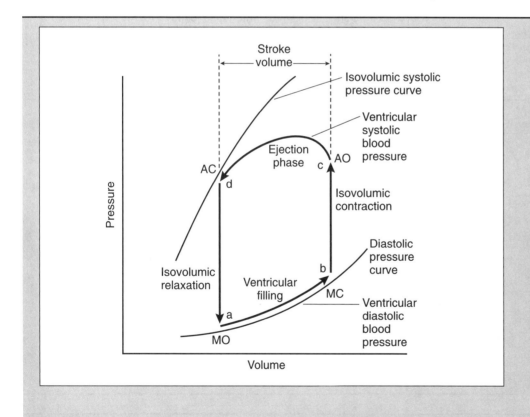

FIG. 1-20
PRESSURE–VOLUME LOOP FOR THE LEFT VENTRICLE. With mitral valve opening (MO), the left ventricle begins to fill following the diastolic pressure curve. The pressure at point *b* represents the preload of the ventricle. At end-diastole, the mitral valve closes (MC) and as the ventricle continues to contract, pressure increases, but volume is constant (isovolumic contraction). Once the ventricular pressure exceeds the aortic pressure, the aortic valve opens (AO), and the ejection phase begins. The pressure at point *c* is the afterload faced by the ventricle. As the ventricle finishes contracting and begins relaxing, the aortic valve closes (AC) when intracavitary pressure drops below aortic pressure. The ventricle continues to relax, and volume remains constant until the mitral valve opens and the cycle repeats. The stroke volume is the difference between the volumes at point *c* and *d*.

At end-diastole, after atrial contraction has just finished, the left ventricle is at its largest volume (point *b*). The pressure at point *b* is a measure of ventricular preload. As systole begins, the mitral valve closes and the pressure in the ventricle increases. The aortic valve does not open until the ventricular pressure exceeds the aortic pressure. Isovolumic contraction, as described above, is the early systolic period after mitral valve closure and before aortic valve opening, in which the ventricular volume is constant (point *b* to point *c*).

When ventricular pressure exceeds aortic pressure, the aortic valve opens and the ejection phase begins. Point *c* is the aortic pressure at aortic valve opening and is a measure of afterload. As systole proceeds, the blood volume in the ventricle is ejected, and the left ventricular volume decreases (point *c* to point *d*). The peak pressure achieved during systole is the systolic arterial pressure. At end-systole, the ventricular pressure falls below the aortic pressure and the aortic valve closes (point *d*). The position of point *d* is determined by the position of the isovolumic systolic pressure curve. The volume of blood ejected during systole, or SV, is the ventricular volume at end-diastole (point *c*) minus the volume at end-systole (point *d*).

Once the aortic valve closes, diastole begins. The ventricular pressure at this point still exceeds left atrial pressure, and the mitral valve remains closed. The myocardium continues to relax and ventricular pressure drops, but the ventricular volume is constant (point *d* to point *a*) since both the aortic and mitral valves are closed. This short period is called the isovolumic relaxation phase of diastole.

As ventricular relaxation continues, the intracavitary left ventricular pressure eventually drops to left atrial pressure, and the mitral valve opens at point *a*. The cycle repeats itself as the left ventricle begins to fill following the left ventricular diastolic pressure curve.

The effects of changes in preload, afterload, and contractility can be graphically illustrated using this pressure–volume relationship (Fig. 1-21). For example, if left ventricular preload is increased (i.e., the left ventricle receives increased venous return, perhaps as a result of reduced venous pooling in the peripheral tissues), there is increased filling of the left ventricle, and if afterload is fixed, SV is increased (see Fig. 1-21A). If contractility is increased (increased intracellular Ca^{2+} concentrations), the isovolumic pressure curve is shifted upward, which also leads to increased SV (see Fig. 1-21B). As a final example, if afterload is increased (increased systemic blood pressure), the SV is decreased, because the left ventricle must generate a higher pressure before blood can be expelled (see Fig. 1-21C).

CO can be increased by:
Increased HR
Increased SV
- Increased preload
- Increased inotropic state
- Decreased afterload

FIG. 1-21
EFFECTS ON STROKE VOLUME (SV) OF CHANGING PRELOAD, INOTROPIC STATE, AND AFTERLOAD. (A) Increased preload moves filling from point *b* to point *b'*, which, if inotropic state and afterload are kept constant, leads to increased SV. (B) If the inotropic state of the left ventricle is increased, at a given preload and afterload, SV increases because during the ejection phase the ventricle contracts to point *d'*. (C) If the afterload is increased and the preload and contractility are kept constant, the SV decreases because the aortic valve does not open until point *c'*.

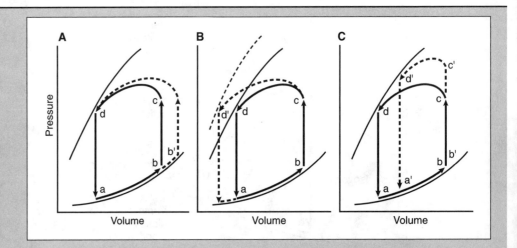

Case Study:
Continued

Mr. Buecheler's heart was exposed to a significant increase in afterload. Can you construct a pressure–volume analysis for Mr. Buecheler's heart?

▌HEART FAILURE

Broadly defined, heart failure is cardiac dysfunction that leads to the inability of the heart to produce a CO that is sufficient to meet the metabolic demands of the body for oxygen and nutrients. Discussion here focuses on heart failure caused by abnormalities of cardiac myocytes that lead to inadequate ventricular function.

Ventricular dysfunction can be the result of either weakness of ventricular contraction (*systolic dysfunction*), abnormal ventricular relaxation (*diastolic dysfunction*), or abnormal thickening of the ventricle that leads to *outflow obstruction*. Heart failure can be caused by failure of the left or the right ventricle, individually or together. Our discussion focuses on the left ventricle, with a final, brief discussion of right ventricular failure.

SYSTOLIC DYSFUNCTION

Pathophysiology. In systolic dysfunction, myocardial contractility is impaired. The specific causes of decreased myocardial contractility are discussed below. However, regardless of etiology, the pathophysiologic impact of reduced contractility can be easily understood by means of the pressure–volume curves.

Reduced myocardial contractility shifts the isovolumic systolic pressure curve to the right and downward, so that a given amount of ventricular filling leads to reduced pressure generated by the ventricle (Fig. 1-22). The fundamental consequence of this shift is that for a given preload and afterload, SV is significantly reduced (Fig. 1-23). The heart can rapidly undergo several compensatory changes in order to maintain SV: *increased preload*, *increased inotropic state*, and *increased HR*. If systolic function is chronically depressed, a final compensatory mechanism is left ventricular hypertrophy and dilatation.

Compensatory Mechanisms in Reduced Contractility
Acute
    Increased preload
    Increased contractility
    Increased HR
Chronic
    Ventricular hypertrophy and dilatation

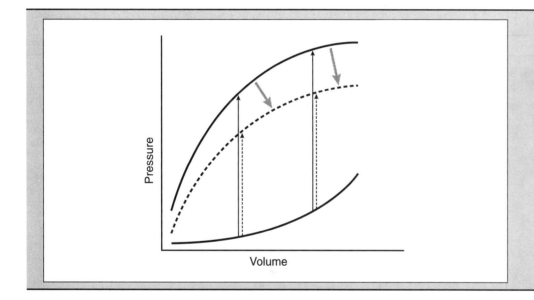

FIG. 1-22
In systolic dysfunction, the isovolumic systolic pressure curve is shifted downward (*dashed line*). For a given amount of filling, the ventricle generates less pressure.

Increased Preload. One of the ways the ventricle can rapidly maintain SV is to increase preload by operating on a rightward portion of the diastolic pressure curve. Fig. 1-24 illustrates this compensatory mechanism. A pressure–volume loop for a ventricle at baseline is shown (loop *abcd*). If the isovolumic systolic pressure curve is suddenly shifted to the right, for a given afterload the SV is suddenly reduced. For that heartbeat, a larger amount of blood remains in the ventricle at end-systole (point *d′*). If the amount of blood entering the ventricle remains constant, the ventricle fills to point *b′*. With this increased amount of filling, SV is maintained (*c–d* is roughly equal to *c′–d′*). On ensuing beats, the ventricle operates on a more rightward region of the diastolic pressure curve (*a′b′c′d′*). The "cost" of increased filling is increased end-diastolic pressure. Remember that point *b′* is a measure of left ventricular and left atrial pressure just before mitral valve closure (end-diastole). Elevated left atrial pressure may cause pressures in the pulmonary capillary bed to increase to a level high enough that fluid is forced into the interstitial spaces and alveolar spaces of the lungs (pulmonary edema). Pulmonary edema makes it hard to expand the lungs with breathing and produces the sensation of breathlessness commonly associated with heart failure.

The consequences of a rightward shift of the isovolumic systolic pressure curve depend on the slope of the diastolic pressure curve. If the ventricle is forced to operate on a steep portion of the diastolic filling curve, increased ventricular filling is associated with a greater increase in end-diastolic pressure.

FIG. 1-23
If the isovolumic systolic pressure curve is shifted downward and afterload and preload are artificially kept constant, the stroke volume (SV) decreases significantly (SV versus SV').

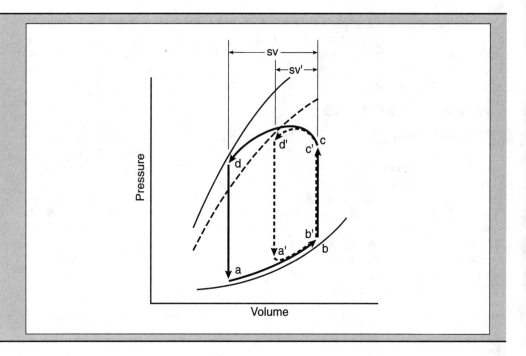

FIG. 1-24
MAINTENANCE OF STROKE VOLUME (SV) BY INCREASING PRELOAD. At baseline the ventricle is operating on volume loop *abcd*. If systolic function is suddenly reduced (shift of the isovolumic systolic pressure curve downward), for the first beat (*dashed arrow*), the heart will empty to point *d'*; if venous return remains constant [(b−a) = (b'−a')], the ventricle will fill to point *b'* and begin operating on pressure–volume loop *a'b'c'd'*. In this way the ventricle can adjust instantly to changes in inotropic state and maintain a constant SV.

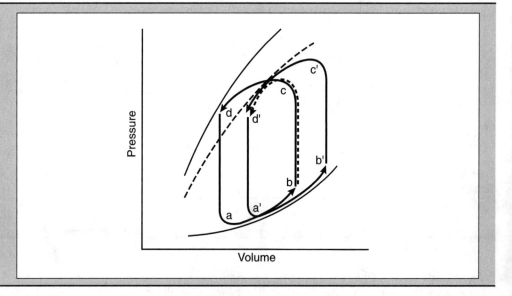

The phrases **concentric** and **eccentric hypertrophy** are derived from the different appearances of the cardiac silhouette on chest radiograph. In concentric hypertrophy, the cardiac silhouette is enlarged but remains in its usual position. In eccentric hypertrophy, the cardiac silhouette is displaced laterally as a result of left ventricular chamber dilatation.

Increased Inotropic State. Another compensatory response to acute systolic dysfunction is an increase in the inotropic or contractile state of the myocardium. As outlined below, one of the acute responses to heart failure is increased sympathetic activation. Stimulation of β-adrenergic receptors in the ventricle causes increased intracellular Ca^{2+} levels, which increase the force generated by a myocardial fiber. As shown in Fig. 1-25, this leads to a small upward and leftward shift of the isovolumic systolic pressure curve and helps maintain SV.

Increased HR. Since CO is the product of SV and HR, increased HR can also be a compensatory mechanism for maintaining CO in a situation of reduced contractility. Stimulation of β-adrenergic receptors in the sinus node (see Chapter 2) leads to an increased HR, which maintains CO.

Ventricular Hypertrophy and Ventricular Dilatation. If decreased contractile function is severe and longstanding, the left ventricle will hypertrophy and dilate in response to the increased stress. Two classic types of left ventricular hypertrophy have been described (Fig. 1-26). In *concentric hypertrophy*, increased systolic pressures stimulate increased synthesis of sarcomeres in a parallel orientation, which causes thickening of the left

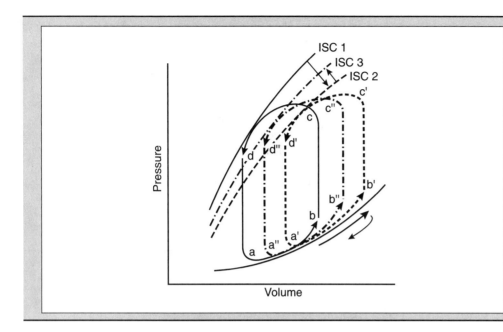

FIG. 1-25
COMPENSATION BY INCREASED INOTROPIC STATE. The baseline pressure volume loop is *abcd*. The isovolumic systolic pressure curve (ISC) is shifted downward: ISC 1 versus ISC 2. The heart initially begins operating on pressure–volume loop *a'b'c'd'*. Within several minutes, inotropic state is increased (ISC 3), and the ventricle begins operating on loop *a"b"c"d"*.

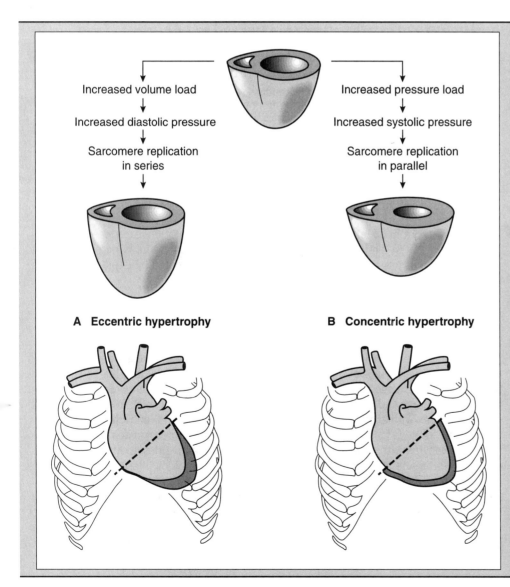

A Eccentric hypertrophy

B Concentric hypertrophy

FIG. 1-26
TWO TYPES OF LEFT VENTRICULAR HYPERTROPHY. (A) Eccentric hypertrophy. If the ventricle is placed under a volume load, diastolic pressure is increased, and the heart increases volume size and wall thickness because of series replication of sarcomeres. Eccentric hypertrophy was originally named because left ventricular enlargement causes the heart to be displaced laterally in the chest cavity. (B) Concentric hypertrophy. If the ventricle is placed under a pressure load, systolic pressure is elevated, and the left ventricle hypertrophies by parallel addition of sarcomeres. Left ventricular wall thickness increases without an increase in cavitary size. In concentric hypertrophy the ventricle remains in its normal position in the chest cavity.

ventricular wall but does not change the interior ventricular diameter. In *eccentric hypertrophy*, increased diastolic pressures cause hypertrophy by increased sarcomeres oriented in series. This leads to a proportional increase in left ventricular wall thickness and chamber size. The pathophysiologic effects of concentric hypertrophy are discussed later. First we focus on eccentric hypertrophy.

Reduced systolic function forces the heart to operate on the rightward portion of the diastolic pressure curve. The left ventricle is exposed to chronically elevated end-diastolic pressures. The actual trigger for eccentric hypertrophy is not well understood. On histologic examination, increased individual sarcomere length and increased sarcomere number oriented in series, which lead to increased myocyte length, have been reported. Initially, eccentric hypertrophy is beneficial. The diastolic filling curve is shifted to the right and downward, which reduces the end-diastolic pressure for a given volume (Fig. 1-27).

FIG. 1-27
ECCENTRIC HYPERTROPHY. (A) Initially, eccentric hypertrophy is beneficial. If the heart has depressed contractility, eccentric hypertrophy shifts the diastolic pressure curve downward (since the ventricular volume is larger), and improves stroke volume *c″–d″* vs. *c′–d′*). (B) Over time, with continued volume overload, the diastolic pressure curve cannot continue to shift downward, and the isovolumic systolic pressure curve continues to shift rightward. This leads to a situation marked by reduced stroke volume (*c*–d**) and low systemic arterial pressures (*c**).

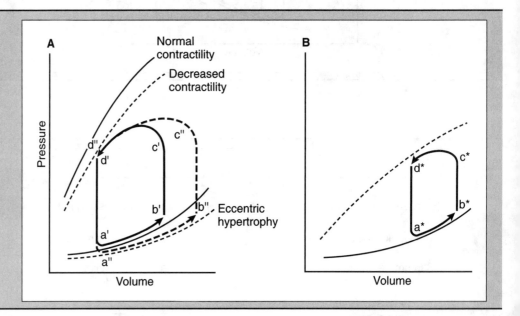

However, continued left ventricular hypertrophy and dilatation leads to a detrimental series of events. At first during eccentric hypertrophy, only slight increases in left ventricular wall stress are observed. Stress can be approximated by Laplace's law for a sphere:

$$\sigma = \frac{p \times r}{2h}$$

where σ is ventricular wall stress, p is left ventricular intracavitary pressure, r is the radius of the endocardial surface of the left ventricle, and h is ventricular wall thickness. When the ventricle is exposed to volume overload, it dilates, which tends to reduce end-diastolic pressure, and the ventricle will thicken to maintain a relatively constant wall stress. However, with exposure to continued volume overload, the ventricle dilates disproportionately, relative to increased wall thickness, because of myocyte death and replacement of myocytes with collagen and other types of connective tissue. Myocyte death is due in part to altered blood supply, since the number of capillaries supplying the hypertrophied ventricle does not increase proportionally. In addition, the proportion of mitochondria to myofibrils decreases, which leads to reduced energy supply in the myocyte. If the isovolumic systolic pressure curve continues to shift rightward, the diastolic pressure curve can no longer shift downward (because of fibrosis), and SV is significantly decreased (see Fig. 1-27). At this point the patient has end-stage heart failure.

Neurohormonal Reflexes in Heart Failure. The systemic response to heart failure is complex and includes the activation of an array of nervous and hormonal systems. The constellation of responses observed in heart failure is referred to as *neurohormonal activation*. Neurohormonal activation includes (1) stimulation of the sympathetic nervous system, (2) suppression of the parasympathetic nervous system, (3) activation of the renin–angiotensin system, and (4) increased release of arginine vasopressin (AVP). In addition, numerous other hormonal responses in heart failure are under investigation, including the release of hormones that are specific to the atrial cardiac chambers, called atrial natriuretic peptides (ANPs). For the purposes of this text, only the changes involving the autonomic nervous system, the renin–angiotensin system, and the AVP hormone systems are discussed.

Sympathetic Nervous System. The first acute neurohormonal response to heart failure is sympathetic nervous system activation. Activation of the sympathetic system causes peripheral arterial vasoconstriction and increased SVR. Sympathetic nervous system arterial vasoconstriction is most prominent in the kidneys, splanchnic organs, skin, and skeletal muscles and tends to preserve blood flow to the heart and brain preferentially. Sympathetic nervous system activation increases venous vascular tone, which tends to increase ventricular filling (and consequently leads to increased preload). Increased vascular tone is useful for maintaining blood pressure, particularly in conditions associated with acute loss of blood (e.g., trauma). However, increased sympathetic activation may have a detrimental effect in chronic heart failure because of the associated increase in afterload.

In addition to these peripheral effects, sympathetic nervous system activation has direct effects on the myocardium. Sympathetic nervous system activation increases the inotropic state of the ventricle, which helps maintain SV. Sympathetic nervous system activation of the sinus node increases HR, which also preserves CO. In heart failure, the parasympathetic nervous system is inhibited; inhibition of parasympathetic nervous activity in the sinus node also causes increased HR.

Renin–Angiotensin System. Within hours after the onset of acute heart failure, juxtaglomerular cells in the kidney begin producing increased renin in response, in part, to reduced renal arteriolar pressure. Renin catalyzes the degradation of angiotensinogen to angiotensin I, which is ultimately converted to angiotensin II (see Chap. 7, Fig. 7-5). Angiotensin II has a number of effects that tend to maintain blood pressure: arterial vasoconstriction, renal Na^+ retention (the result of increased aldosterone secretion), and increased inotropy of cardiac myocytes. Like activation of the sympathetic nervous system, the effects of angiotensin II are useful for maintaining blood pressure in the setting of acute blood loss but may be detrimental in the patient with heart failure.

AVP System. In heart failure, the posterior portion of the pituitary gland secretes increased AVP. AVP is a powerful vasoconstrictor and promotes reabsorption of water in the renal tubules.

Despite the immediate benefits of neurohormonal activation for maintaining venous return to the heart and thereby maintaining ventricular preload, it is generally believed that these changes have deleterious effects in the long run. For example, circulating levels of norepinephrine correlate with the magnitude of the neurohormonal activation, and norepinephrine levels correlate directly with mortality in patients with heart failure. In addition, blocking neurohormonal activation with various drugs improves cardiac function and patient outcomes. Treatment of heart failure patients with drugs such as angiotensin-converting enzyme (ACE) inhibitors (see Chap. 7), which reduce production of angiotensin II, and β-adrenergic receptor blockers significantly reduces mortality.

Causes of Systolic Dysfunction. The multiple causes of systolic dysfunction are summarized in Table 1-2.

Myocardial Ischemia and Infarction. The most common cardiac disease in the United States is coronary artery disease. The most common form of coronary artery disease is the development of an atherosclerotic plaque within the lumen of the vessel, which limits myocardial blood supply (Fig. 1-28) [see Chap. 3]. Reduced myocardial blood supply can

Neurohormonal Activation Associated with Heart Failure
Sympathetic nervous system activation
Parasympathetic nervous system inhibition
Renin–angiotensin system activation
Increased AVP secretion

Table 1-2
Causes of Systolic Dysfunction

1. Coronary artery disease
   Myocardial ischemia
   Myocardial infarction
2. Infection
   Virus (coxsackie B)
   Bacteria (Lyme disease)
   Protozoa (Chagas' disease)
3. Toxicity (alcohol, anthracyclines, cobalt, lead)
4. Idiopathic
5. Metabolic conditions (diabetes mellitus)
6. Altered loads
   Valvular abnormalities
   Longstanding hypertension
7. Peripartum disorders
8. Neuromuscular disorders
   Muscular dystrophy
   Myotonic dystrophy
9. Collagen vascular diseases

FIG. 1-28
The coronary arteries arise from the aorta as the first arterial branches. They course over the surface of the heart and supply blood to the cardiac myocytes. Blockage of the coronary arteries causes ischemia to the area of heart subtended by that artery. If blood flow is limited for a long period, irreversible myocardial damage occurs (myocardial infarction).

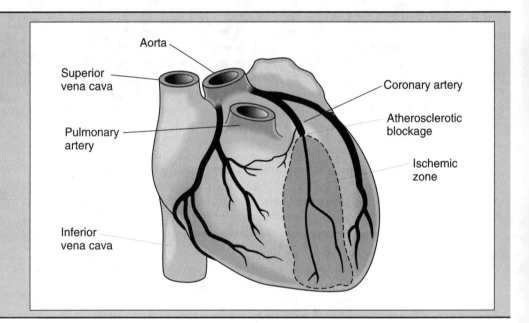

Consequences of Ischemia
Depletion of ATP and CP
Accumulation of lactate
Acidosis
Loss of contractility

cause systolic dysfunction by two mechanisms. *Myocardial ischemia* refers to an oxygen deficiency relative to the oxygen demands of the myocyte that results in cardiac dysfunction without permanent damage. *Myocardial infarction* refers to oxygen deprivation that results in cell death and necrosis and, therefore, permanent myocardial damage.

In myocardial ischemia, if an artery is suddenly occluded, the reduced oxygen tension of myocytes subtended by the occluded artery causes several characteristic changes. The first effect of ischemia is rapid breakdown of high-energy phosphates (creatine phosphate [CP] and ATP), which leads to increased intracellular concentrations of inorganic phosphate. Inorganic phosphate stimulates glycolysis, but the ATP produced by anaerobic glycolysis is insufficient to meet the demands of the myocyte. Lactate produced by glycolysis accumulates in the cell and leads to acidosis.

While the precise mechanism by which ischemia causes systolic dysfunction is not completely known, it appears that intracellular accumulation of phosphate and acidosis may reduce myocyte contractility. In experimental preparations, acidosis decreases the sensitivity of the contractile myofilaments to Ca^{2+}, and inorganic phosphate inhibits cross-bridging between the myosin head and actin. Abnormal myocyte contractility can be observed within seconds of occluding blood flow. Interestingly, loss of myocyte contractility can be observed before depletion of intracellular high-energy phosphates.

The systolic dysfunction caused by myocardial ischemia resolves with restoration of oxygen delivery. If the time of tissue ischemia is short (several minutes), systolic function normalizes relatively quickly. However, if ischemia is prolonged (5–20 min), even when blood flow is restored, recovery of mechanical function of the injured area can take hours, days, or weeks to recover. This phenomenon is called *myocardial stunning*. The exact mechanism of myocardial stunning is not known. Such possibilities as slow resynthesis of proteins damaged during ischemia, membrane damage by the production of oxygen-free radicals, and impaired handling of intracellular Ca^{2+} have been forwarded by various investigators.

Prolonged low-level ischemia can cause long-term contractile dysfunction. This condition is called *myocardial hibernation*. Myocardial hibernation is typically caused by gradual reduction in blood flow to approximately 15%–20% of normal by a *slowly* progressive severe narrowing of the coronary artery that is present for an extended period of time. It has been demonstrated that in such conditions, myocardial cells can dramatically down-regulate cellular energy utilization and thereby avoid cell death. With restoration of myocardial blood supply, hibernating myocardium slowly regains systolic function. The sequelae of coronary artery occlusion are summarized in Table 1-3.

Table 1-3
Sequelae of Coronary Artery Occlusion

DURATION OF OCCLUSION	EFFECT
Sudden and total coronary artery occlusion	
< 2 min	Myocardial ischemia without stunning
2–20 min	Myocardial ischemia with stunning
> 20 min	Myocardial infarction
Gradual and significant reduction in coronary artery flow	Myocardial hibernation

In myocardial infarction, if an artery is suddenly occluded for a prolonged period (greater than 20 min) and the myocyte does not receive blood from other vascular beds (collateral circulation), irreversible cell death occurs. If collateral circulation can only provide a small portion of blood flow (10%–15% of normal), irreversible cell death is delayed but still begins within 40–60 minutes. Irreversible damage is signaled by several histologic findings including diffuse mitochondrial swelling, accumulation of calcium phosphate precipitates within the mitochondria, and small breaks in the cytoplasmic membrane and membranes of intracellular organelles. Excess Ca^{2+} accumulates in the cytoplasm, activating intracellular phospholipases, which further reduce the integrity of the cell membrane and inhibit mitochondrial energy production. The cells eventually burst, and large necrotic regions can be observed by light microscopy.

The healing process following infarction begins within the first day. Neutrophils appear in the injured region during the first week, and during the second week macrophages begin to accumulate. During the third week, fibroblasts appear in the region and deposit large amounts of extracellular collagen, which forms a dense matrix around the few remaining viable myocytes. Loss of viable myocytes causes thinning of the wall at the region of the myocardial infarction. The scarred myocardium does not contract or contracts very poorly, and consequently systolic function of the left ventricle is reduced. The severity of systolic dysfunction is related to the size of the myocardial infarction. Large myocardial infarctions obviously are associated with a greater reduction in systolic function than small myocardial infarctions. In addition, large myocardial infarctions are more likely to be associated with progressive left ventricular dilatation as a result of a complex process called *remodeling*.

In the postinfarction patient, remodeling refers to the architectural changes in left ventricular size and mass that occur as a result of myocardial necrosis. Changes are observed both in the region of the heart containing the myocardial infarction and in regions of the heart that are distant from it. In patients with larger myocardial infarctions, particularly those that involve the apex, gradual expansion of the infarcted region can be observed. Expansion occurs most rapidly during the first several weeks after a myocardial infarction, and in some cases a 50% increase in size of the infarcted region can be observed during this period. It is important to keep in mind that this increase in size does not involve additional myocardial necrosis and appears to be due to "slippage" between the remaining viable myocytes and to myocyte "stretching." Expansion continues until structural integrity of the myocardium can be restored by fibroblast production of collagen and other types of connective tissue. It appears that increased wall stress is an important factor for stimulating infarct expansion. Since the left ventricle has an ellipsoid shape, despite being the thinnest portion of the heart, normally the apex has reduced wall stress because of the very small radius (Fig. 1-29). However, if a myocardial infarction involves the apex, the increased radius causes increased wall stress and favors further expansion of the region.

FIG. 1-29
(A) The apex normally has the thinnest walls (h_{apex} *versus* h_{mid}). However, wall stress is not elevated because the radius at the apex is also small (R_{apex} versus R_{mid}. (B) With an infarction involving the apex, however, the wall thins further and the radius increases. By Laplace's law these architectural changes cause an increase in wall stress. Increased wall stress causes the region to dilate further (infarct expansion). The expansion stops when enough scar tissue has been produced to restore structural integrity to the region.

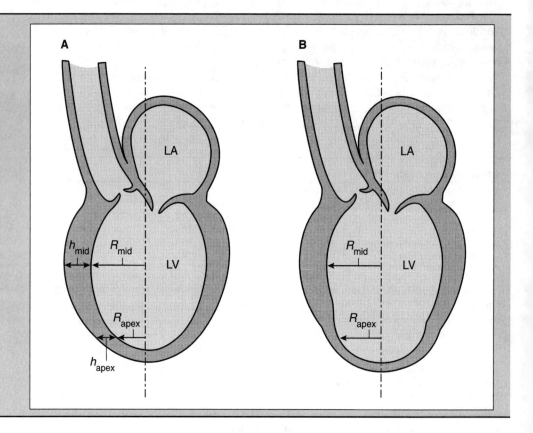

After the period of early expansion of the infarcted region, another phase of remodeling that involves global ventricular enlargement can also be observed (Fig. 1-30). After myocardial infarction, the remaining living myocytes remote from the infarction begin to hypertrophy to compensate for the loss of systolic function. In patients with a significant reduction in systolic function, eccentric hypertrophy resulting from chronic volume overload can be observed. In the short term, left ventricular enlargement helps maintain SV despite the presence of reduced systolic function (see Fig. 1-27). Eventually continued left ventricular enlargement increases wall stress to a "point of no return." The capillary microvasculature does not increase in proportion to myocyte hypertrophy; this condition may be responsible for the reduced proportion of mitochondria observed in the hypertrophied cells and may cause relative "energy starvation" of the myocytes. Progressive dilatation leads to a severe reduction in systolic function, and the patient is described as having an *ischemic cardiomyopathy*. It appears that angiotensin II is an important growth factor for stimulating hypertrophy of the ventricular cells after myocardial infarction. Treatment of patients with ACE inhibitors soon after a myocardial infarction appears to inhibit subsequent eccentric hypertrophy of the left ventricle.

Infection. Several different types of organisms are associated with myocardial damage and inflammation (myocarditis). Myocarditis is commonly associated with reduced systolic function resulting from reduced myocyte contractility. Viruses, particularly the coxsackie B virus and the adenovirus family, have been found to be associated with myocarditis. Several bacterial infections can cause myocarditis. The best-known cause is

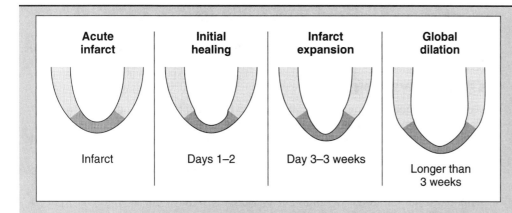

FIG. 1-30
PROGRESSION OF LEFT VEN-TRICULAR SHAPE AND SIZE AF-TER A LARGE MYOCARDIAL IN-FARCTION INVOLVING THE APEX. The infarct does not cause any initial architectural changes. The infarcted area begins to thin, and if wall stress is high enough, infarct expansion occurs as a result of myocyte "slippage" and "stretching." The noninfarcted areas begin to dilate and thicken by eccentric hypertrophy.

Lyme disease, which is due to infection with the spirochete *Borrelia burgdorferi*. While the most common manifestation of Lyme disease is atrioventricular (AV) node heart block (see Chapter 2), isolated cases of generalized myocarditis and heart failure have been described. Two protozoal infections have also been associated with myocarditis and systolic dysfunction. Infection with *Trypanosoma cruzi* and *Toxoplasma gondii* have been associated with myocarditis.

It is thought that these organisms cause an adverse immune response. Histologic evaluation of myocytes from patients with myocarditis caused by infection has revealed macrophage and T-lymphocyte infiltration of myocardial tissue.

The association between viral infection and myocardial damage has been difficult to study because most patients present well after the acute infection has passed. In those patients who do present acutely, inflammation consistent with viral infection and intra-myocyte virus can be demonstrated by biopsy. This clearly indicates that viral infections do cause cardiomyopathy. However, in patients who present late following an infection, no residual evidence of infection remains. Therefore, patients who present with global systolic dysfunction for which no other etiology can be identified may have had a previous viral infection, although this often cannot be firmly established. The condition of global systolic dysfunction for which a cause cannot be established is termed an *idiopathic cardiomyopathy*.

Idiopathic indicates a condition that is due to an unknown cause.

Toxicity. Exposure to toxic substances can cause myocardial damage and, therefore, systolic dysfunction. Chronic alcohol abuse results in direct myocardial toxicity, myocardial cell injury and death, and thus global systolic dysfunction. As a result of the prevalence of alcohol abuse, *alcoholic cardiomyopathy* is the second most common cause of cardiomyopathy in the United States (after ischemic cardiomyopathy). The exact mechanism of alcohol-induced cardiomyopathy is not known. Alcohol may depress contractility by inhibiting the interaction between Ca^{2+} and the myofilaments. Other toxins that are associated with cardiomyopathy include the anthracycline chemotherapeutic agents (doxorubicin, daunorubicin), cobalt, and cocaine. In many patients, removal of the offending agent results in little or no recovery of cardiac function. However, in some patients, improvement and even normalization of systolic function can occur.

Other Causes. Cardiomyopathy can also be the end result of severe, chronic stress experienced by the myocardium. For example, severe, life-long hypertension or aortic stenosis places sustained stress on the myocardium of the left ventricle by elevating the afterload, the pressure against which the muscle must work. Hypertrophy is the initial compensatory response. After many years of exposure to high afterload, however, the left ventricle dilates, and systolic function deteriorates. Longstanding severe regurgitation of the heart valves can also cause systolic dysfunction. The pathophysiology of valvular dysfunction and hypertension are discussed in Chapters 4 and 7.

Reduced systolic dysfunction can be due to a number of causes. It is also important to remember that this discussion is not exhaustive: collagen vascular diseases, other autoimmune causes, and metabolic abnormalities like diabetes mellitus can all lead to systolic dysfunction. Regardless of etiology, the final, common pathophysiologic circumstance is failure of compensatory responses that ultimately results in an enlarged, "baggy" ventricle that is associated with pulmonary edema (*dilated* or *congestive cardiomyopathy*).

DIASTOLIC DYSFUNCTION

Most commonly, heart failure is associated with reduced contractile function. However, it is important to remember that William Harvey described the motion of the heart as cyclic "swallowing and transfusion of the blood from the veins to the arteries." His description emphasizes the interrelated but separate functions of filling (diastole) and contraction (systole). It is now clear that approximately one-third of patients who manifest symptoms of heart failure actually have normal left ventricular function, and symptoms in this group of patients are due to abnormal filling of the left ventricle, which is commonly called diastolic dysfunction.

Pathophysiology. In diastolic dysfunction the ventricle fills abnormally. While abnormal filling can be due to extramyocardial abnormalities (pericardial diseases and abnormalities of the mitral valve), the discussion here focuses on abnormal filling caused by abnormalities of the myocardium. Commonly, abnormal filling is due to reduced compliance or abnormal distensibility of the left ventricle. The effects of abnormal filling resulting from abnormal ventricular compliance and abnormal ventricular distensibility can be understood by studying pressure–volume loops (Fig. 1-31). As the normal ventricle fills during diastole, there is very little increase in pressure as left ventricular volume increases. In other words, the diastolic pressure curve is generally rather flat. However, a ventricle with reduced compliance is associated with an increased pressure for a specific volume during diastole. Graphically, in the pressure–volume loop, the slope of the diastolic pressure curve becomes steeper. In the figure, the pressure–volume loop for a normal ventricle is represented by the loop *abcd*. If the ventricle becomes less compliant, the left ventricle begins filling at point *a'*. If venous return is kept constant, the ventricle fills to point *b'*. The elevated end-diastolic pressure at *b'* also causes elevated left atrial pressure in the same manner described for systolic dysfunction. The difference between ventricular compliance and distensibility can also be understood by evaluating pressure–volume loops. In Fig. 1-31B, decreased distensibility (a higher pressure is required to fill the ventricle to a given volume) causes an upward shift of the diastolic pressure curve. The slope of the diastolic pressure curve, which is equal to 1/compliance (compliance = $\Delta V/\Delta P$), remains unchanged. Regardless of whether abnormal ventricular filling is due to reduced compliance or distensibility, the end result is the same: an elevated end-

Heart Failure Resulting from Myocardial Muscle Abnormalities
Abnormal contraction
Abnormal ventricular filling
Obstruction

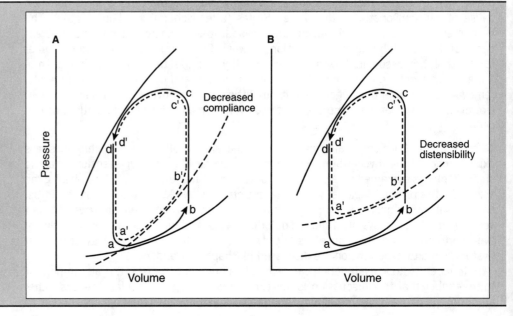

FIG. 1-31
PRESSURE-VOLUME LOOPS IN DIASTOLIC DYSFUNCTION. (A) Reduced compliance of the left ventricle causes the diastolic filling curve to become steeper (slope = 1/compliance). (B) Distensibility of the left ventricle is reduced, which causes a parallel upward shift of the diastolic pressure curve. Neither decreased compliance nor decreased distensibility is associated with reduced stroke volume (c–d = c'–d'), but both cause elevated end-diastolic pressures (points b'). Generally most clinical cases of diastolic dysfunction are associated with reduced distensibility and reduced compliance.

diastolic pressure. Elevated end-diastolic pressure is the pathophysiologic basis for the similar symptoms observed in heart failure resulting from diastolic dysfunction and systolic dysfunction.

Causes of Diastolic Dysfunction. The causes of diastolic dysfunction are listed in Table 1-4, and some of the more common causes are discussed in the following paragraphs.

Coronary artery disease
Myocardial ischemia
Infiltrative diseases
Amyloidosis
Sarcoidosis
Hemochromatosis
Hypertrophy in response to an abnormal load
Aortic stenosis
Hypertension
Primary or genetic conditions (hypertrophic cardiomyopathy)

Table 1-4
Causes of Diastolic Dysfunction

Hypertension (Increased Afterload). If the left ventricle is exposed to a chronic increase in afterload (e.g., systemic arterial hypertension), the constant increase in systolic wall tension leads to myocyte hypertrophy by parallel replication of sarcomeres. This leads to thickening of the ventricular wall without an accompanying increase in chamber size, or concentric hypertrophy. The basis for concentric hypertrophy can be understood by Laplace's law:

$$\sigma = \frac{p \times r}{2h}$$

where σ is wall stress, p is intraventricular pressure, r is the radius of the endocardial surface of the ventricle, and h is ventricular thickness. In this case, the ventricle is exposed to continued pressure overload, and to maintain wall stress constant in the setting of increased pressure, wall thickness increases without an accompanying increase in the intracavitary radius. As in the case of eccentric hypertrophy, the actual mechanism for concentric hypertrophy is not well understood.

Thickening of the left ventricle reduces the distensibility and compliance of the left ventricle. Considerable remodeling occurs in ventricles exposed to chronic pressure overload. Individual myocytes become separated by an extensive branching network of collagen. In addition, several experimental models have shown that the high-energy phosphate content in the pressure-overloaded heart is decreased. In the hypertrophied heart, diastolic dysfunction is observed before systolic dysfunction. During systole, Ca^{2+} is rapidly released from the sarcoplasmic reticulum down its electrochemical gradient. Conversely, during diastole, extrusion of Ca^{2+} through the sarcolemma and reuptake of Ca^{2+} into the sarcoplasmic reticulum are both energy-requiring processes. The removal of intracellular Ca^{2+} can occur only 1/100,000 as fast as Ca^{2+} entry, which suggests that there is a smaller reserve for myocyte relaxation.

Primary Hypertrophy of the Ventricle. Hypertrophy of the ventricle can be due to a family of genetic disorders collectively called hypertrophic cardiomyopathy. Since some forms of hypertrophic cardiomyopathy are associated with abnormal septal hypertrophy causing a left ventricular outflow gradient, these diseases are discussed extensively under outflow obstruction. However, it is important to remember that all forms of hypertrophic cardiomyopathy are associated with abnormal ventricular filling.

Ischemia. Another important cause of diastolic dysfunction is ischemia. Since myocyte relaxation is an energy-requiring process, reduced high-energy phosphate concentrations resulting from ischemia result in relatively high concentrations of intracellular Ca^{2+} and residual cross-linking between actin and myosin myofilaments. In this way, ischemia causes reduced ventricular distensibility and reduced ventricular compliance.

Infiltrative Cardiomyopathies. A number of disease states result in infiltration of the myocardium by abnormal and, usually, noncardiac substances. The infiltration occurs in the intracellular space and results in stiffening of the myocardium and, therefore, impaired diastolic function. Sarcoidosis, amyloidosis, and hemochromatosis are the most common of these cardiomyopathies.

Case Study:
Continued

Mr. Buecheler had extremely elevated blood pressure, which placed a significant after-load on his heart. To maintain SV, his heart had to fill along a steeper portion of the diastolic pressure curve (Fig. 1-32). This led to increased end-diastolic pressure and the accumulation of fluid in his lungs. To make matters worse, over time his heart thickened in response to the elevated blood pressure (concentric hypertrophy), which shifted his diastolic pressure curve upward. This resulted in an even higher increase in left ventricular end-diastolic pressure and an accompanying elevation in pulmonary venous pressure.

FIG. 1-32
MR. BUECHELER'S PRESSURE–VOLUME CURVE. Systemic hypertension has caused increased afterload (the left ventricle must reach greater pressures before the aortic valve can open [*dashed lines*]). End-diastolic pressure is elevated because of the upward and steeper shift of his diastolic pressure curve. A pressure–volume loop from a normal heart is shown for comparison (*solid lines*).

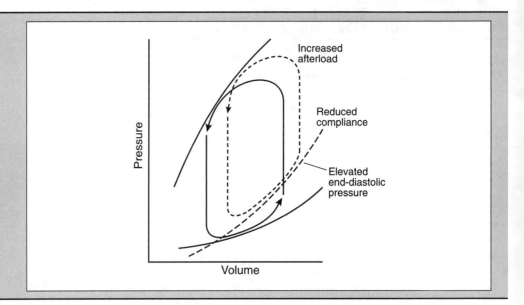

HYPERTROPHIC CARDIOMYOPATHY (OUTFLOW OBSTRUCTION)

Hypertrophic cardiomyopathy is an autosomal dominant disease that is characterized by left ventricular hypertrophy in the absence of any abnormal external loads (e.g., hypertension). The pathologic findings associated with hypertrophic cardiomyopathy were originally described by two French pathologists in the mid-19th century. However, it was not until Teare's description in 1958 that hypertrophic cardiomyopathy was clearly recognized as a separate entity. Hypertrophic cardiomyopathy is relatively rare, with an occurrence rate of approximately 0.1%. However, like any genetic disease, it shows significant familial clustering.

Anatomy and Histology. Hypertrophic cardiomyopathy has been classified by the anatomic pattern of hypertrophy observed in the left ventricle (Table 1-5). Often hypertrophy is asymmetric and is frequently most prominent in the ventricular septum. On histologic examination, the individual myocytes are arranged in a haphazard, disorganized pattern, instead of having the usual parallel structure. In addition, the myocardial walls are characterized by a significant amount of fibrosis.

Pathophysiology. Clinically, hypertrophic cardiomyopathy is most commonly classified by whether obstruction of the left ventricular outflow tract is present.

In approximately 25% of patients with hypertrophic cardiomyopathy, hypertrophy of the septum causes obstruction of the left ventricular outflow tract during ventricular

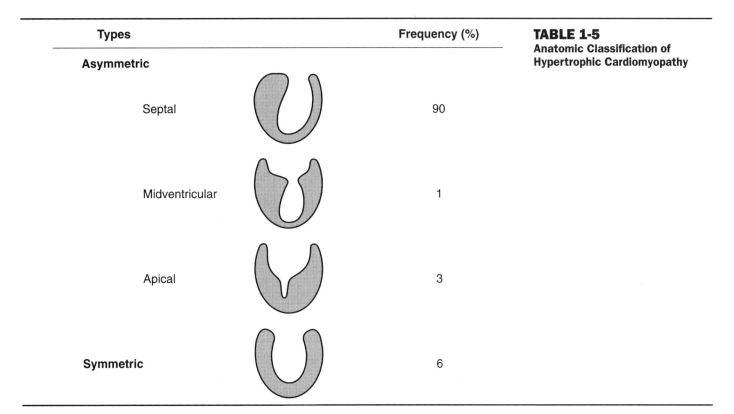

Types		Frequency (%)
Asymmetric		
Septal		90
Midventricular		1
Apical		3
Symmetric		6

TABLE 1-5
Anatomic Classification of Hypertrophic Cardiomyopathy

contraction (Fig. 1-33). The precise mechanism is still not known, but it is generally thought that septal hypertrophy results in a narrowed left ventricular outflow tract and a rapid ejection velocity. The path of ejection is relatively close to the anterior mitral leaflet and may pull the anterior leaflet toward the septum by a Venturi effect. The anterior leaflet is brought close to or may even touch the septum, which creates a dynamic obstruction to flow out of the heart. The obstruction is usually most prominent during mid- or late systole. The obstruction during mid-to-late systole places a large afterload on the ventricle, as shown in the pressure–volume curve in Fig. 1-34. In some cases, the

Venturi effect is named after Gianni Venturi, an Italian physicist who studied flow of liquids. If liquid flows through a narrowed tube, as velocity of flow increases, pressure within the tube decreases.

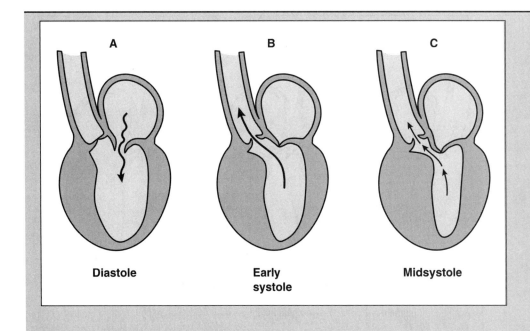

A   B   C

Diastole   Early systole   Midsystole

FIG. 1-33
MECHANISM OF THE OUTFLOW TRACT GRADIENT. (A) During diastole, the ventricle fills through the mitral valve. Ventricular filling is abnormal (*wavy arrow*) because of the thickened ventricular wall. (B) During the early portion of the ejection period, blood flows through the aortic valve. Flow of blood through the left ventricular outflow tract is directed abnormally close to the mitral valve. (C) During midsystole, continued septal thickening and a Venturi effect cause the anterior leaflet of the mitral valve to be pulled toward the septum, which creates a dynamic obstruction in the outflow tract. Blood flow through the aortic valve is significantly reduced despite a markedly elevated intracavitary pressure.

FIG. 1-34
PRESSURE–VOLUME RELATION-SHIP IN HYPERTROPHIC CAR-DIOMYOPATHY WITH OUTFLOW TRACT OBSTRUCTION. The diastolic pressure curve is shifted upward and is steeper because of reduced compliance and distensibility, and the isovolumic systolic pressure curve is shifted upward slightly as a result of the hypertrophy. The heart is exposed to a sudden increase in afterload when the midsystolic gradient is created. Stroke volume is reduced, and end-diastolic pressures can be markedly elevated.

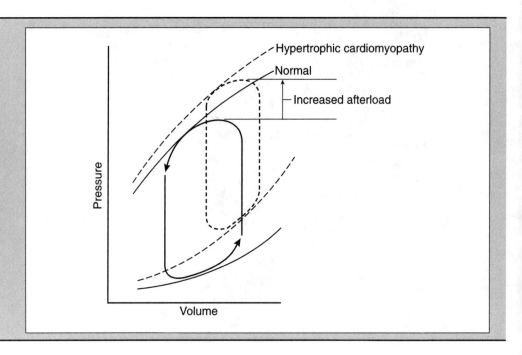

cyclic contact of the anterior leaflet to the septum causes a localized region of fibrosis in the septum of the outflow tract. The turbulent flow from the dynamic obstruction causes a midsystolic murmur. Murmurs are relatively prolonged sounds resulting from turbulent flow within the heart or the great vessels. The causes of heart murmurs are reviewed in greater detail in Chapter 4 and in Appendix I. The heart murmur associated with left ventricular outflow tract obstruction is also dynamic (Fig. 1-35). Maneuvers that increase ventricular size (such as leg raising, which increases venous return) cause the left ventricular outflow obstruction to lessen and the murmur becomes softer. Conversely, maneuvers that decrease ventricular size (such as sudden standing, which decreases venous return) cause the left ventricular outflow obstruction to increase and the murmur becomes louder.

FIG. 1-35
Since the obstruction in the outflow tract is dynamic, the murmur created by turbulent flow through the outflow tract can change in intensity. (A) Normal filling creates a moderate outflow tract obstruction. A murmur can be appreciated between the first (S_1) and second) (S_2) heart sounds (during systole). (B) Increased ventricular filling by maneuvers that increase venous return (e.g., leg raising) causes increased filling and increased ventricular size, which reduces the gradient and the intensity of the murmur. (C) Conversely, by decreasing venous return (sudden standing), smaller ventricular size leads to a severe outflow obstruction, and the murmur is intensified.

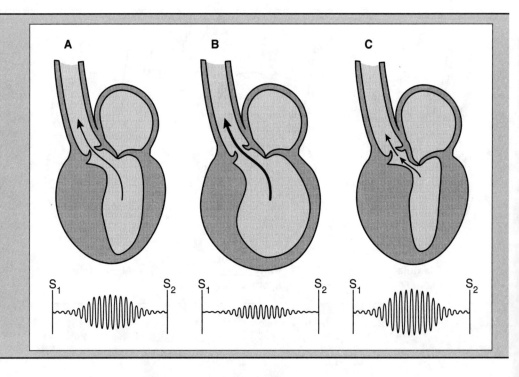

Regardless of whether outflow obstruction is present, abnormalities of ventricular filling are observed in most patients with hypertrophic cardiomyopathy. Abnormal filling is due to decreased distensibility and compliance of the thickened and fibrotic ventricle. In addition, myocardial relaxation is abnormal in patients with hypertrophic cardiomyopathy. On pressure–volume analysis, the diastolic pressure curve is shifted upward and is steeper than normal.

Approximately 10%–15% of patients with longstanding hypertrophic cardiomyopathy develop systolic dysfunction. In these patients, the left ventricle enlarges and the walls thin. If a left ventricular gradient is present, it often is reduced and sometimes resolves completely. Pathophysiologically, the ventricle becomes similar to one in dilated cardiomyopathy. Pathologically, the ventricle is characterized by diffuse scarring.

Genetics. Molecular biology techniques have greatly expanded our knowledge of hypertrophic cardiomyopathy. It is now clear that hypertrophic cardiomyopathy is genetically heterogeneous. Approximately 50%–70% of cases are inherited as an autosomal dominant disorder with variable penetrance; the remainder of cases appear to be sporadic. To date, abnormalities on chromosomes 1, 11, 14, and 15 have been described in this disorder. The *β-MHC* gene exists on chromosome 14. The *β-MHC* gene is constituted of 40 exons that transcribe a 6-kb mRNA, which then can be translated into the 220-kD β-MHC protein. Remember that the β-MHC protein is the central component for the thick filament in adults. More than 36 different mutations of the *β-MHC* gene have been identified. The abnormal myosin proteins form abnormal sarcomeres. *β-MHC* mutations account for 20%–40% of cases of hypertrophic cardiomyopathy. Mutations in the *troponin-T* gene (chromosome 1) and *tropomyosin gene* (chromosome 15) account for some of the remaining cases, but clearly a number of other mutation types will be identified in the future. All of these mutations appear to cause abnormal sarcomere architecture and function. The final common pathway appears to be compensatory hypertrophy of the left ventricle. The reason that septal hypertrophy is favored in the great majority of patients is not known.

SIGNS AND SYMPTOMS OF HEART FAILURE

Dyspnea (Breathlessness). Both the systolic dysfunction and diastolic dysfunction forms of heart failure are associated with elevated end-diastolic pressures in the left ventricle. This increased pressure can be transmitted to the left atrium, the pulmonary veins, and the pulmonary capillaries. If the elevated pressure is high enough to overcome the plasma oncotic pressure, fluid tends to move from the capillaries to the interstitial spaces and alveoli (pulmonary edema). Normally plasma oncotic pressure is 25–30 mm Hg so that significant increases in hydrostatic pressure must occur before flow out of the capillaries is favored.

If elevated pulmonary capillary pressures cause net flow of fluid into the interstitial spaces, initially the lymphatic system can drain the surplus fluid. However, as the flow of fluid from the capillaries increases, fluid begins collecting in the interstitial spaces, which causes hypoxia and tachypnea because of ventilation–perfusion mismatches, reactive bronchoconstriction, and interstitial fluid causing direct compression of small bronchioles. Eventually, if interstitial fluid accumulation is great enough, fluid begins to accumulate in the alveoli.

Acute episodes of ischemia can cause sudden shortness of breath due to pulmonary edema. Ischemia can cause pulmonary edema by diastolic and systolic dysfunction. Chronic shortness of breath associated with heart failure is most likely due to increased pulmonary "dead space" and chronic ventilation–perfusion mismatches.

One of the characteristics of dyspnea associated with heart failure is that the shortness of breath is worse in the supine position (orthopnea). In addition, patients frequently complain that they can go to sleep normally but wake up in the night "gasping for breath" (paroxysmal nocturnal dyspnea). Both of these characteristics are probably due to increased venous return on lying flat, which causes an increase in end-diastolic pressure.

Auscultation of the lungs can be very revealing in the patient with heart failure. Laënnec, who developed the stethoscope in the early 1800s, described "rattling" sounds during inspiration in very ill patients. He was the first to use the phrase *rales* (which means "rattle" in French), which is still in common use today. Rales are fine or coarse crackling sounds heard during late inspiration. It has traditionally been thought that these sounds are due to movement of air through fluid-filled passages; recently it has been suggested that the sounds are more likely due to sudden opening of small airways associated with thoracic expansion. Rales can be heard in a number of pathophysiologic states such as chronic bronchitis, asbestosis, and sarcoidosis; however, the presence of rales should always arouse suspicion of heart failure.

Fatigue. Patients with heart failure frequently complain of generalized fatigue. Traditionally, fatigue in the presence of heart failure has been thought to be due to inadequate delivery of oxygen to the peripheral tissues, which has led to the buildup of anaerobic by-products. Recent investigations suggest that the process is much more complex. Impaired vasodilation of muscle arterioles, reduced oxidative capacity of peripheral muscles, and impaired muscle strength have been reported in patients with heart failure. The important implication of these findings is that symptoms of fatigue in patients with heart failure may be alleviated by exercise training.

Third and Fourth Heart Sounds. Auscultation of the heart is one of the most important skills for the physician to acquire. Physicians have classified the sounds produced by the heart into two general categories: *heart murmurs*, which are relatively prolonged sounds due to turbulent flow, and *heart sounds*, which are short sounds that are produced by sudden opening or closing of valves or abnormal ventricular filling (Fig. 1-36). The *first heart sound (S_1)* is a high-frequency sound that is due to closure of the mitral and tricuspid valves. S_1 corresponds to end-diastole. The ventricles contract and eject blood, and the *second heart sound (S_2)* is produced when the aortic and pulmonic

FIG. 1-36
PHONOCARDIOGRAM (WHICH ALLOWS RECORDING OF THE HEART SOUNDS AND MURMURS) AND PRESSURE TRACINGS FOR THE LEFT VENTRICLE AND LEFT ATRIUM. In all three phonocardiograms, notice that the first heart sound (S_1) coincides with mitral valve closure (MC) and tricuspid valve closure (TC). The second heart sound (S_2) corresponds to aortic valve closure (AC) and pulmonic valve closure (PC). (A) A phonocardiogram showing a normal heart is illustrated. Only the high-frequency S_1 and S_2 can be heard. (B) In this example, a low-frequency third heart sound (S_3) can be heard after the mitral valve opens (MO) and is due to sudden "checking" of blood when a dilated left ventricle reaches its elastic limit. (C) The fourth heart sound (S_4) corresponds to atrial contraction. This low-frequency sound is due to additional blood being forced (by atrial contraction) into a noncompliant chamber.

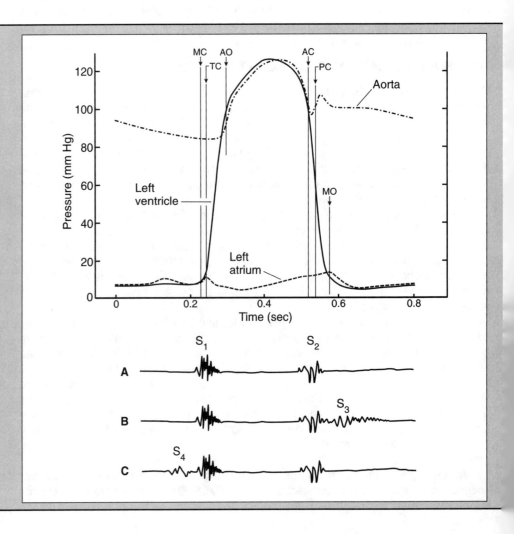

valves close at end-systole. Since systole is shorter than diastole, S_2 follows relatively soon after S_1, and the two heart sounds together are often described by the popular, descriptive phrase "lub-dub."

In some cases, low-frequency heart sounds resulting from abnormal ventricular filling can be appreciated. In patients with dilated hearts, a *third heart sound* (S_3) can be heard in early diastole. When the mitral valve opens, the blood that has accumulated in the left atrium suddenly flows into the left ventricle. S_3 is due to sudden deceleration of blood when the heart reaches its elastic limits. In patients with left ventricular hypertrophy, a *fourth heart sound* (S_4) can be heard in late diastole. S_4 is due to blood being pushed into a noncompliant left ventricle by atrial contraction. Both S_3 and S_4 are short, low-frequency sounds and are best appreciated using the bell of the stethoscope. They are distinguished by their position in the cardiac cycle. As a general rule (which is broken often) S_3 is more commonly associated with systolic dysfunction, and S_4 is more commonly associated with diastolic dysfunction. The student must remember that there are many exceptions to this "rule." A longer discussion on the mechanisms and causes of S_3 and S_4 is provided in Appendix I.

S_1 = "lub"; S_2 = "dub"; S_3 = "lub-dub-**da**'"; S_4 = "**da**'-lub-dub."

Sustained Apical Impulse.

If the hand is placed on the chest, pulsations from the heart can be readily appreciated. Physicians have been carefully evaluating precordial motion since the Middle Ages. The most important pulsation for the student of medicine to recognize is the apical impulse. The apical impulse is due to the outward motion of the left ventricular apex during systole. The apical impulse can normally be felt in the left chest at the midclavicular line at approximately the fourth or fifth intercostal interspace. The timing, location, and size of the apical impulse should be considered separately.

The apical impulse normally coincides with S_1 (beginning of isovolumic contraction) and before the carotid upstroke (during the isovolumic contraction period). If the apical impulse occurs at the same time as or later than the carotid upstroke, the apical impulse is termed "sustained." A sustained apical impulse can be observed in left ventricular hypertrophy and depressed left ventricular systolic function. However, patients with left ventricular dilatation (which often accompanies depressed left ventricular function) frequently have a laterally displaced apical impulse. The normal apical impulse can be palpated in an area the size of a quarter. If the apical impulse can be felt over a relatively large area (a half-dollar for example), an increase in left ventricular size should be suspected.

Evaluation of the Apical Impulse
Timing
Position
Size

Elevated Jugular Venous Pressure (JVP).

Evaluation of the venous pulse is an important part of the cardiac evaluation. Most commonly the venous pulsations of the internal jugular vein are evaluated, since the JVP is a close approximation to the central venous pressure and right atrial pressure (Fig. 1-37). The experienced examiner evaluates both the height of the meniscus and the individual waveforms. For the evaluation of a patient with heart failure, meniscus height, which estimates right atrial pressure, is most critical and is the focus of this discussion.

Before we discuss the JVP, it is important to remember that other venous systems can be used to estimate right atrial pressure. For example, the veins on the back of your hand are relatively prominent if your hand is below your heart as you read this chapter. Now slowly lift your hand; the point where the veins in your hands collapse is an estimate of your right atrial pressure. The sternal angle of Louis, which is approximately 5 cm above your right atrium, is a convenient landmark. If the vessels on the back of your hand flatten when you reach the angle of Louis on your sternum, your right atrial pressure is approximately 5 cm. Unfortunately this method actually estimates peripheral venous pressure rather than central venous pressure (pressure within the inferior or superior vena cava) and is significantly affected by venous tone.

The internal jugular vein is most commonly used for estimating central venous pressure, since it is directly connected to the superior vena cava. In most patients, the meniscus of the internal jugular vein is observed when the patient is positioned at approximately 30 degrees (see Fig. 1-37); the patient with severe elevation of central venous pressure will have to be positioned at an increased angle to observe the meniscus. Again, the angle of Louis can be used as a landmark.

Evaluation of JVP
Meniscus height
Waveform morphology

FIG. 1-37
ESTIMATING RIGHT ATRIAL PRESSURE FROM THE JUGULAR VENOUS PULSATION. (A) In a normal patient, the meniscus of the jugular vein can usually be observed when the patient is placed at a 30-degree angle. The angle of Louis is a convenient landmark, since it is usually 5 cm above the right atrium (RA) independent of the body angle. The meniscus of the jugular venous pulsation is at the level of the angle of Louis, which suggests that jugular venous pressure is approximately 5 cm of water. (B) In this patient, the jugular venous meniscus can only be observed when the patient is positioned at an 80-degree angle; jugular venous pressure is markedly elevated at approximately 13 cm of water. RV = right ventricle.

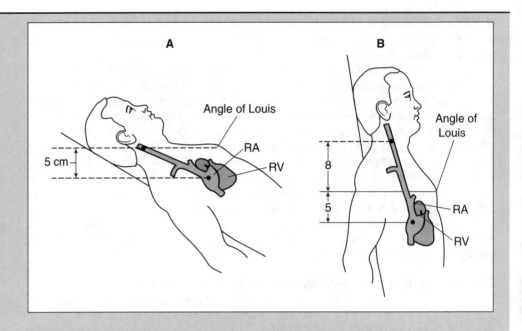

Elevated central venous pressure can be observed in any condition associated with elevated right atrial pressure. Elevated right atrial pressure is most commonly due to right ventricular failure. The most common cause of right ventricular failure is left ventricular failure. Thus the central venous pressure can provide an estimate of preload of the ventricles.

Case Study:
Continued

Elevated pulmonary venous pressures cause increased pressure of plasma into the interstitial spaces and the alveolar spaces of the lung. This abnormal flow was responsible for the symptoms of shortness of breath and the rales on Mr. Buecheler's lung examination. Mr. Buecheler's thickened and noncompliant left ventricle had become very dependent on atrial filling. The sound of blood being forced into the left ventricle was responsible for S_4.

RIGHT HEART FAILURE

To this point, the pathophysiology of heart failure has been described in terms of systolic and diastolic dysfunction of the left ventricle. Failure of the right ventricle is analogous to left ventricular failure in many ways. It occurs principally in the form of systolic dysfunction. The most common cause of right ventricular failure is pressure overload resulting from elevated pulmonary artery pressures (termed *pulmonary hypertension*).

The most common cause of pulmonary hypertension that leads to right heart failure is left heart failure. Left heart failure results in increased left-sided filling pressures (e.g., increased left atrial pressure), which are transmitted through the pulmonary vasculature to the right heart. The right heart then fails in the face of increased afterload in a way analogous to that described for left heart failure. Frank-Starling curves and pressure–volume loops described above for left ventricular systolic failure apply directly in describing the hemodynamics of right heart failure.

Almost any severe pulmonary disease (e.g., chronic obstructive pulmonary disease, idiopathic pulmonary fibrosis, chronic pulmonary emboli,) can cause damage to the pulmonary vasculature in its advanced stage. As such, all of these diseases can cause pulmonary hypertension and subsequently right heart failure. When right heart failure results from pulmonary hypertension caused by a primary pulmonary disease, it is termed *cor pulmonale.*

Over time, if Mr. Buecheler's high blood pressure had been left untreated, his left ventricle would have begun to decompensate, causing his isovolumic systolic pressure curve to shift to the right and a significant decrease in SV, which would force the heart to operate on an ever steeper portion of the diastolic pressure curve and cause even more symptoms (Fig. 1-38). Longstanding untreated high blood pressure can cause heart failure by first producing diastolic dysfunction and then systolic dysfunction. In addition, hypertension is a significant risk factor for the development of atherosclerotic lesions in the coronary arteries (see Chap. 3). Commonly, atherosclerotic lesions can rupture, forming occlusive thrombi in the coronary artery, leading to myocardial infarction. Damage to the myocardium can cause systolic dysfunction, and transient ischemia can worsen diastolic dysfunction.

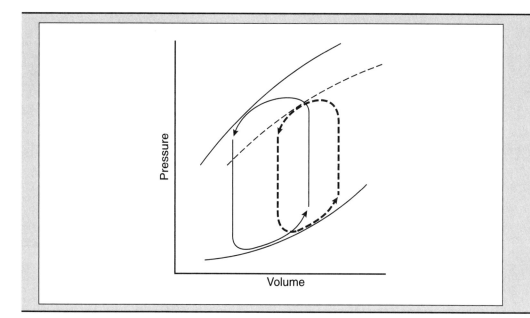

FIG. 1-38
Mr. Buecheler's isovolumic systolic pressure curve has shifted rightward (*dashed line*). Stroke volume is markedly reduced, and left ventricular end-diastolic pressure is extremely elevated.

▮ SUMMARY

The heart is a pump that supplies blood to all tissues of the body. When the heart is unable to perform this basic function, the patient is described as having *heart failure*, which is often manifested by profound shortness of breath and fatigue. Abnormalities of the cardiac muscle can cause heart failure by reducing contractile function (systolic dysfunction), reducing ventricular compliance (diastolic dysfunction), and obstructing flow. The distinction among these types of heart failure is important because they produce different physical examination findings and often require very different treatment strategies. In addition, once the pathophysiologic type of heart failure is identified, the specific etiology must be determined. For example, if a patient presents with severe systolic dysfunction, it is critical to distinguish between hibernating myocardium due to coronary artery disease and cardiomyopathy due to alcohol abuse. Although systolic dysfunction due to any cause is treated acutely by reducing afterload and preload, the best long-term treatment of hibernating myocardium is reestablishment of blood flow to the ischemic myocardium, while alcoholic cardiomyopathy may resolve with abstention from alcohol consumption.

The ability to diagnose, evaluate, and treat heart failure is one of the most important skills for the student to learn during his or her training. A comprehensive understanding of the basic pathophysiology of heart failure is necessary for accomplishing this goal.

KEY POINTS

- Cardiac output is dependent on HR and SV. SV is affected by three different factors: preload, inotropic state, and afterload.
- Pressure–volume curves can graphically distinguish the different pathophysiologic mechanisms of heart failure (decreased cardiac output). *Systolic dysfunction* is indicated by downward and rightward shift of the isovolumic pressure curve. *Diastolic dysfunction* is associated with an upward shift of the diastolic pressure curve. *Outflow tract obstruction* cause increased afterload.
- The heart has two types of hypertrophic responses, depending on the abnormal load. Volume overload of the heart (which increases diastolic pressure) leads to eccentric hypertrophy (increase in both left ventricular volume and thickness). Pressure overload of the heart is associated with concentric hypertrophy (increased ventricular thickness without an accompanying increase in volume).
- Symptoms of heart failure are dyspnea (particularly orthopnea) and fatigue. Signs of heart failure can be outlined as:

1. **Systolic dysfunction**
   S_3
   Rales
   Elevated JVP
   Sustained and displaced apical impulse

2. **Diastolic dysfunction**
   S_4
   Rales
   Elevated JVP
   Sustained apical impulse

3. **Obstruction**
   S_4
   Rales
   Elevated JVP
   Sustained apical impulse
   Systolic murmur

- As an introduction to the pathophysiology of heart failure resulting from cardiomyopathies, the distinction among systolic dysfunction, diastolic dysfunction, and outflow obstruction is useful educationally and clinically. It is important for the student to remember that many patients with heart failure have both systolic and diastolic dysfunction.

Case Study:
Resolution

Mr. Buecheler was admitted and given furosemide, which is a potent diuretic. Stimulating the kidney to produce additional urine is a rapid and effective way to reduce preload. In addition, he was started on intravenous nitroglycerin, which causes venous vasodilation (reduced preload) and arterial vasodilation (reduced afterload). Nitroglycerin is converted to nitric oxide, which causes smooth muscle relaxation in the vascular wall.

Aggressive treatment of his hypertension led to prompt improvement in his shortness of breath, and complete resolution of his rales and S_4. He was discharged after a 48-hour hospitalization on lisinopril, which is an ACE inhibitor. As discussed in Chap. 7, inhibiting ACE causes peripheral arterial vasodilation and is a very effective method for controlling blood pressure.

■ REVIEW QUESTIONS

1. Ms. Isabel Figueredo is a 72-year-old woman who has had several myocardial infarctions. She now comes to the physician's office complaining of shortness of breath, which is worse when she lies down. An echocardiogram shows that her left ventricle is dilated and has an ejection fraction of 20%. Which of the following physical examination findings is likely?

   (A) The meniscus of her jugular venous pulse can be observed when the patient is lying flat.
   (B) The systolic murmur becomes louder with standing and softer with passive leg raise.
   (C) A third heart sound (S_3) can be heard.
   (D) An apical impulse can be felt before the carotid upstroke.

2. Which one of the following statements about compliance is true?

   (A) Compliance is equal to $\Delta P/\Delta V$.
   (B) The right ventricle is normally less compliant than the left ventricle.
   (C) The systemic arterial system is more compliant than the pulmonary artery circulation.
   (D) Compliance is an important determinant of the diastolic pressure curve.
   (E) A compliant left ventricle is usually associated with a fourth heart sound (S_4).

3. Stroke volume (SV) can be increased by

   (A) increased heart rate (HR)
   (B) increased preload
   (C) increased afterload
   (D) decreased inotropic state

4. Which of the following statements about cell physiology is true?

   (A) Reduced cytosolic calcium ion (Ca^{2+}) promotes sarcomere contraction.
   (B) Contraction occurs when the globular head of myosin can interact with the tropomyosin-binding site.
   (C) The troponin complex is important for the regulation of contraction.
   (D) Muscle relaxation does not require active energy since the thick filaments passively slide across thin filaments.
   (E) Increased intracellular Ca^{2+} during myocyte contraction is predominantly due to passive Ca^{2+} inflow across the sarcolemma via specialized channels.

■ ANSWERS AND EXPLANATIONS

1. The answer is C. Ms. Figueredo has symptoms very suggestive of heart failure (shortness of breath, worse when lying down). The history of multiple myocardial infarctions should arouse suspicion for heart failure due to systolic dysfunction. The echocardiogram, which is very helpful in this situation, uses sound waves to construct a two-dimensional picture of the heart (see Appendix II). The normal heart fills with approximately 120–130 mL of blood and ejects approximately 65–75 mL of blood with each heartbeat (stroke volume, SV). The ejection fraction is the ratio of the SV to the end-diastolic volume; the normal ejection fraction is greater than 55%. In Ms. Figueredo's case, significant direct ischemic damage to her cardiac myocytes and ventricular remodeling have left her with an enlarged heart with an ejection fraction of only 20%. In this case, a S_3 is commonly heard since we expect her end-diastolic pressure to be fairly elevated. A dynamic murmur that increased with intensity on standing and decreased with passive leg raise would not be expected. This murmur is characteristic of a left ventricular outflow tract obstruction. This murmur is noted in patients with hypertrophic cardiomyopathy where normal or vigorous contraction of the left ventricle in association with a hypertrophied interventricular septum causes obstruction of the left ventricular outflow tract. Patients with severe systolic dysfunction have a sustained apical impulse. Instead of occurring during the isovolumic period of systole, the apical impulse is felt during midsystole and is coincident with or occurs after the carotid upstroke. Patients with systolic dysfunction usually have an elevated jugular venous pressure; the meniscus is observed when the patient is in a more upright position.

2. The answer is D. Compliance is $\Delta V/\Delta P$ and is an important determinant of the position of the diastolic pressure curve. The thin-walled right ventricle is much more compliant than the left ventricle. The pulmonary arterial system, with its very dense lung capillary network necessary for efficient gas exchange, is significantly more compliant than the systemic arterial circulation. A S_4 from audible filling of the left ventricle from atrial contraction is expected in patients with a thickened and noncompliant left ventricle.

3. The answer is B. Remember that cardiac output is the product of HR and SV, and SV is a function of preload, afterload, and inotropic state. Increased SV can be achieved by increasing the preload, decreasing the afterload, or increasing the inotropic state of the cardiac muscle.

4. The answer is C. Contraction of the sarcomere occurs when membrane depolarization causes a small amount of Ca^{2+} to enter the cytoplasm across the sarcolemma. This small increase in cytoplasmic Ca^{2+} stimulates the release of a large amount of Ca^{2+} from the sarcoplasmic reticulum. Ca^{2+} diffuses into the sarcomere and binds to one of the proteins of the troponin complex (troponin-C), which exposes a myosin-binding site on the actin molecule. The myosin head binds to actin, and the sarcomere contracts. Relaxation is an energy-requiring process. Ca^{2+} is resequestered in the sarcoplasmic reticulum by the action of a Ca^{2+}-ATPase.

■ REFERENCES

Deedwania PC: Congestive heart failure. *Cardiol Clin* 12:280–287, 1994.

Grossman E, Messerli FH: Diabetic and hypertensive heart disease. *Ann Intern Med* 125:304–310, 1996.

Lenihan DJ, Gerson MC, Hoit BD, et al: Mechanisms, diagnosis, and treatment of diastolic heart failure. *Am Heart J* 130:153–166, 1995.

Marian AJ, Roberts R: Molecular genetics of hypertrophic cardiomyopathy. *Ann Rev Med* 46:213–222, 1995.

Pfeffer MA: Left ventricular remodeling after acute myocardial infarction. *Ann Rev Med* 46:455–466, 1995.

Schlant RC, Sonnenblick EH: Pathophysiology of heart failure. In *Hurst's the Heart*, 8th ed. Edited by Sclant RC, Alexander RW, O'Rourke RA, et al. New York, NY: McGraw-Hill, 1994, pp 515–555.

Chapter 2

ARRHYTHMIAS

Fred M. Kusumoto, M.D.

■ CHAPTER OUTLINE

Case Study: *Introduction*	*Ms. Sally Augusta Eswine was a 28-year-old woman with no significant medical history who had experienced episodes of palpitations since she was 5 years old. The episodes could occur at any time. Initially, she felt "a fluttering" in her chest, and then her heart would suddenly "race." The episodes usually resolved spontaneously after 5–10 minutes, but they could last for several hours. When her heart began to "race," Ms. Eswine felt lightheaded but did not lose consciousness. On physical examination her vital signs were normal, and her cardiac examination was unremarkable. A baseline electrocardiogram (ECG) and an ECG of an episode of her rapid heart rhythm are shown in Fig. 2-1.*

■ INTRODUCTION

Philosopher scientists from Egypt (c. 1550 B.C.), China (c. 500 B.C.), and Greece (c. 300 B.C.) realized that the pattern of the peripheral pulse was an indicator of health and disease and was somehow associated with the heart. Using a capillary electrometer, A. D. Waller was able to demonstrate unequivocally the presence of cardiac electrical currents generated in man. Soon afterward, Willem Einthoven systematically studied the electrical activity of the human heart and, with clinical input from Sir Thomas Lewis, laid the foundation of electrocardiography. Over the last several decades, our understanding and knowledge of cardiac electrophysiology have increased dramatically. It is now known that cyclic changes in ion permeability of the membrane are responsible for the electrical activity of the cardiac cell and heart. It is critical for the student of medicine to understand the physiologic basis of cardiac activity to understand pathophysiologic conditions that give rise to abnormal heart rhythms.

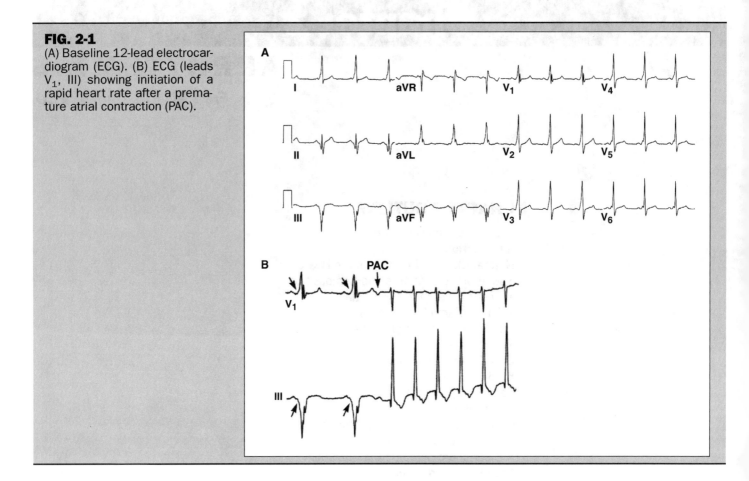

FIG. 2-1
(A) Baseline 12-lead electrocardiogram (ECG). (B) ECG (leads V_1, III) showing initiation of a rapid heart rate after a premature atrial contraction (PAC).

This chapter is divided into two sections. In the first, basic electrophysiology of the heart is reviewed; in the second, the pathophysiology of abnormal heart rhythms is discussed. Abnormal heart rhythms can be simply classified as those that are too slow (bradycardias) and those that are too fast (tachycardias).

■ NORMAL ELECTRICAL ACTIVITY OF THE HEART

MEMBRANE STRUCTURE AND COMPOSITION

The cell membranes that separate the interior of the cell from the extracellular fluid play an important role in determining the electrical function of cardiovascular tissue. In particular, cell membranes provide a barrier that limits the movement of charged ions. The cell membrane is composed of a phospholipid bilayer approximately 50–70 Angström units thick (Fig. 2-2). The phospholipids are formed from a glycerol backbone with a charged phosphate group attached to one end and several fatty acids attached to the other end. The charged phosphate ions face outward, and the hydrophobic fatty acid tails are aligned inward. In animals, a high concentration of cholesterol molecules is inserted between the phospholipid molecules, thereby reducing the fluidity of the membrane. Ions and water move poorly through the membrane bilayer, but proteins that span the bilayer will allow ion and water movement under tightly regulated conditions (Table 2-1). These transmembrane proteins can function either as "channels" that allow passive flow of specific ions in response to receptor binding or voltage changes, as "pumps" that actively transport ions against their concentration gradient using energy derived from the hydrolysis of adenosine triphosphate (ATP), or as "exchangers" that simultaneously transport different ions extracellularly and intracellularly.

Recently, the molecular structure of several important membrane proteins has been partially elucidated. While crystallography is necessary to determine the exact three-dimensional structure of proteins, informed guesses on protein structure can be made by analyzing the amino acid sequence. Regions of protein with a high content of hydro-

Proteins act as channels, pumps, and exchangers.

PROTEIN	CHARACTERISTICS	
Pumps		**Table 2-1** **Membrane Proteins**
Na^+–K^+-ATPase	Three intracellular Na^+ are extruded in exchange for uptake of two extracellular K^+ with hydrolysis of ATP. Important for maintaining the resting concentration differences between the intracellular and extracellular space.	
Ca^{2+}-ATPase	Extrudes one Ca^{2+} from the intracellular space with hydrolysis of ATP. High concentrations in the sarcoplasmic reticulum.	
Channels		
Na^+ channels		
Fast Na^+ (I_{Na})	When open, allows Na^+ to flow down its concentration gradient, which depolarizes the cell and produces the phrase 0 rapid upstroke.	
Funny Na^+ (I_f)	A current produced by slow inward flow of Na^+ that is responsible for diastolic depolarization (phase 4) in His-Purkinje tissue. This current is also present in sinus node and atrioventricular node cells; however, the contribution of this current to diastolic depolarization in these cells is controversial.	
Ca^{2+} channels		
Ca^{2+}-L	The "long-lasting" Ca^{2+} channels open during phase 0 and through the plateau phase (phase 2) of fast-response tissue. Responsible for depolarization in slow-response tissue. Allows Ca^{2+} to flow inward down its electrochemical gradient.	
Ca^{2+}-T	The "transient-opening" Ca^{2+} channels open during the latter part of diastolic depolarization. Responsible in part for the pacemaker activity. Present only in slow-response tissues. Allows Ca^{2+} to flow inward down its electrochemical gradient.	
K^+ channels		
Inward rectifier (I_{K1})	Open at rest. Important for allowing K^+ to equilibrate at rest to a value predicted by the Nernst equation. Turns off when the cell becomes depolarized. Present only in fast-response tissues.	
Transient outward (I_{to})	Opens after cell depolarization in fast-response tissues. Responsible for the phase 1 notch seen in certain tissues. Allows outward flow of K^+ and tends to return the membrane potential to the resting membrane potential.	
Delayed rectifier (I_K)	Opens slowly after depolarization, allowing outward flow of K^+. Responsible for repolarization (phase 3) of the cell. Gradual decay of this current is thought to be partially responsible for the spontaneous diastolic depolarization (phase 4) seen in slow-response tissues.	
Exchangers		
Na^+–Ca^{2+}-exchanger	Extrudes one intracellular Ca^{2+} in exchange for the intracellular transport of three Na^+. Facilitated by ATP, but the energy for this exchange is derived by Na^+ flowing down its concentration gradient. This background current is in part responsible for the slight deviation of the actual resting potential from the potential predicted by the Nernst equation.	

Note. ATP = adenosine triphosphate; Ca^{2+} = calcium ion; K^+ = potassium ion; Na^+ = sodium ion.

phobic amino acids are probably located within the membrane bilayer, while regions of protein with a high concentration of hydrophilic amino acids are probably located on the outer or inner surfaces of the membrane.

The sodium–potassium adenosine triphosphatase (Na^+–K^+-ATPase) "pump" has been purified; it is composed of a larger α-subunit of approximately 1000 amino acids (110,000 daltons [D]) and a smaller β-subunit (50,000 D) [Fig. 2-3]. At least five isoforms of the Na^+–K^+-ATPase α-subunit genes have been cloned and sequenced; the isoforms differ in their sensitivity to digitalis and also are variably expressed, depending on tissue type. All isoforms appear to form seven or eight transmembrane segments; the binding sites for ATP, sodium (Na^+), and potassium (K^+) ions are incompletely characterized at this time. The β-subunit appears to have one transmembrane segment that is attached to the α-subunit by a disulfide bond.

The amino acid sequences of several of the ion channels have also been determined, and a hypothesis on overall structure of these proteins has been postulated (Figs. 2-4 and 2-5). One type of K^+ channel appears to be formed from four subunits. Each subunit is

FIG. 2-2
SCHEMATIC OF THE CELL MEMBRANE. The phospholipid bilayer is shown with the hydrophilic charged phosphate "heads" aligned outward and the hydrophobic fatty acid tails aligned inward. Proteins "float" in the lipid bilayer. Some proteins have "pores" that allow ions to pass through the membrane under tightly controlled conditions.

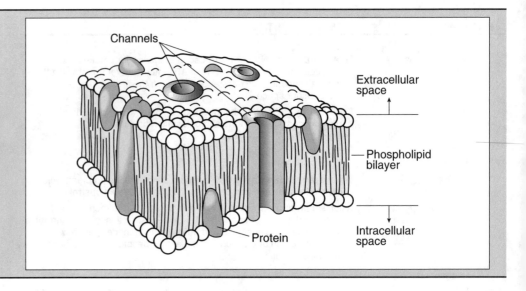

FIG. 2-3
HYPOTHETICAL MODEL OF THE NA+–K+-ATPase PUMP. The larger α-protein with eight transmembrane segments and the smaller β-protein with one transmembrane segment are shown. The putative binding site for adenosine triphosphate (ATP) is indicated by ATP in the figure.

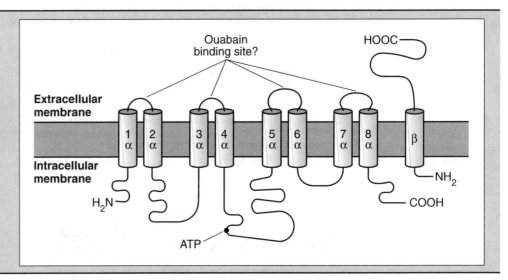

composed of approximately 500–1000 amino acids arranged in several strings of hydrophobic amino acids, which form six membrane-spanning helices. Calcium (Ca^{2+}) and Na^+ channels are more complex and appear to be made up of a large α-protein associated with one to three other proteins (see Fig. 2-5). The α-protein appears to be sufficient to form a functional channel and is composed of four homologous domains (I–IV), each consisting of six transmembrane spanning segments (1–6). There is considerable homology between the domains of the α-subunits of the Ca^{2+} and Na^+ ion channels and the individual K^+ ion channel subunits, which suggests that they are derived from a single ancestral gene. The K^+ channels appear to be the most primitive form of ion channel and are present in yeast. Ca^{2+} channels first appear in higher protozoa, and Na^+ channels are present only in multicellular organisms.

RESTING MEMBRANE POTENTIAL

If a microelectrode is implanted into the interior of a cardiac cell, a voltage potential difference can be measured, with the interior of the cell approximately 90 mV lower than the exterior of the cell. This voltage difference arises because of differing ion concentrations and permeabilities. Under normal conditions, the myocardial cell can maintain an intracellular ion concentration that is markedly different from the extracellular fluid (Fig. 2-6). Extracellular fluid ion concentration is very similar to that of blood plasma: Na^+ and Ca^{2+} concentrations are high, and K^+ concentration is low. Conversely, in the intracellular space, Na^+ and Ca^{2+} concentrations are relatively low, and K^+ concentration is high.

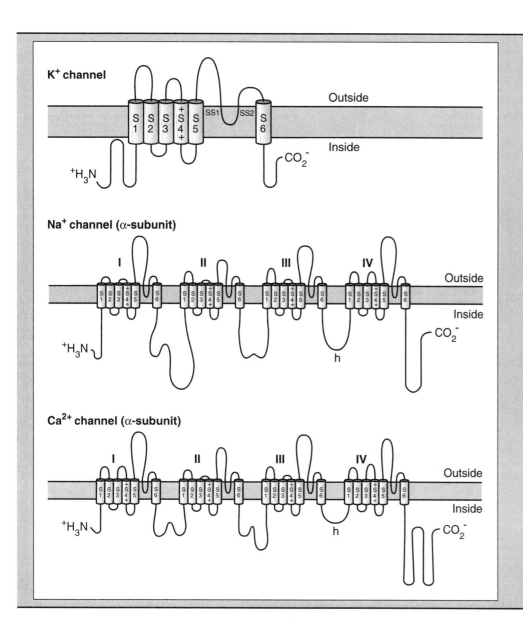

FIG. 2-4
HYPOTHETICAL MODELS OF THE ION CHANNELS OF CARDIAC CELLS. Na^+ and Ca^{2+} channel α-subunit proteins show striking similarities in structure, with four domains (I–IV) composed of six transmembranous segments (1–6). The K^+ channel is made up of four separate subunit proteins, each with six transmembranous segments, which combine to form a channel. The K^+ channel subunit is very similar to a single domain from Na^+ or Ca^{2+} channels. h = gate.

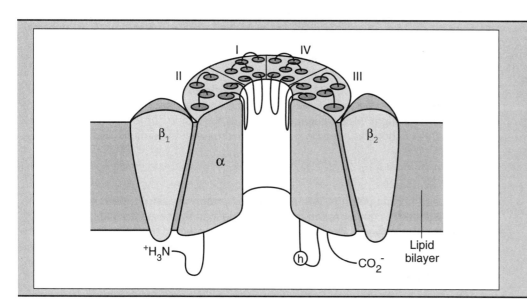

FIG. 2-5
Hypothetical model showing how the Na^+ channel α-protein is thought to be aligned in the cell membrane to form a pore. β_1- and β_2-subunits are smaller proteins with a single transmembrane domain whose functions are poorly understood. h = gate.

FIG. 2-6
Ion pumps and exchangers establish different ion concentrations in the extracellular and intracellular space. The intracellular space has low Na$^+$ and Ca^{2+} concentrations and high K$^+$ concentrations relative to the extracellular space.

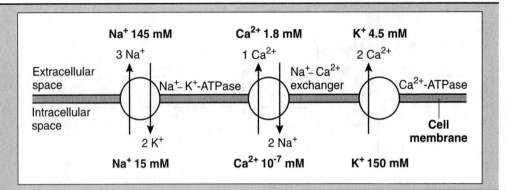

While the membrane serves as a relatively impermeable barrier to the flow of ions and water, several specialized proteins are necessary for establishing and maintaining the different ion gradients between the intracellular and extracellular space. First, the Na$^+$–K$^+$-ATPase, whose molecular structure was briefly discussed above, extrudes three Na$^+$ in exchange for the uptake of two K$^+$. The energy required for transporting both of these ions against their concentration gradients comes from the hydrolysis of ATP. Second, a Na$^+$–Ca^{2+}-exchanger extrudes one Ca^{2+} in exchange for the uptake of three Na$^+$. While this exchange is facilitated by ATP, the energy necessary for this process appears to come from Na$^+$ flowing down its concentration gradient. Third, a Ca^{2+}-ATPase, which is the same protein found in the sarcoplasmic reticulum (see Chap. 1), actively extrudes two Ca^{2+} against their concentration gradient by utilizing energy derived from the hydrolysis of ATP. These proteins, particularly the Na$^+$–K$^+$-ATPase, are important for establishing and maintaining the relative ion concentration differences between the interior and exterior of the cell. If the Na$^+$–K$^+$-ATPase is blocked or inactivated, initially there will be only a very small change in the membrane potential. However, over time the ionic gradients gradually dissipate, the membrane potential becomes less negative, and eventually the cardiac cell loses excitability.

The magnitude of the resting membrane potential (E_m) is determined by the Goldman-Hodgkin-Katz equation:

$$E_m = \frac{RT}{F} \ln \frac{gK^+[K^+]_0 + gNa^+[Na^+]_0 + gCa^{2+}[Ca^{2+}]_0}{gK^+[K^+]_i + gNa^+[Na^+]_i + gCa^{2+}[Ca^{2+}]_i},$$

where R and F are constants; T is temperature; $[K^+]_o$, $[K^+]_i$, $[Na^{++}]_o$, $[Na^+]_i$, $[Ca^{2+}]_o$, and $[Ca^{2+}]_i$ are extracellular and intracellular concentrations of K$^+$, Na$^+$, and Ca^{2+}, respectively; and gK$^+$, gNa$^+$, gCa^{2+} are membrane conductances for K$^+$, Na$^+$, and Ca^{2+}. While large electrochemical gradients exist for Na$^+$ and Ca^{2+}, at the resting state the membrane is relatively impermeable to Na$^+$ and Ca^{2+} (i.e., gNa$^+$ and gCa^{2+} are very small), so that the contribution of Na$^+$ and Ca^{2+} to the resting membrane voltage potential is minimal (Fig. 2-7). However, at the resting state, the membrane is relatively permeable to K$^+$ via specialized K$^+$ channels (I_{K1}, or inwardly rectifying K$^+$ current). Since intracellular anions are relatively large nondiffusable proteins, efflux of K$^+$ ions down its concentration gradient is not accompanied by a corresponding efflux of anions, which results in a slight excess negative charge on the inside of the cell. The Goldman-Hodgkin-Katz equation can then be simplified to the Nernst equation:

$$E_m = \frac{RT}{F} \ln \frac{[K^+]_0}{[K^+]_i}.$$

At this equilibrium potential, the net passive flux of K$^+$ is zero, since outward flow of K$^+$ ions down the K$^+$ concentration gradient is balanced by the electrical forces tending to have K$^+$ ions flow inward. The membrane potential predicted by the Nernst equation is very close to the actual measured potential (Fig. 2-8). The actual membrane potential is slightly positive to that predicted by the Nernst equation because of an inward "leak" of Na$^+$ ions that enter via the Na$^+$–Ca^{2+}-exchanger and other, poorly described channels.

The resting K$^+$ current has the interesting property of inward rectification. Rectification describes the voltage dependence of resistance to ion flow. Ohmic or nonrectifying

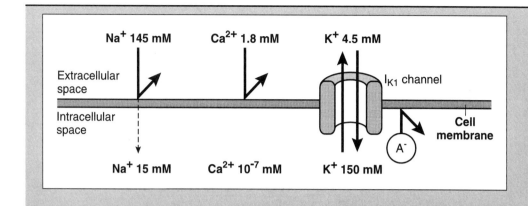

FIG. 2-7
At baseline, the membrane is relatively impermeable to Na^+ and Ca^{2+}. K^+ flows freely through ion channels at a baseline equilibrium potential where outward flow of K^+ (favored by the concentration gradients) is just balanced by inward flow of K^+ (favored by the electrical gradient). The electrical gradient is formed because the relatively large protein anions (A^-) cannot flow through the membrane. A small inward leak of Na^+ (*dashed arrow*) occurs because of the Na^+–Ca^{2+}-exchanger and other, poorly described channels.

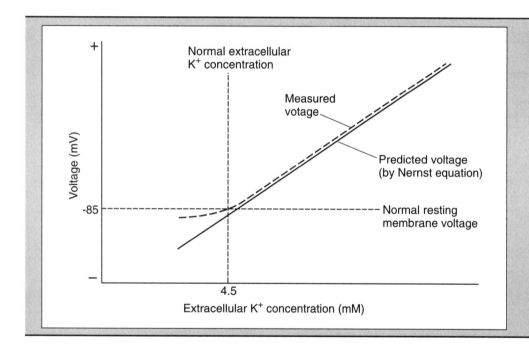

FIG. 2-8
The *solid line* shows the voltage predicted by the Nernst equation for varying concentrations of extracellular K^+. The actual measured resting state membrane voltage (*dashed line*) is slightly positive to the voltage predicted by the Nernst equation because of a relatively small inward "leak" of Na^+ ions.

current obeys Ohm's law (IR = V), which states that current (I) is linearly dependent on voltage (V), if resistance (R) is constant (Fig. 2-9). For an inwardly rectifying current, conductance decreases (resistance increases) with progressive membrane depolarization. For an outwardly rectifying current, conductance increases (resistance decreases) with progressive membrane depolarization. As we will see, this inwardly rectifying property is important for "turning off" the relatively large resting K^+ current (I_{K1}) when the cell is depolarized.

Whereas K^+ equilibrium determines the magnitude of the resting membrane potential, different extracellular and intracellular ion concentrations are established by the Na^+–K^+-ATPase.

CARDIAC ACTION POTENTIALS

If an excitatory impulse is applied to a cardiac cell, the cell membrane depolarizes and initiates a sequence of changes in membrane permeability to various ions, which changes the voltage of the cell in a predictable and reproducible fashion. In general, inward movement of positive ions depolarizes the cell (relative accumulation of intracellular positive charge), and outward flow of positive ions repolarizes the cell (relative accumulation of intracellular negative charge). Cardiac action potentials can be broadly classified into two types, termed "fast-response" and "slow-response" potentials, depending on the presence or absence of fast Na^+ channels (Table 2-2; Fig. 2-10). Atrial,

There are two types of **cardiac action potentials: fast response** and **slow response.**

FIG. 2-9
CURRENT–VOLTAGE RELATION-SHIP FOR VARIOUS TYPES OF CURRENTS. In Ohmic current, resistance is constant, and voltage and current are linearly related (slope = 1/R). For an inwardly rectifying current (I_{K1}), resistance increases at more positive voltages and decreases at voltages negative to the equilibrium potential. For an outwardly rectifying current (I_{to}), resistance decreases at more positive voltages.

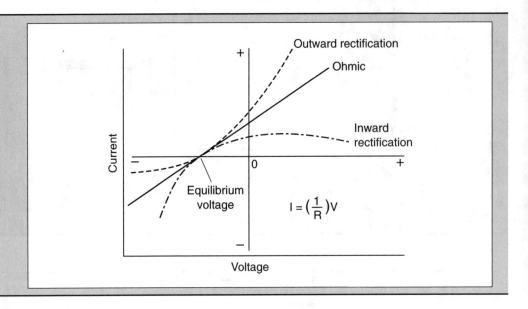

Table 2-2
Action Potentials of Different Tissues

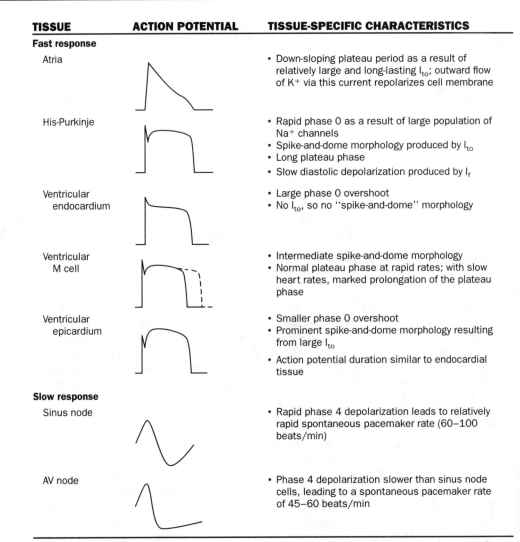

TISSUE	ACTION POTENTIAL	TISSUE-SPECIFIC CHARACTERISTICS
Fast response		
Atria		• Down-sloping plateau period as a result of relatively large and long-lasting I_{to}; outward flow of K^+ via this current repolarizes cell membrane
His-Purkinje		• Rapid phase 0 as a result of large population of Na^+ channels • Spike-and-dome morphology produced by I_{to} • Long plateau phase • Slow diastolic depolarization produced by I_f
Ventricular endocardium		• Large phase 0 overshoot • No I_{to}, so no "spike-and-dome" morphology
Ventricular M cell		• Intermediate spike-and-dome morphology • Normal plateau phase at rapid rates; with slow heart rates, marked prolongation of the plateau phase
Ventricular epicardium		• Smaller phase 0 overshoot • Prominent spike-and-dome morphology resulting from large I_{to} • Action potential duration similar to endocardial tissue
Slow response		
Sinus node		• Rapid phase 4 depolarization leads to relatively rapid spontaneous pacemaker rate (60–100 beats/min)
AV node		• Phase 4 depolarization slower than sinus node cells, leading to a spontaneous pacemaker rate of 45–60 beats/min

Note. AV = atrioventricular; K^+ = potassium ion; Na^+ = sodium ion; I_f = funny current; I_{to} = transient outward current.

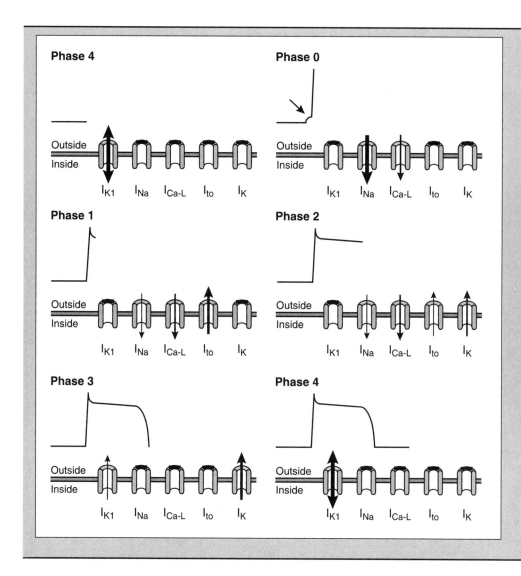

ventricular, and His-Purkinje cells have fast-response action potentials, and sinus node and atrioventricular (AV) node cells have slow-response action potentials.

Fast-Response Action Potentials. In a response similar to that of nerve and skeletal muscle, when atrial, ventricular, or His-Purkinje myocytes are stimulated and reach threshold level (approximately −70 mV), Na^+ channels on the cell surface membrane (sarcolemma) open, and Na^+ flows down its electrochemical gradient into the cell. This sudden inward surge of ions is responsible for the sharp upstroke of the myocyte action potential (phase 0) [Fig. 2-11; see Fig. 2-10]. The maximum rate of rise of the upstroke (V_{max}) reflects the magnitude of I_{Na}. For example, His-Purkinje tissue, which has the highest V_{max} (500–700 V/sec), also has the highest density of Na^+ channels.

Understanding the pattern in which ion channels open and close (*gating characteristics*) is essential for the student to understand how ion channels function. A mathematical model was developed in the 1950s that explains the gating action of Na^+ channels. It appears that this model can apply to many types of ion channels. The model suggests that the ion channel can exist in three different states: *resting, activated,* and *inactivated.* Transition among these states appears to occur through protein conformational changes and the opening and closing of activation (m) and inactivation (h) gates (Fig. 2-12). In the resting state, the m gate is closed, and the h gate is open. When the membrane is depolarized to a threshold level, the m gate opens, and ions can flow in the direction of their electrochemical gradient (activated state). After a variable period of time, the h gate will close, thus stopping ion flow (inactivated state). Finally, the m gate will close, and the h gate will open, returning the ion channel to its resting state. As illustrated in Fig. 2-13, the proportion of gates that are in a given state in Na+ channels is voltage-dependent and changes over time.

FIG. 2-11
TIME COURSE OF CHANGES IN MEMBRANE POTENTIAL AND ION PERMEABILITY DURING THE VARIOUS PHASES OF THE ACTION POTENTIAL. Permeabilities of Na+ (gNa+), Ca2+ (gCa2+), and K+ (gK+) change dramatically over time. I_K = delayed rectifier current; I_{K1} = inward rectifier current; I_{to} = transient outward current.

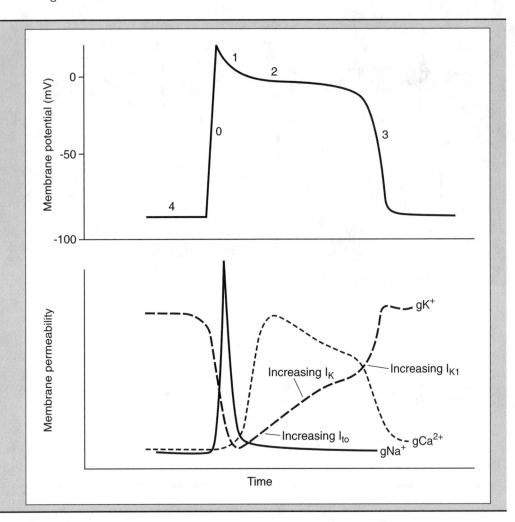

FIG. 2-12
HYPOTHETICAL GATES THAT CONTROL OPENING AND CLOSING OF ION CHANNELS. At the resting state, the m gate is closed, and the h gate is open. When the cell is depolarized, voltage-sensitive regions of the channel protein lead to the opening of the m gate, and ions can flow in the direction favored by their electrochemical gradient (e.g., inward Na+ flow). The channel then changes to the inactivated state when the h gate closes, while the m gate remains open. Finally, in this example, the cardiac cell repolarizes, and as the membrane voltage returns to baseline, the m gate closes, the h gate opens, and the ion channel returns to the resting state.

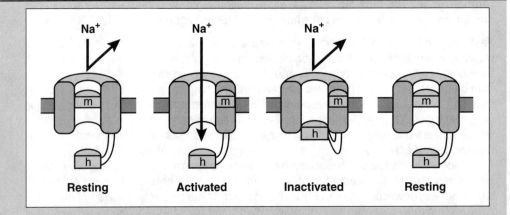

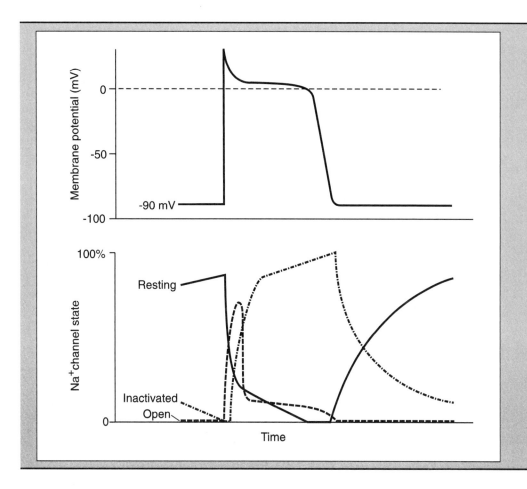

FIG. 2-13
CHANGES IN SODIUM (NA+) CHANNEL STATE OVER TIME. At the resting potential, the great percentage of Na+ channels are in the resting state. During phase 0 there is a sudden increase in the percentage of cells in the open state and accompanying decrease in the number of channels in the resting state. Fairly quickly, most open channels become inactivated. As the cell begins to repolarize, channels begin to change from the inactivated state to the resting state.

Recently, some of the molecular mechanisms for channel activation and inactivation have become partially elucidated and are summarized in Figs. 2-4 and 2-5. The fourth transmembrane segment of each of the four domains of the α-protein is currently thought to be the voltage sensor. This segment contains repeating motifs of a positively charged amino acid separated by two hydrophobic amino acids. Changes in membrane voltage appear to cause poorly described conformational changes in the protein, which allows ions to flow. The actual pore appears to be formed from a large loop between the fifth and sixth segment of each of the four domains. Changes in the amino acids of this region have dramatic effects on ion selectivity. For example, mutation of a critical lysine and alanine residue to glutamine is sufficient to make a Na+ channel become highly selective for Ca^{2+}. Finally, the inactivation gate appears to be a highly conserved intracellular loop that separates the third and the fourth domains (h in Fig. 2-5). Inactivation appears to occur when this loop acts as a "hinged lid" for the intracellular entrance of the ion pore.

After depolarization, a complex interplay of ion currents ensues. Membrane depolarization inactivates the relatively large I_{K1}, and relatively small currents can significantly affect the membrane voltage (see Figs. 2-10 and 2-11). First, the action potential goes from its peak to the plateau value (phase 1). This change is mediated by the transient outward current (I_{to}). While this current appears to involve the flow of several different ions, at least one component is outward K+ flow, which tends to make the potential more negative (closer to the K+ equilibrium potential). The action potential then maintains a relatively positive membrane potential (10–20 mV) for a relatively long period of time (plateau phase, or phase 2). The plateau phase is maintained by the following: (1) *Inward flow of Ca^{2+}* is via Ca^{2+}-L channels (L for "long-lasting"). The Ca^{2+}-L channels open when the membrane potential is approximately −45 to −40 mV and take a relatively long time to reach peak flows (5–10 msec). (2) While most of the Na+ channels are rapidly inactivated, a subpopulation of Na+ channels will inactivate slowly. Thus, *inward flow of Na+ (I_{Na})* also occurs during the plateau phase. (3) These inward currents are balanced

Membrane depolarization markedly reduces K+ permeability.

by *outward K+ flow* via the previously mentioned I_{to} current and slow activation of the delayed rectifier current (I_K). The I_K activates slowly in response to membrane depolarization and has outward rectification properties. The I_K actually has several components, which are characterized by slow activation in response to membrane depolarization.

Repolarization (phase 3) begins as the I_K increases, and the Ca^{2+}-L channels and slowly inactivating Na^+ channels close. As the membrane potential approaches the resting potential, the I_{K1} channels open, and the membrane voltage returns to the resting potential. The fundamentals of the action potential can be understood by taking these five currents into account (fast inward Na^+ current, slow inward Ca^{2+} current, and the three outward K^+ currents). However, the situation is actually much more complex. First, there are several other currents that we have not described here. Second, some currents such as the I_K and I_{to} currents are known to have several components with different pharmacokinetic properties.

Since Na^+ and Ca^{2+} channels go through an inactivated state before returning to the resting state, the cardiac cell will not recover excitability until after a specific period of time (Fig. 2-14). Initially the cell will not be excitable regardless of the stimulus strength; this period is called the *absolute refractory period*. After time, some of the Na^+ and Ca^{2+} channels recover, so that a stimulus causes local depolarization of the cell membrane, but the response will not propagate. The sum of the absolute refractory period and this interval is called the *effective refractory period*, since no self-sustaining electrical activity can be produced. At the end of the effective refractory period, the *relative refractory period* begins, in which a larger-than-normal stimulus depolarizes the membrane and leads to a propagating response. Finally, after most of the channels have recovered, a normal stimulus will lead to a propagating response, and the relative refractory period ends. In fast-response tissue, the refractoriness of tissue is voltage-dependent. In practical terms, once a fast-response cell has returned to its resting voltage it can be fully excited. In contrast, the refractoriness of slow-response tissue is time-dependent. Slow-response cells often display a period of postrepolarization refractoriness during which the cell will not be fully excitable, despite the return to baseline potentials.

The action potentials of various fast-response cells vary slightly from tissue to tissue. These differences are summarized in Table 2-2. Most of the differences relate to differences in repolarization: atrial action potentials have the shortest plateau phase, His-Purkinje cells have the longest plateau periods, and ventricular tissue usually shows some median value. These differences may be due to the specific populations of the different K^+ channels in each tissue type. For example, the down-sloping action potential of atrial tissue appears to arise from a large and relatively long-lasting I_{to} as compared to other myocardial tissue. This outward flow of K^+ tends to return the membrane voltage to the K^+ equilibrium level predicted by the Nernst equation. Similarly, the spike-and-dome morphology of ventricular epicardial tissue and His-Purkinje tissue appears to be due to the presence of I_{to} in these cell populations; in contrast, ventricular endocardial tissue does not have a large population of I_{to} channels.

Slow-Response Action Potentials. The action potential of slow-response cells (sinus node, AV node) is different from that described for ventricular, atrial, and His-Purkinje myocytes. Fast Na^+ channels are absent, so rapid phase 0 depolarization is not observed. Depolarization appears to be solely due to the influx of Ca^{2+} through specialized Ca^{2+} channels (Ca^{2+}-L). As in fast-response cells, repolarization appears to be due to K^+ efflux through the I_K after Ca^{2+} influx has stopped. Cells with slow-response action potentials do not return to a constant resting membrane potential but, instead, display gradual depolarization.

The slow-response cardiac tissue of the sinus node and AV node and one fast-response tissue type (His-Purkinje) do not have a fixed resting potential but rather demonstrate gradual depolarization during phase 4. In the sinus node and AV node, this dynamic change in membrane potential arises from the interplay of several ion currents (Fig. 2-15). These tissues do not have an I_{K1}, and for this reason, the membrane potential does not return to the K^+ equilibrium potential predicted by the Nernst equation (-85 mV). Instead, these tissues reach a maximum diastolic potential of -65 mV, and three currents then appear to be initially responsible for the net inward current required for diastolic depolarization. These are: (1) Decay of the outward K^+ current (I_K,

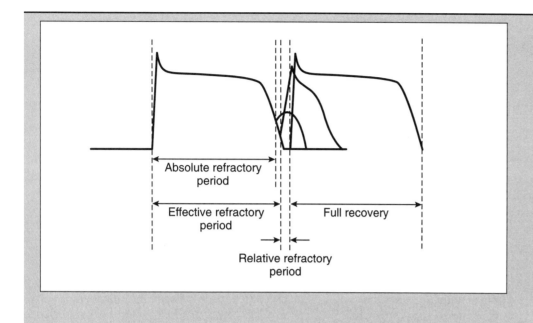

FIG. 2-14
Since most sodium (Na^+) channels are inactivated during the plateau phase, the cardiac cell cannot be reactivated for a specific period of time, called the *absolute refractory period*. After the absolute refractory period, a stimulus may cause some cellular depolarization but does not lead to a propagated response; the sum of this period and the absolute refractory period are termed the *effective refractory period*. After the effective refractory period, a larger-than-normal stimulus causes activation of the cell and leads to a propagating response; this interval is termed the *relative refractory period*. Finally, the tissue recovers full excitability.

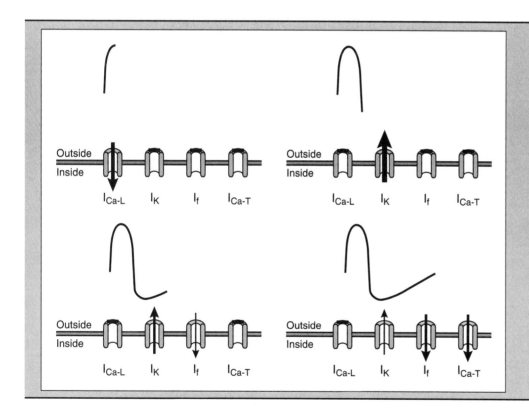

FIG. 2-15
ION FLOWS IN SLOW-RESPONSE TISSUES. Since no sodium (Na^+) channels exist in slow-response tissues, a slower upstroke resulting solely from calcium (Ca^{2+}) inflow is observed. Repolarization occurs when the delayed rectifier current (I_K) begins. Since slow-response tissues have no inwardly rectifying K^+ (I_{K1}) current, the maximum diastolic potential ranges only between -55 and -75 mV. The membrane potential shows gradual depolarization as a result of decay of the delayed rectifier current (I_K) and to inward flow of Na^+ and Ca^{2+} via the I_f (f for "funny") and Ca^{2+}-T currents (T for transient opening). Ca^{2+}-L = long-lasting calcium. I_f = inward Na^+ current.

or delayed rectifier current) in the presence of a background current of gradual inward Na^+ leaks, resulting from the Na^+–Ca^{2+}-exchanger; (2) activation of a small inward Na^+ current called I_f (f stands for "funny" because of the unusual properties of this current); and (3) midway through diastole, Ca^{2+} begins to flow inward through specialized activation of Ca^{2+}-T channels (T stands for "transient opening"), which are found only on slow-response tissues. Depolarization of slow-response tissue occurs when the cell reaches threshold (approximately -45 to -40 mV) and Ca^{2+}-L channels open. Sinus node tissue has a faster pacemaker rate than AV node tissue because it reaches a less negative maximum diastolic potential and has a steeper slope during diastolic depolarization

(Table 2-2). The specific channel mechanisms responsible for this difference are unknown.

His-Purkinje tissue also displays gradual phase 4 depolarization. However, His-Purkinje tissue reaches a maximum diastolic potential that is similar to other fast-response tissues (−85 to −90 mV), and the change in membrane potential appears to be solely mediated by the I_f (Na+ current). The pacemaker rate for His-Purkinje tissue is low, approximately 30–40 beats/min.

ELECTRICAL ACTIVATION OF THE HEART

Electrical Activation of the Heart

Sinus node
↓
Atria
↓
Atrioventricular node
↓
His-Purkinje system
↓
Ventricles

The left and right atria and ventricles contract in coordinated fashion to pump blood to the body and lungs. An electrical impulse is initiated in the sinus node, which activates the right and left atria. The electrical impulse then travels through the AV node, where conduction delay allows the ventricles to fill optimally. The impulse then travels rapidly through the His bundle and the left and right bundles to activate the ventricles rapidly and almost simultaneously (Fig. 2-16). The atria and ventricles are separated by a fibrous framework (annulus) that is electrically inert so that the AV node and the contiguous His bundle form the only electrical connection between the atria and ventricles under normal conditions. This arrangement allows the atria and ventricles to beat in a synchronized fashion and minimizes the chance of electrical feedback between the chambers.

FIG. 2-16
CONDUCTING SYSTEM OF THE HEART SHOWING THE ACTION POTENTIALS OF VARIOUS TISSUE TYPES AND THEIR CORRELATION WITH THE ELECTROCARDIOGRAM (ECG).

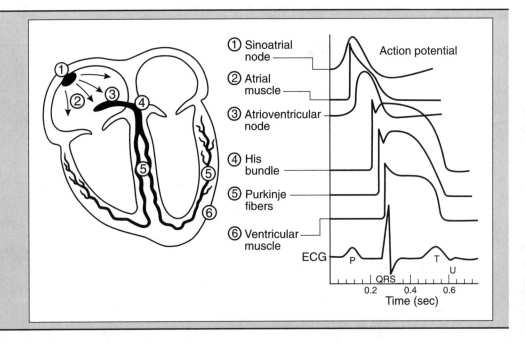

Sinus Node. Since the time of Hippocrates, there has been interest in how the heartbeat is activated. During the 17th century, anatomists thought that the nervous system initiated the cardiac impulse. In the 18th century, Haller proposed that the atria initiated the cardiac beat, but it was not until the pioneering work by Keith and Flack in 1907 that the sinus node was identified as the source of the cardiac impulse. The sinus node lies subepicardially in the groove formed by the junction of the right atrial appendage and the superior vena cava (Fig. 2-17). It is an amorphous, cigar-like structure (1.5 cm long and 0.3–0.5 cm wide) that extends down along the lateral wall of the right atrium, although it can sometimes extend superiorly, forming a "saddle." The sinus node usually receives blood via a prominent central sinus node artery. Within the sinus node, there are nests of pacemaker cells that are smaller than atrial myocytes and set within a fibrous matrix. With age, cell number decreases, and collagen content increases.

These small pacemaker cells lack fast-response Na+ channels and thus have a slow rate of rise of the action potential, which is dependent on inward flow of Ca^{2+}. Pacemaker

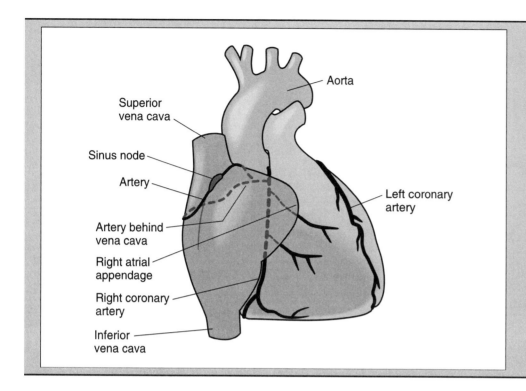

FIG. 2-17
DIAGRAM SHOWING THE LOCA-
TION OF THE SINUS NODE AND
ITS ARTERIAL BLOOD SUPPLY.

cells also have a relatively rapid phase 4 spontaneous depolarization, which leads to a spontaneous pacemaker rate of 60–100 beats/min.

The sinus node is richly innervated by both sympathetic and parasympathetic fibers, which allow the central nervous system (CNS) to modulate the sinus rate closely, depending on need (Fig. 2-18). Sympathetic stimulation causes an increased upstroke velocity in pacemaker cells by increasing I_{Ca-L}. This change is mediated by increased cyclic adenosine monophosphate (cAMP) and protein kinase A activity, which leads to phosphorylation of the Ca^{2+}-L channels. Sympathetic stimulation also increases I_K, which shortens the action potential duration and starts the pacemaker cycle earlier. Finally, sympathetic stimulation increases I_f, which results in the faster development of inward current and increases the rate of diastolic depolarization. Parasympathetic stimulation, via the vagus nerve, has the opposite effect. Increases in acetylcholine (ACh) activate a G protein, which inhibits adenylate cyclase and leads to reduced concentrations of cAMP and reduced I_{Ca-L}, I_K, and I_f. In addition, there is a K^+ current ($I_{K(ACh)}$) that is activated in the presence of ACh, which slows the rate of diastolic depolarization.

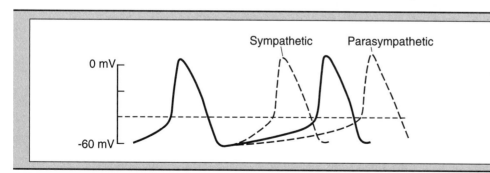

FIG. 2-18
EFFECTS OF SYMPATHETIC AND
PARASYMPATHETIC STIMULA-
TION ON SINUS NODE AUTOMA-
TICITY. Sympathetic activity
increases inward Na^+ current
(funny current) and transient
opening Ca^{2+} current and
speeds decay of delayed rectifier current.

Atria. After initiation in the sinus node, the electrical impulse activates the atria (Fig. 2-19). The atria are a fast-response type tissue and conduct electrical activity at a rate of approximately 1 m/sec. Since the sinus node is in the right atrium, the right atrium is usually completely activated within 60–70 msec. Activation of the left atrium begins within 30–60 msec of impulse initiation anteriorly over Bachmann's bundle and posteriorly at the medial aspect of the inferior vena cava. The two wavefronts converge in the posterior portion of the left atrium within 100–130 msec.

FIG. 2-19
SCHEMATIC OF ATRIAL ACTIVA-TION IN HUMANS. Both the anterior and posterior aspects are shown. The cardiac impulse is initiated in the sulcus terminalis at the junction of the right atrial appendage (RAA) and the superior vena cava (SVC). The right atrium is activated from superior to inferior, with activation complete within 60 msec. The left atrium is activated anteriorly over Bachmann's bundle and inferiorly near the inferior vena cava (IVC). The two waves collide in the lateral left atrium (LA) near the left lower pulmonary vein (PV) after 110–120 msec. MV = mitral valve; TV = tricuspid valve.

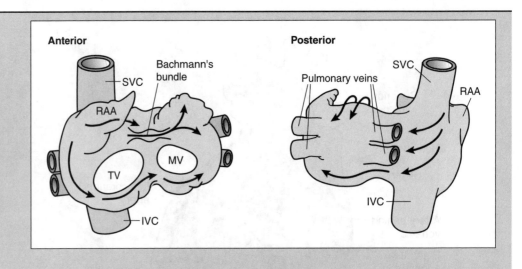

Historically, there has been considerable controversy over how the atria are activated. Some investigators have described specialized atrial conduction tracts analogous to the His-Purkinje tissue (sometimes called James fibers). Other investigators have suggested that, while preferential conduction routes exist, no specialized tracts connect the sinus node and AV node. Most data available today suggest that the atria are activated over preferential routes of conduction that are composed of normal atrial tissue.

Rapid conduction through cardiac tissue occurs through specialized cell-to-cell connections called gap junctions. Gap junctions are formed from six proteins called connexons, which are arranged to form a central pore (1.6–2.0 nm in diameter) and are associated with a similar structure on an adjacent cell (Fig. 2-20). These aqueous channels allow direct cell-to-cell transfer of current and small molecules. The distribution and density of gap junctions are tissue-dependent and are summarized in Fig. 2-21. Gap junctions in sinus node and AV node tissues are relatively sparse, which may in part be responsible for the slow conduction properties observed in these tissues. In atrial and ventricular tissue, most gap junctions are observed at the longitudinal "ends" of the cells rather than the "sides." This spatial difference in density is responsible for the greater velocity observed in the longitudinal direction (3–12 times higher) of the cell compared to the horizontal direction. Orientation of atrial cells and different densities of gap junctions are probably the main reason for the preferential routes of activation observed in the atria.

AV Node. The atria are insulated from the ventricles by the fibrous annulus. Normally, there is only one electrically active pathway between the atria and ventricles, the AV node, which was originally described by Sunao Tawara in 1906. This pathway is located in the triangle of Koch, a region defined superiorly by the tendon of Todaro, inferiorly by the tricuspid annulus, and posteriorly by the coronary sinus (Fig. 2-22). The atrial portion of the AV node is a large, amorphous region composed of "transitional" cells. Several types of transitional cells have been identified, but in general, they are cells with action potentials similar to atrial tissue with a phase 0 upstroke (Fig. 2-23). The finger-like projections of transitional cells lead to an oval of cells set in fibrous tissue called the compact AV node. Cells of the compact AV node have an action potential characterized by the absence of a phase 0 upstroke and a spontaneous phase 4 depolarization (with a spontaneous pacemaker rate of 40–60 beats/min). As with sinus node cells, the slow upstroke is thought to be due to Ca^{2+}-L channels and the absence of fast Na^+ channels. The mechanism for spontaneous phase 4 depolarization is thought to be analogous to the sinus node, but this has not been well studied. Action potentials of AV node cells have a more negative maximum diastolic potential and slower rate of diastolic depolarization than do sinus node cells. As mentioned earlier, AV nodal tissue has a very low density of

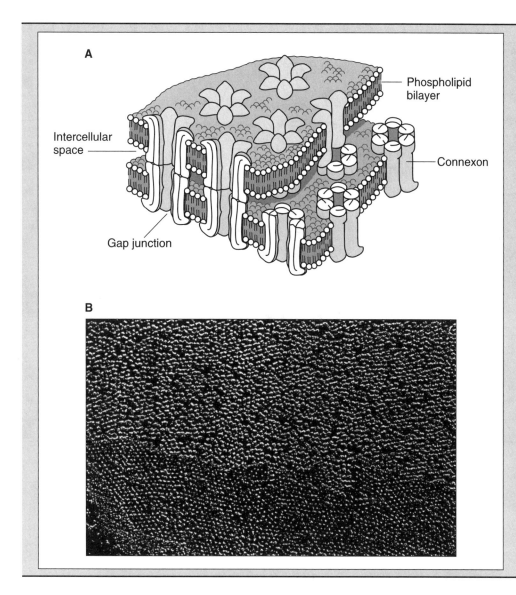

FIG. 2-20
(A) Drawing showing the structure of gap junctions. Six similar proteins, called connexons, are aligned with a similar structure in the membrane of an adjacent cell. Gap junctions provide relatively low-resistance connections between cells. (B) Freeze-fractured electron micrograph showing actual gap junctions from atrial tissue. (*Source:* Reprinted with permission from Page E: Cardiac gap junctions. In *The Heart and Cardiovascular System: Scientific Foundations*, 2nd ed. Edited by Fozzard HA, et al. New York, NY: Raven Press, 1991, p 1005.)

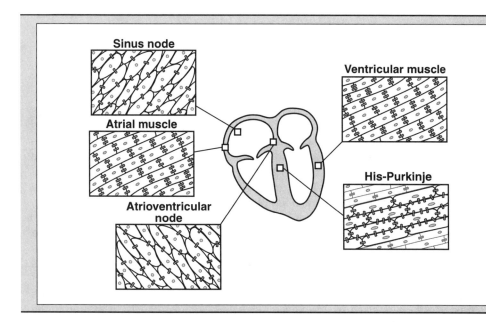

FIG. 2-21
DISTRIBUTION OF GAP JUNCTIONS IN DIFFERENT CARDIAC TISSUES. In atrial and ventricular tissue, gap junctions are concentrated at the "ends" of the cells. In His-Purkinje tissue there are large numbers of gap junctions on all cell surfaces between His-Purkinje tissues. In atrioventricular (AV) node cells, gap junctions are sparsely scattered over the cell membrane.

FIG. 2-22
**RIGHT ATRIUM WITH THE ANTE-
RIOR SURFACE REMOVED.** The
triangle of Koch is formed by
the coronary sinus, the tricuspid annulus, and the tendon
of Todaro. The transitional portion of the atrioventricular (AV)
node is in this tissue, and the
compact AV node is located at
the vertex formed by the tendon of Todaro and the tricuspid
annulus.

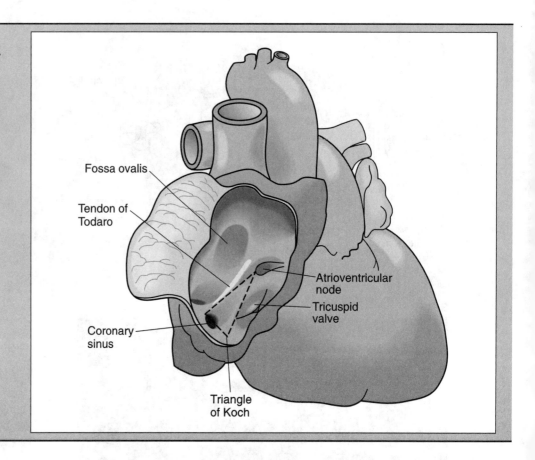

Fossa ovalis

Tendon of
Todaro

Coronary
sinus

Atrioventricular
node

Tricuspid
valve

Triangle
of Koch

gap junctions, which are randomly distributed over the cell (see Fig. 2-21). The slow
conduction properties (0.05 m/sec) displayed by the AV node are probably due to a
combination of both cellular (an action potential that is due solely to the I_{Ca-L}) and
intercellular (low gap-junction density) properties.

A comparison of conduction velocities of the different tissues is offered in Table 2-3.

Table 2-3
**Comparison of Conduction
Velocities by Tissue**

TISSUE TYPE	CONDUCTION VELOCITY (m/sec)
Atria	1
Atrioventricular node	0.05
His-Purkinje tissue	4–5
Ventricles	1

His-Purkinje System. From the compact AV node, myocytes encased by a fibrous sheath
(penetrating bundle) enter the fibrous annulus and become the His bundle (see Fig.
2-23). Originally described by Wilhelm His in the early 1900s, the His bundle begins
imperceptibly at the anterior extension of the AV node and travels through the fibrous
annulus to emerge at the summit of the muscular ventricular septum just below the
membranous septum. The common bundle then splits into a relatively broad fan-like
band of fibers that activates the septum and left ventricle (left bundle) and a slender
(1 mm diameter) right bundle that activates the right ventricle. Both bundles densely
branch out to all regions of the right and left ventricles. The common bundle, left bundle,
right bundle, and their distal branches are collectively called the Purkinje system.

The action potentials from myocytes of the His bundle and Purkinje system are
similar and are characterized by a rapid phase 0 depolarization, a long plateau period,
and very slow diastolic depolarization. The rapid phase 0 depolarization that occurs is
due to an extremely high density of fast Na+ channels. The long plateau period (phase 2)
is thought to arise because of the relatively late inactivation of Ca^{2+} channels or late
activation of K+ channels. The slow phase 4 depolarization is thought to arise from the

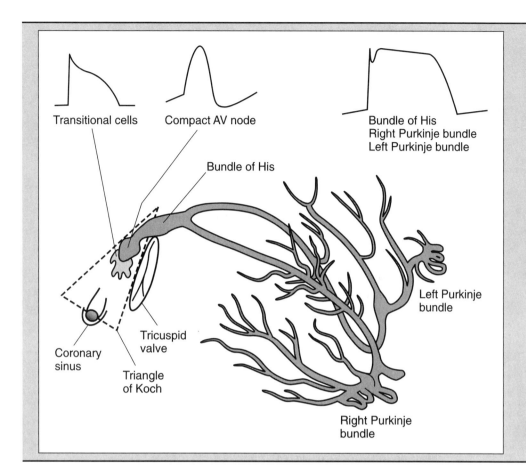

Transitional cells

Compact AV node

Bundle of His
Right Purkinje bundle
Left Purkinje bundle

Bundle of His

Left Purkinje
bundle

Coronary
sinus

Tricuspid
valve

Triangle
of Koch

Right Purkinje
bundle

FIG. 2-23
Schematic showing the relative anatomic locations of the transitional atrioventricular (AV) node, the compact AV node, the His bundle, the right and left bundle branches, and the branching Purkinje tissue. The tricuspid valve and coronary sinus are shown to provide anatomic reference. Action potentials of various conduction tissues are also shown.

slow inward flow of Na+ (I_f). The rapid conduction properties of the His-Purkinje system (large cells arranged in parallel with low intercellular resistance and rapid phase 0 depolarization) result in rapid and almost simultaneous activation of the ventricles. In addition, while adjacent His-Purkinje cells are connected by a very high concentration of gap junctions (see Fig. 2-21), there are relatively few gap junctions between His-Purkinje tissue and adjacent connective tissue or ventricular myocardium. This arrangement might help isolate His-Purkinje tissue and allow the electrical impulse to proceed more rapidly, preventing the voltage from dissipating into adjacent ventricular tissue too quickly.

Ventricles. It has recently been found that ventricular myocytes are electrophysiologically heterogeneous. Regional differences in the action potentials among epicardial, endocardial, and midmyocardial (M cells) cells have been identified (see Table 2-2). These differences appear to arise because cells from each of these regions have different populations of K+ channels, which in turn lead to differences in the plateau phase and repolarization. While all three types of cells have rapid phase 0 upstrokes, epicardial cells have the lowest phase 0 overshoot. Epicardial cells also have distinct spike-and-dome morphology (prominent phase 1), which is thought to be secondary to the presence of transient outward type ion channels (I_{to}).

Several investigators have identified an electrophysiologically distinct population of cells (M cells) located in the midmyocardium. M cells have a smaller phase 1 notch than do epicardial cells, but they are mainly characterized by a dramatic increase in the plateau phase at slow heart rates. Preliminary studies suggest that M cells have a significantly smaller I_K compared to epicardial or endocardial cells.

ELECTROCARDIOGRAPHY

Physical Basis of the ECG. The electrical activity of the heart can be "measured" from the body surface at 12 standardized positions. The standardized positions are shown in Fig. 2-24 and can be divided into those in the frontal plane and those in the horizontal

Actually, the ECG measures the electrical field changes generated by the heart.

or transverse plane. In the frontal plane, electrical activity is measured along six separate axes (leads). In lead I, the voltage difference that exists between the left and right arm is measured, with the positive electrode on the left arm by convention. In lead II, the voltage difference between the right arm and left leg is measured, with the positive electrode on the left leg. In lead III, the voltage difference between the left arm and left leg is measured, with the positive electrode at the left leg. Besides the three bipolar leads (I, II, and III), which measure the potential voltage difference between two sites, there are three augmented unipolar leads (i.e., aVR, aVL, aVF). These leads are referred to as augmented because their value must be multiplied by 1.15 to normalize them to the standard bipolar leads. They are unipolar because the potential recorded is compared to a zero reference electrode.

The six leads recorded in the transverse plane are augmented unipolar leads arranged around the anterior and left chest wall using easily recognized and learned landmarks. These leads are labeled V_1 (located just to the right of the sternum at the fourth intercostal space) through V_6 (located at the midaxillary line in the fifth intercostal space).

The frontal leads can be organized into a hexaxial system, with the negative electrode positioned in the center (Fig. 2-25), which allows a clear understanding of how these leads are related. By convention, the vector formed by lead I is defined as zero degrees;

FIG. 2-24
(A) Location of the standard positions of the ECG electrodes. (B) Close-up of the chest lead positions relative to the rib cage. V_1 is located just to the right of the sternum in the fourth intercostal space. V_2 is also in the fourth intercostal space but to the left of the sternum. V_4 is in the midclavicular line of the fifth intercostal space. V_3 is located halfway between V_2 and V_4. V_5 is located in the anterior axillary line of the fifth intercostal space, and V_6 is located in the midaxillary line of the fifth intercostal space. (C) The limb leads of the frontal axis, with the *arrows* showing the direction of the positive vector.

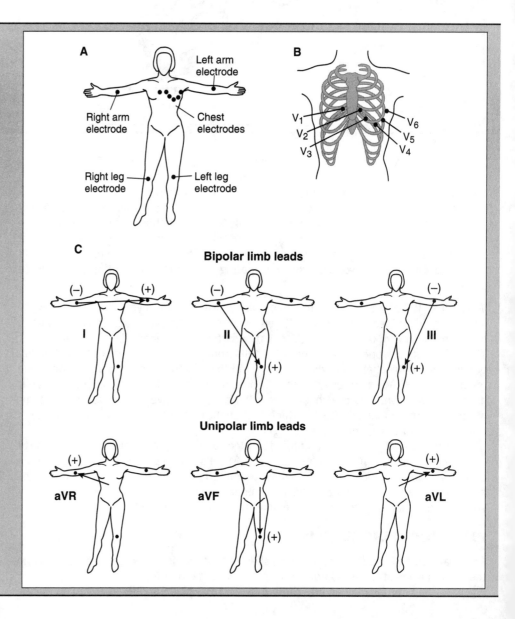

clockwise motion is positive, and counterclockwise motion is negative. For example, lead aVR is oriented with the positive electrode at −150 degrees, and lead II is oriented at 60 degrees. The horizontal leads (V_1 through V_6) can be arranged in a similar fashion.

The Dutch physiologist Willem Einthoven studied and developed the physical basis of electrocardiography in the early 1900s. As described below, he noted that the wave of cardiac depolarization could be modeled as a dipole, with a closely spaced negative surface (depolarized cells, which have just experienced a rapid influx of Na^+) and positive surface (resting cells, which have a negative charge in the intracellular space). The shape and size of the ECG signal depend on the direction and charge of the depolarizing current and the location of the measuring electrodes. These important points are illustrated in Fig. 2-26. A single myocardial cell with three pairs of measuring electrodes is shown (A, B, C). In the resting state, while the inside of the cell is negative relative to the outside, since the surface is homogeneously positively charged, no voltage is recorded in any of the lead systems. A depolarizing current is delivered on one end of the cell, and the cell is progressively depolarized. The depolarizing current causes rapid influx of Na^+, which makes the surface of this region of the cell have a relatively negative charge when compared to regions of the cell that are still in their resting state. At any instant an electrical field will be measured because of the potential difference between those parts of the cell that are depolarized (10 mV, surface relatively negatively charged) and those regions that are still in the resting state (−90mV, surface relatively positively charged). The wavefront of activation that separates the depolarized and resting membrane can be modeled as a dipole with a negative pole (depolarized portion with a negative surface charge) and a positive pole (resting membrane with a positive surface charge). By convention, a positive deflection is measured when the positive electrode of a measuring system faces an approaching positive pole, and a negative deflection is recorded when the positive electrode faces the negative surface. In the example, a positive deflection is recorded in the lead system with the positive electrode on the right (A), a negative deflection is recorded in the lead system with the positive electrode on the left (B), and a biphasic signal is recorded in lead system C as depolarization first goes toward and then goes away from the positive electrode. While the cell is completely depolarized (the plateau phase of the action potential), there are no potential differences between different regions of the cell, and the signal in all three lead systems is isoelectric. During repolarization, positive charge reaccumulates on the surface on the left side of the cell. Since the surface of the left side of the cell is positive relative to the right side, as repolarization proceeds from left to right, a positive deflection is observed in lead system B, and a negative deflection is observed in lead system A.

This model can now be applied to recording cardiac activity on the 12 surface ECG leads. The surface ECG simply measures the sum of cardiac action potentials at a given time. If the net direction of cardiac depolarization is directed toward the positive electrode of a specific lead, a positive deflection is inscribed. Conversely, if depolarization is oriented away from the positive electrode, a negative signal is recorded. The ECG is a simple method that measures the amount and direction of instantaneous electrical activity of the heart.

Normally the ECG is calibrated so that a 1 mV signal produces a 10 mm deflection, and paper speed is 25 mm/sec. Since ECG paper is divided into 1-mm square boxes, in the horizontal direction, each box represents 0.04 seconds. The 1-mm square boxes are grouped into larger boxes that are 5 mm by 5 mm. In the horizontal direction, one large box (5 mm) represents 0.20 seconds, and in the vertical direction, one large box represents 0.5 mV.

Normal ECG. On the normal ECG, the first identifiable electrical activity is the P wave, which represents the depolarization of atrial tissue, since the atria are the first chambers to be activated during the cardiac cycle (Figs. 2-27 and 2-28). Given its small size, the electrical activity of the sinus node is not seen on the surface ECG. Since the sinus node is located at the junction of the superior vena cava and the right atrium, the atria are activated from superior to inferior and from right to left. Thus the P wave is usually positive in lead II (since the positive electrode is at 60 degrees) and negative in aVR (since the positive electrode is directed to −150 degrees). Since, as previously mentioned, atrial depolarization is completed in 100–130 msec, the P wave is normally

Dipole is an object that is oppositely charged at two poles.

FIG. 2-25
(A) Hexaxial system of the frontal leads with the negative electrodes aligned to a central point. The heart is shown for reference. The leads are then described relative to the vector of lead I. Lead I is defined as 0 degrees; counterclockwise is defined as the negative direction and clockwise the positive direction. (B) Hexaxial system of the horizontal leads with the negative electrodes positioned to a central point. The heart is shown for reference.

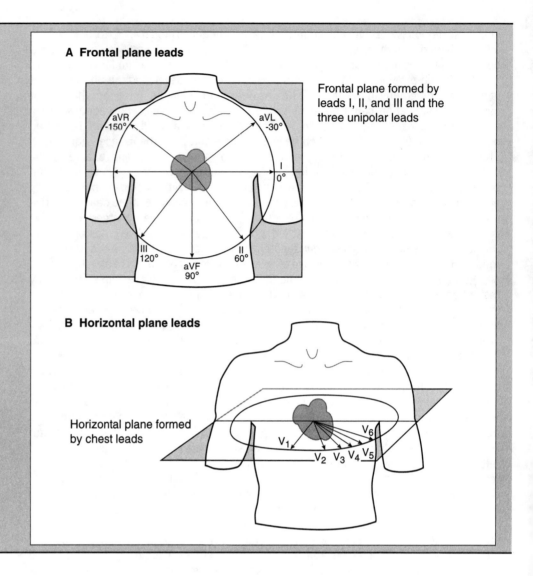

A Frontal plane leads

aVR -150°
aVL -30°
I 0°
III 120°
aVF 90°
II 60°

Frontal plane formed by leads I, II, and III and the three unipolar leads

B Horizontal plane leads

Horizontal plane formed by chest leads

V_1 V_2 V_3 V_4 V_5 V_6

approximately 3 mm wide. The interval between the beginning of the P wave and the second identifiable wave (the QRS complex) is called the PR interval. The PR interval represents intra-atrial conduction and conduction through the AV node and the His bundle. Since the AV node is located in the septum separating the right and left atria, during the terminal portion of the P wave there is simultaneous activation of the left atrium and the proximal portion of the AV node. The isoelectric portion of the PR interval represents the conduction time through the AV node and His bundle after the left atrium has been completely activated. This interval is isoelectric, since no large voltage gradients exist in the heart. (The atria are in the plateau phase, and the ventricles have not yet been depolarized.) As with the sinus node, the electrical activity of the small AV node normally cannot be measured from the surface. The normal PR interval is approximately 0.12–0.20 seconds (three to four small boxes).

The second deflection observed in the ECG, the QRS complex, represents ventricular depolarization. Normal ventricular depolarization occurs via conduction through the Purkinje system, which rapidly and simultaneously activates the right and left ventricles. Since ventricular activation is usually complete within 60–100 msec, normally the QRS complex is narrow (less than 3 mm wide); because the mass of ventricular tissue is larger than that of the atria, the QRS complex normally has a higher amplitude than the P wave. Ventricular depolarization occurs first in the septum, in a left-to-right direction. After septal depolarization, since the left ventricle normally has more tissue mass than the right ventricle, the mean summation of electrical activity proceeds from right to left (Fig. 2-29). In the horizontal plane, this activation pattern characteristically yields a small

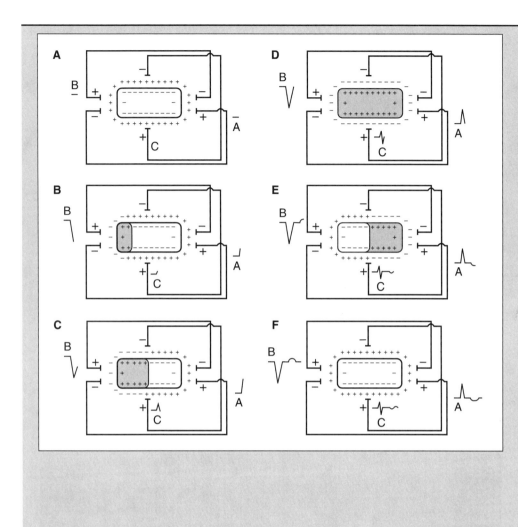

FIG. 2-26
SIMPLE MODEL SHOWING THE PHYSICS INVOLVED WITH THE ECG. (A) At baseline the interior of the cell is negative relative to the exterior. No potential differences exist, so the voltage recorded is zero or isoelectric. (B) If a depolarizing pulse is applied to the left side of the cell, the inside of the cell becomes positive relative to the outside. A potential difference is now recorded (C). By convention, a positive signal is recorded on the positive electrode when it faces the positive surface (lead system A), and a negative potential is recorded when the negative surface faces the positive electrode (lead system B). In practical terms, this means that a positive signal will be recorded in the positive electrode that faces an oncoming wave of depolarization, and a negative signal is recorded if the wave of depolarization is going away from the positive electrode. As the cell becomes depolarized the recorded currents become larger, and when the cell is completely depolarized (D), the voltage recorded returns to zero (in all lead systems) since no current now flows. Since the cell remains depolarized (in the plateau phase) for a specific period of time, an isoelectric ST segment is recorded (E). As the tissue begins to repolarize, a deflection in the opposite direction is recorded (F).

positive deflection followed by a predominantly negative QRS complex in lead V_1, since the activation forces are going "away" from lead V_1, which is located on the right side of the sternum. Conversely, in lead V_6 there is a small negative deflection followed by a predominantly positive QRS complex. In the frontal plane, the predominant force of left ventricular activation is directed downward and toward the left so that a large positive QRS complex is normally recorded in lead II and a predominantly negative QRS complex is recorded in aVR. However, the orientation of the heart in the chest cavity greatly affects the shape and size of the QRS complexes recorded in the frontal plane. For example, a tall, thin person may have a relatively vertically oriented heart, which could cause the largest QRS complex to be seen in lead aVF. The angle of the predominant forces of the QRS complex in the frontal plane is frequently referred to as the cardiac axis.

After the ventricular cells have been depolarized, they enter the plateau phase. Since at this time no large voltage differences exist in the heart, the QRS complex is followed by an isoelectric period called the ST segment. Repolarization of the different parts of the left and right ventricles occurs in a more heterogeneous pattern than does depolarization, which leads to a broader, lower-amplitude T wave. In humans, repolarization usually occurs in a direction opposite to that of depolarization, so the T-wave deflection is normally in the same direction as the QRS complex. For example, in lead V_6 or lead II where the QRS is positive, the T wave is also usually positive. The QT interval is measured

Normal ECG Intervals
- PR interval: beginning of the P wave to the beginning of the QRS complex
- QRS complex: beginning of the QRS complex to the end of the QRS complex
- QT interval: beginning of the QRS complex to the end of the T wave

FIG. 2-27
NORMAL ELECTROCARDIO-GRAM SHOWING THE P WAVE, QRS COMPLEX, AND T WAVE. (A) The PR interval is defined as the beginning of the P wave to the beginning of the QRS. This interval measures the amount of time for intra-atrial conduction and conduction via the AV node and proximal His-Purkinje system. The QRS complex measures the amount of time required to activate the ventricles over the more distal His-Purkinje system. The QT interval, which is measured from the beginning QRS to the end of the T wave, represents the duration of the ventricular action potential. (B) Activation of the sinus node occurs before the P wave. Electrical activity from this small structure cannot be measured from the surface ECG. The P wave represents atrial activation. The interval just after the P wave represents the period of time when the electrical impulse is delayed in the AV node and the atria are in their plateau phase. For this reason, this period is normally isoelectric, since no potential voltage differences exist in the heart. Electrical activation proceeds down the His-Purkinje system to activate the ventricles, and the QRS complex is inscribed. During this period the atria repolarize, but this relatively small amount of electrical activity is obscured by the QRS complex. After the QRS, an isoelectric period ensues as the ventricular cells are in the plateau phase. Finally the ventricular cells repolarize, and the T wave is inscribed. (Compare with Fig. 2-1A.)

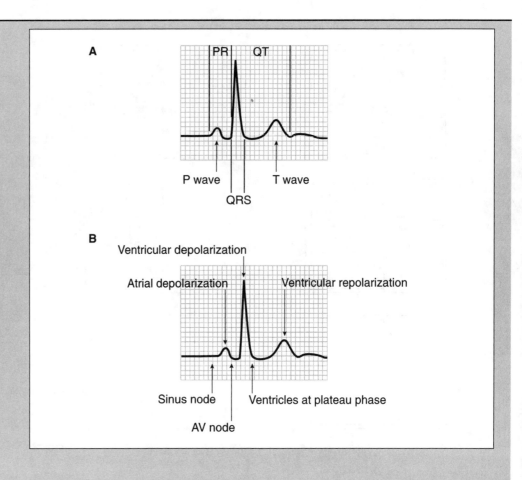

from the beginning of the QRS complex to the terminal portion of the T wave. This interval is important because it approximates the time that ventricular cells are depolarized. The normal QT interval is rate-dependent, longer at slower heart rates and shorter at faster heart rates. Some conditions are associated with a prolonged period of ventricular depolarization, normally because of extension of the plateau phase (phase 2). This condition, called the "long QT syndrome," is associated with significant arrhythmias and is explored more fully later.

In some cases, after the T wave, another, usually smaller wave can sometimes be observed. Einthoven originally described the U wave in 1903. The U wave probably arises from late repolarization of certain areas of the ventricle such as His-Purkinje tissue or M cells.

Finally, the heart rate can be calculated from the ECG. The interval from P wave to P

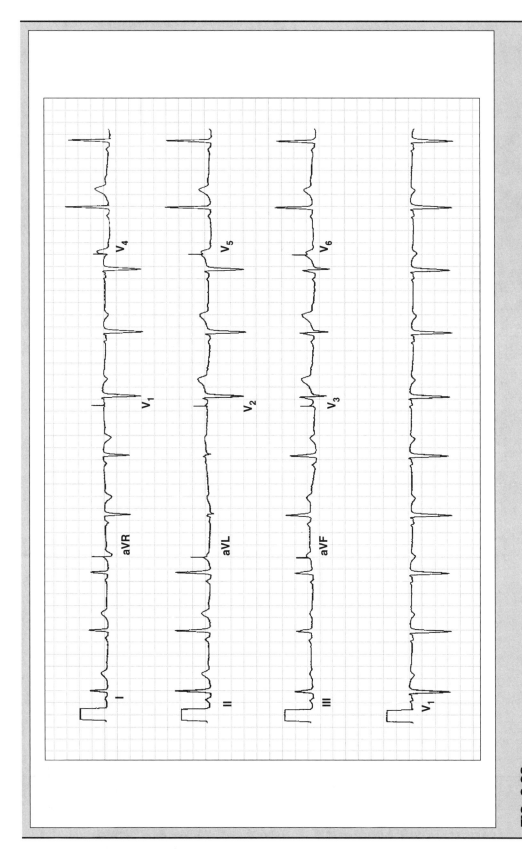

FIG. 2-28

NORMAL ELECTROCARDIOGRAM (ECG). Note the standardized recording positions (see Fig. 2-25; see also Figs. 2-16 and 2-27). The first deflection observed is the P wave, resulting from atrial activation. Since the sinus node is located at the junction of the right atrium and the superior vena cava, the atria are activated from right to left and from superior to inferior. This leads to a P wave that is negative in aVR (since atrial activation is traveling away from the right arm), and a positive deflection in the inferior leads (II, III, aVF). The P wave is relatively small, since the atria are relatively thin-walled. After the atria are activated, conduction occurs through the AV node. At this time the atria are at their plateau phase, and the discrete electrical activity at the AV node cannot be seen by the surface leads so the PR interval is isoelectric in all lead systems. The activation then spreads quickly through the His-Purkinje system, which leads to rapid depolarization of ventricular tissue, recorded as a sharp, narrow QRS complex. Since the mass of ventricular tissue is larger, the QRS is larger than the P wave. Since the left ventricle normally has a greater mass than the right, the QRS complex is usually negative in aVR. All the ventricular cells then are in plateau phase, and an isoelectric ST segment ensues. The ventricular tissue then repolarizes, and the T wave is inscribed on the surface ECG. Repolarization is much more heterogeneous and occurs more slowly, and for this reason the T wave is normally broad-based and of lower amplitude. Interestingly, while depolarization of ventricular tissue travels from endocardium to epicardium, repolarization travels from epicardium to endocardium. For this reason, as a general rule (which is often broken), the normal T wave will usually be in the same direction as the QRS complex.

FIG. 2-29
(A) Lead V_1 is located in the fourth intercostal space just to the right of the sternum, and V_6 is located in the fifth intercostal space at the midaxillary line. The first portion of the ventricles to be activated is the septum, and this normally occurs from left to right (*thin arrow*). This causes a small positive deflection in lead V_1 and a small negative deflection in V_6. The remainder of the ventricle depolarizes from right to left (*broad arrow*), which then leads to a large negative deflection in lead V_1 and a large positive deflection in lead V_6. (B) The ventricular cells are then at the plateau phase, and the isoelectric ST segment is recorded. (C) The ventricle then repolarizes from left to right (*broad arrow*) and a negative T wave and positive T wave are recorded in lead V_1 and lead V_6, respectively.

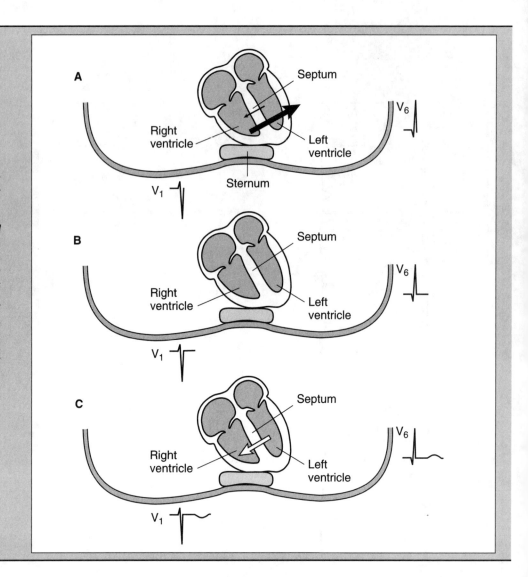

wave usually represents the rate of spontaneous depolarization of the sinus node. In general, instead of calculating the number of seconds between P waves, clinicians are used to thinking in terms of beats per minute. At standard speed, a simple rule can be used to estimate the heart rate:

$$\text{Heart rate (beats/min)} = \frac{300}{\text{Number of large boxes between QRS complexes or P waves}}$$

In Fig. 2-28, the P waves are separated by five boxes so that the sinus rate is approximately 60 beats/min. In this case, conduction through the AV node is constant so the ventricles are also activated at a rate of 60 beats/min.

Case Study:
Continued

Reexamine and compare Ms. Eswine's ECG in Fig. 2-1A to the normal ECG in Fig. 2-28. The P wave in Ms. Eswine's ECG is followed almost immediately by the QRS complex, which suggests that the normal delay in the AV node is not occurring. In addition, in Ms. Eswine's ECG the QRS complex in lead V_1 is predominantly positive and is very wide, which suggests that Ms. Eswine's ventricles are not being activated in the normal manner.

■ BRADYCARDIAS

Slow heart rates (bradycardias) can arise from one of two reasons. Either impulse formation can be abnormally decreased, or there can be blocked conduction.

Since the sinus node has the fastest pacemaker rate, it tends to be the normal source for impulse formation. Abnormal impulse formation in the sinus node can occur for several reasons. *Intrinsic causes* of sinus node dysfunction include replacement of the pacemaker cells by fibrosis resulting from age, inflammation (e.g., from collagen vascular diseases or viral infection), and ischemia. In addition, direct damage to the sinus node during cardiac surgery, particularly for congenital abnormalities that involve the atria, has been reported. Numerous *extrinsic causes* of sinus node dysfunction have been reported. Low temperature, electrolyte disturbances, hypothyroidism, and eating disorders have been reported to affect sinus node function without causing any structural damage to the sinus node itself. The most common cause of extrinsic sinus node dysfunction is the use of cardiac drugs such as β-blockers, calcium channel blockers, and digitalis. Drugs used for psychiatric problems, such as phenothiazines, lithium, and amitriptyline, have been associated with sinus node dysfunction. Finally, autonomic effects such as significant vagotonia have been associated with prolonged sinus pauses and sinus bradycardia.

Electrocardiographically, abnormal impulse formation in the sinus node is manifested by loss of the P wave; since the sinus node does not fire, the atria are not activated, and no P wave is observed. Usually a subsidiary pacemaker such as the AV node then fires as the slower phase 4 depolarization of AV nodal tissue reaches threshold. On the ECG, this is represented by a normal-appearing QRS complex without a preceding P wave (Fig. 2-30).

Causes of bradycardia include reduced automaticity or blocked conduction.

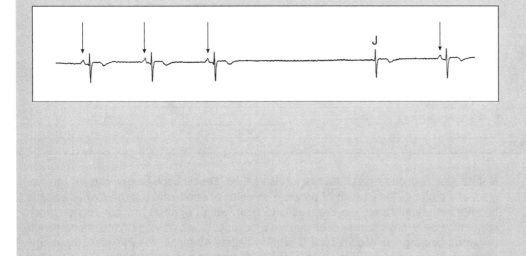

FIG. 2-30
SLOW HEART RATE RESULTING FROM REDUCED AUTOMATICITY. The sinus node activates for the first three beats (*arrows*), which leads to P waves and subsequent QRS complexes (produced by activation via the AV node and His-Purkinje system). However, for uncertain reasons, the sinus node stops firing, and after a prolonged interval (since the phase 4 slope is slower for junctional cells), a QRS complex generated from the AV node is recorded (J for junctional beat). This system of subsidiary pacemakers prevents complete pauses if the sinus mechanism fails.

Blocked conduction normally occurs in the region of the AV node. Normally, the AV node serves as the only area that connects the atria and ventricles. In other regions of the heart the atria and ventricles are separated by the fibrous annulus. This arrangement reduces the chance of electrical feedback, but it also means that the AV node and His bundle are especially vulnerable to blocked conduction.

Electrocardiographically, several forms of AV block have been identified (Fig. 2-31). Normally, the PR interval is shorter than 200 msec. In *first-degree AV block*, there is a one-to-one relationship between the P wave and the QRS complex; that is, activation of the atria leads to activation of the ventricles. However, the PR interval is prolonged (> 220 msec), suggesting that some sort of additional delay is occurring in the AV node or His bundle. In *second-degree AV block*, some—but not all—atrial activity leads to ventricular activity. Two types of second-degree heart block have been characterized. In

FIG. 2-31
EXAMPLES OF CONDUCTION BLOCK THROUGH THE AV NODE. (A) Normal AV node conduction of each activation of the atria leads to activation of the ventricles. (B) In first-degree AV block, a one-to-one relationship still exists between the atria and ventricles, but because of delay in the AV node, the PR interval is prolonged (> 0.22 sec). (C) In second-degree AV block a one-to-one relationship no longer exists between atrial and ventricular activity. There are two types of second-degree AV block. In type I, or Wenckebach, AV block, conduction in the AV node is gradually prolonged until a beat is completely blocked. This leads to gradual prolongation of the PR interval until there is a P wave that is not followed by a QRS complex. (D) In type II second-degree AV block, no gradual prolongation of the PR interval exists. There is a sudden dropped beat. Type II second-degree AV block is far less common and is often associated with block in the His bundle, whereas type I second-degree AV block is usually associated with block in the AV node. (E) In complete or third-degree AV block, no relationship exists between atrial and ventricular activity.

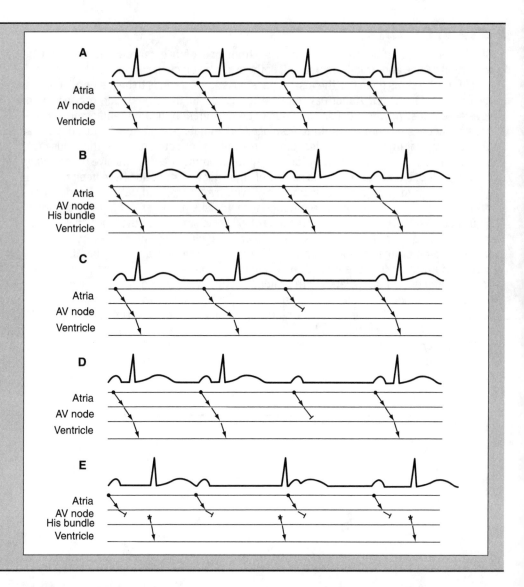

Mobitz type I second-degree AV block (also called Wenckebach block), the PR interval gradually prolongs (as a result of progressive delay of conduction in the AV node or His bundle) until finally there is a dropped QRS beat, which signifies that conduction block rather than delay has occurred. The pattern then repeats, which leads to the phenomenon of "group beating." In Mobitz type II second-degree AV block, the PR interval remains constant, but there is a sudden drop of the QRS complex. In general, the more common Mobitz type I second-degree AV block is thought to represent a block in the compact AV node region, while Mobitz type II second-degree AV block is associated with abnormalities in the His bundle. In *third-degree AV block*, no relationship exists between atrial and ventricular activity. The atria are depolarized, but conduction is completely blocked in the AV node or His bundle. The ventricles are activated by a subsidiary pacemaker distal to the site of the block.

The other region where the electrical impulse can be frequently blocked or delayed is the bundle branches. Block in the bundle branches does not necessarily lead to a slow heart rate, since the ventricles can usually be activated by the contralateral bundle. However, since the ventricles are now activated sequentially rather than simultaneously, the QRS is widened to greater than 120 msec (> 3 mm) [Fig. 2-32].

Two characteristic ECG patterns have been identified, depending on whether conduction through the right or left bundle is blocked (Fig. 2-33). In *right bundle branch block* (*RBBB*), since the septum is normally activated by the left bundle, initial activation of the septum and the left ventricle is unchanged. However, late activation of the right ventricle produces a relatively late rightward force. On the ECG, a late positive wave in V_1

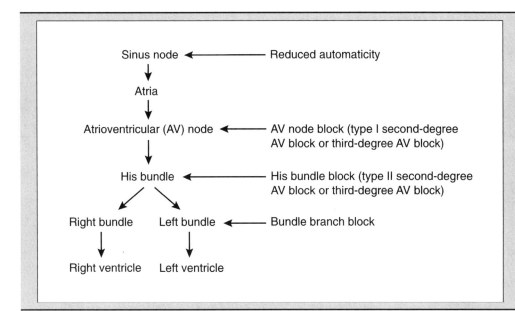

FIG. 2-32
CAUSES AND MECHANISTIC SITES OF BRADYCARDIA OR ABNORMAL VENTRICULAR ACTIVATION.

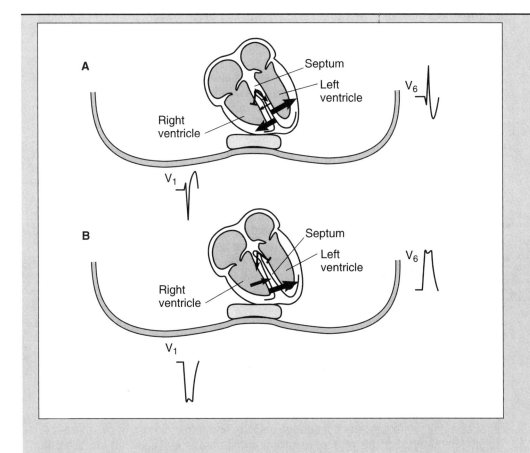

FIG. 2-33
ELECTROCARDIOGRAM IN LEFT AND RIGHT BUNDLE BRANCH BLOCK. Please refer to Fig. 2-29 and note the differences. (A) In right bundle branch block, septal activation occurs normally from left to right (*thin arrow*), which leads to a positive septal wave in lead V_1 and a negative wave in V_6. The left ventricle is activated normally, which causes a negative wave in V_1 and a positive wave in V_6 (*top broad arrow*). The right ventricle is activated late, so a late positive wave is inscribed in V_1 and a late negative wave in V_6 (*bottom broad arrow*). Since the ventricles are now activated sequentially rather than simultaneously, the QRS complex is usually wide (> 120 msec). (B) In left bundle branch block, septal activation now predominantly occurs from right to left (*top broad arrow*), and left ventricular activation is late (*bottom broad arrow*). This leads to a wide complex negative QRS in lead V_1 and a wide complex positive QRS in V_6.

and a late negative wave in V_6 are observed. In *left bundle branch block* (*LBBB*), the septum is activated from right to left, and the left ventricle is activated rather late. This leads to a wide QRS complex that is predominantly negative in V_1 and positive in V_6. Since the septum is now activated abnormally, the small positive septal wave in V_1 and small negative septal wave in V_6 are frequently not seen. RBBB is more common than LBBB since the right bundle is relatively thin compared to the left bundle. The left bundle actually divides into anterior and posterior fascicles. Specific ECG patterns have been described for individual fascicular block; description of these patterns is beyond the scope of this text.

Case Study: *Continued*	*In Ms. Eswine's case, while the baseline QRS is widened and has some similar morphologic similarities to RBBB, the PR interval is extremely short. In patients with RBBB, the PR interval should be normal (since AV node conduction is unchanged).*

■ TACHYCARDIAS

Abnormally fast heart rates (tachycardias) can be classified scientifically either by cellular mechanism or anatomically (Table 2-4). From a clinical standpoint, tachycardias are classified by their ECG appearance.

ELECTROPHYSIOLOGIC CLASSIFICATION

Mechanisms for Tachycardia
- Increased automaticity
- Triggered activity
- Reentry

Tachycardia can arise from three basic cellular or tissue mechanisms as illustrated in Fig. 2-34.

First, *increased automaticity* from more rapid phase 4 depolarization can cause a more rapid heart rate. For example, the phase 4 depolarization of the sinus node depends on inward Na^+ (I_f) and Ca^{2+} (Ca^{2+}-T) currents and decay of outward K^+ current (I_K). Adrenergic stimulation causes, among other things, phosphorylation of the Na^+ channels responsible for the I_f current, which leads to increased inward flow of Na^+ and more rapid phase 4 depolarization.

Second, spontaneous depolarizations can sometimes occur in phase 3 or phase 4 of an action potential. These depolarizations are classified by their location in the action potential. Early afterdepolarizations (EADs) occur during the plateau or repolarization phase. EADs can appear whenever the duration of the action potential is prolonged. Prolongation of the action potential can be observed if there is persistent inward current during the plateau phase (from I_{Ca-L} for example) or if outward current is delayed (decreased I_K). Delayed afterdepolarizations (DADs) occur after repolarization is complete and appear to be mediated by intracellular Ca^{2+} overload. Increased intracellular Ca^{2+} could lead to a positive inward current via the Na^+–Ca^{2+}-exchanger or other Ca^{2+}-dependent channels. If early or delayed depolarizations reach threshold, Na^+ and Ca^{2+} channels may reactivate and cause repetitive depolarization of the cardiac cell and lead to *triggered activity*. This mechanism of tachycardia is termed "triggered" because it depends on the existence of a preceding action potential and is not self-initiating.

Third, and most commonly, tachycardia can arise from a *reentrant circuit* in abnormal cardiac tissue. Any condition that gives rise to adjacent regions with different conduction velocities (such as the border zone of a myocardial infarction) and refractory periods can serve as the substrate for a reentrant circuit. In regions with heterogeneous electrophysiologic properties, activation usually occurs simultaneously in both pathways. However, a premature stimulus (such as a spontaneous premature atrial or ventricular contraction) can occur during the absolute or effective refractory period in one of the pathways. The impulse is blocked in this pathway and conducts solely down the second pathway. If the first pathway has recovered (i.e., the effective refractory period has elapsed), electrical activation may proceed retrogradely and initiate reentry. Reentry requires a delicate balance of conduction velocity and refractoriness in two electrically isolated pathways. For this reason, reentrant arrhythmias are usually not incessant but occur sporadically. However, reentrant mechanisms are the most common cause of rapid heart rates that physicians encounter.

ANATOMIC CLASSIFICATION

While it is important to understand the underlying cellular mechanisms, tachycardias are more commonly classified by anatomic location (Fig. 2-35). In atrial tachycardias, whether the result of reentry, triggered activity, or automaticity, only atrial tissue is involved. In junctional tachycardias, whether the result of reentry, triggered activity, or

Table 2-4
Classification of Tachycardias

TISSUE CLASSIFICATION	CELLULAR MECHANISM	ELECTRO-CARDIOGRAPHIC CHARACTERISTICS	CLINICAL CHARACTERISTICS
Atrial			
Atrial tachycardia	Automaticity, triggered activity, or reentry	Rapid, regular, narrow QRS complexes; P waves usually observed before each QRS complex; P waves are similar	Results from a single focus in either atria; fairly uncommon
Multifocal atrial tachycardia	Automatic or triggered activity	Rapid, irregular, narrow QRS complexes; P waves seen before each QRS, but the P waves have at least three different forms	Result of several rapidly firing foci in the atria; usually associated with severe pulmonary disease or other systemic problems
Atrial fibrillation	Wandering wavelets	Fine irregular atrial activity; narrow QRS complexes, very irregular	Most common atrial arrhythmia, results from multiple wavelets activating the atria in random fashion
Atrial flutter	Reentry	Regular "sawtooth" pattern; narrow QRS complexes usually regular	Results from a stable reentrant circuit in the right atrium; the "slow zone" is frequently the isthmus formed by the tricuspid annulus and the inferior vena cava
Junctional			
Atrioventricular node reentrant tachycardia	Reentry	Rapid, regular, narrow QRS complexes; P waves often not seen	Common cause of tachycardias
Junctional tachycardia	Triggered activity or automaticity	Rapid, regular, narrow QRS complexes; P waves often not seen	Relatively uncommon; sometimes observed after open heart surgery or in the newborn
Ventricular			
Ventricular tachy-cardia	Usually reentry. In very rare cases result of auto-maticity or triggered activity	Rapid, wide QRS complexes of normal amplitude; in mono-morphic ventricular tachycardia, QRS complexes are uniform, and in polymorphic ventricular tachycardia, the QRS complexes have differing form	Life-threatening; normally results from reentrant circuit that uses a region of slow conduction secondary to damaged tissue
Ventricular fibrillation	Multiple wandering wavelets in ventric-ular tissue	Rapid irregular low amplitude QRS complexes	Life-threatening
Accessory-pathway–mediated			
Orthodromic tachy-cardia	Reentry	Narrow, complex, regular	Most common tachycardia associated with accessory pathways
Antidromic tachy-cardia	Reentry	Wide complex, regular	Very uncommon
Atrial tachycardia	Same mechanisms as atrial tachycardias	Wide complex, regular or irregular depending on mechanism of atrial tachycardia	May lead to ventricular fibrillation

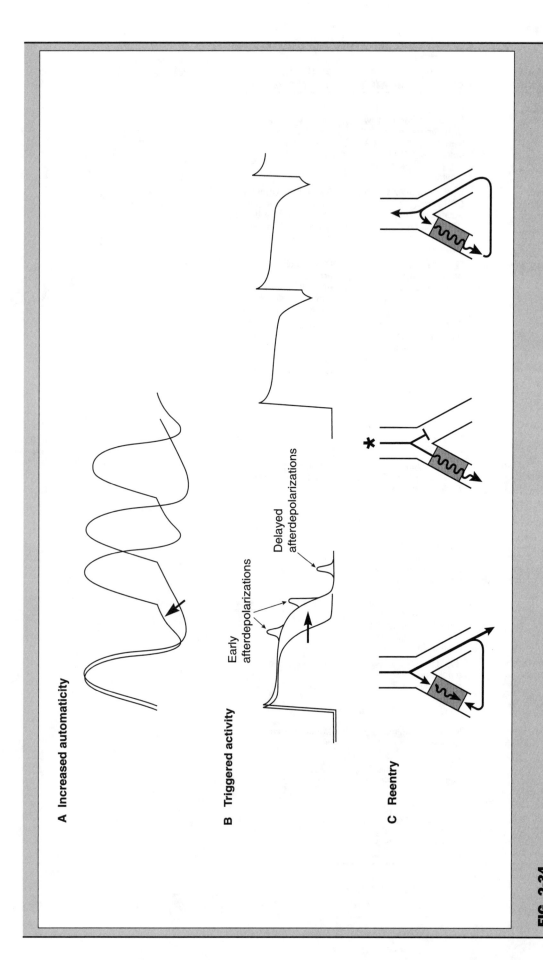

FIG. 2-34

THREE CELLULAR MECHANISMS FOR RAPID HEART RATES. (A) Increased automaticity from more rapid phase 4 depolarization causes an increased heart rate. This is the way sympathetic stimulation increases the heart rate. (B) Triggered activity. If the plateau phase is prolonged from any mechanism, reactivation of sodium or potassium channels can lead to early afterdepolarizations that, if they reach threshold, can cause a rapid heart rate from triggered activity. In addition, afterdepolarizations can occur after the cell has returned to its baseline potential (delayed afterdepolarizations) and also cause triggered activity. (C) Reentry is the most common mechanism for tachycardia. For reentry to occur, there must be two electrophysiologically separate pathways for conduction (*left*). One pathway must have slower conduction properties (*gray*), and the two pathways must have different refractory periods. Normally conduction proceeds down the pathway that has more rapid conduction properties. Conduction down the second pathway is normally blocked when it reaches refractory tissue. A premature beat can block in the "fast" pathway (as a result of fast pathway refractoriness) and proceed slowly down the "slow" pathway (which must have a shorter refractory period) [*center*]. If enough time has elapsed, the fast pathway may be activated in a retrograde fashion, and a reentrant circuit may be initiated (*right*).

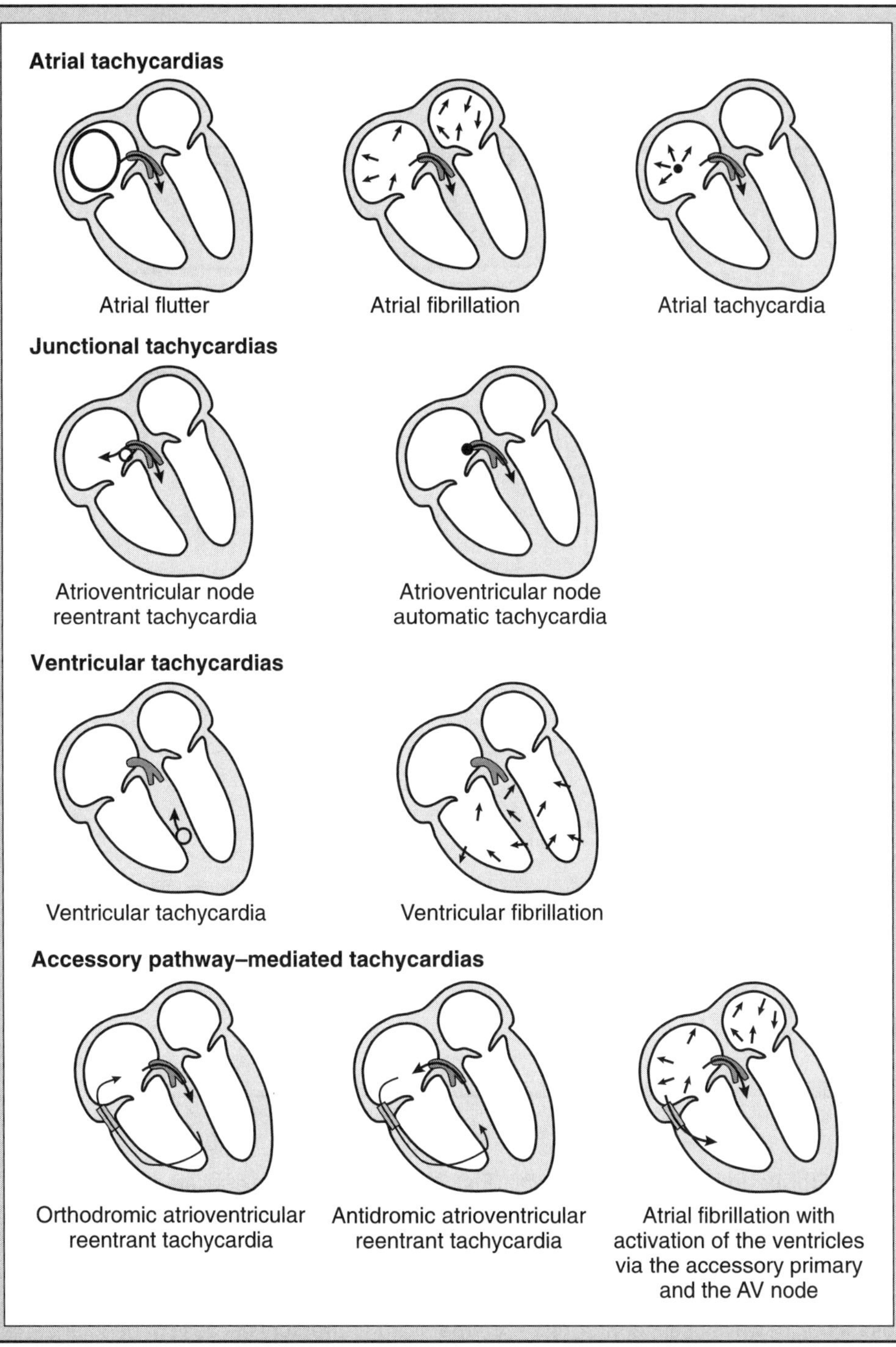

FIG. 2-35
TISSUE CLASSIFICATION OF
TACHYARRHYTHMIAS.

Atrial tachycardias

Atrial flutter   Atrial fibrillation   Atrial tachycardia

Junctional tachycardias

Atrioventricular node
reentrant tachycardia

Atrioventricular node
automatic tachycardia

Ventricular tachycardias

Ventricular tachycardia   Ventricular fibrillation

Accessory pathway–mediated tachycardias

Orthodromic atrioventricular
reentrant tachycardia

Antidromic atrioventricular
reentrant tachycardia

Atrial fibrillation with
activation of the ventricles
via the accessory primary
and the AV node

automaticity, the arrhythmia substrate is located wholly or partly in the AV node. In ventricular tachycardia, the arrhythmia arises from ventricular tissue alone. Finally, in accessory-pathway–mediated tachycardia, an abnormal connection between the atrium and ventricles forms the substrate for stable reentrant circuits.

Atrial Tachycardias. There are several types of tachycardias in which the arrhythmic focus or circuit is located solely in atrial tissue (see Fig. 2-35).

Ectopic Atrial Tachycardias. First, and most commonly, a patient can have a premature atrial contraction (PAC) resulting from early activation from a focus in the atrium other than the sinus node (Fig. 2-36). Isolated PACs are a common finding in all hearts. If this focus fires repetitively, a *unifocal atrial tachycardia* can ensue (Fig. 2-37A). If several competing atrial foci are firing, the arrhythmia is termed *multifocal atrial tachycardia*

(Fig. 2-37B). These abnormal foci are usually due to increased automaticity or triggered activity. Multifocal atrial tachycardia is usually seen in the setting of severe pulmonary disease or infection.

FIG. 2-36
PREMATURE ATRIAL CONTRACTION. An ectopic focus in the atrium activates the atria (*arrow*) and the ventricles early.

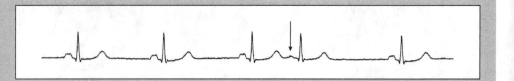

FIG. 2-37
(A) ELECTROCARDIOGRAPHIC (ECG) APPEARANCE OF ATRIAL TACHYCARDIA. An abnormal atrial focus fires repetitively (*arrows*). The P wave is inverted in lead aVF, which suggests that the ectopic focus is in the inferior portion of the atrium. Since the atria are firing relatively rapidly, the atrioventricular (AV) node allows conduction of every other or every third atrial beat. Slow conduction properties of the AV node "protect" the ventricles from being exposed to very rapid rates.

(B) ECG APPEARANCE OF MULTIFOCAL TACHYCARDIA. In this strip, at least three different P-wave forms (which suggests at least three different atrial foci) can be identified. Rapid irregular activation of the atria leads to rapid and irregular activation of the ventricles.

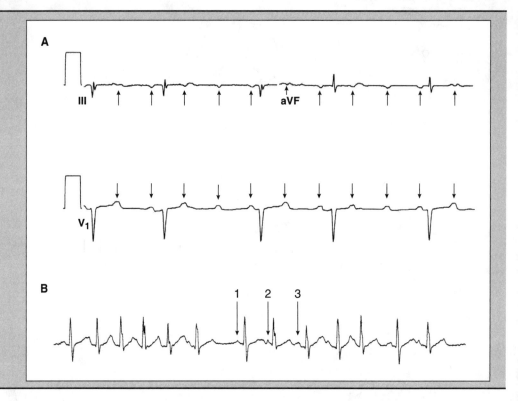

Atrial Fibrillation. In *atrial fibrillation* (Fig. 2-38), the atria are activated by a number of wavelets that wander randomly through atrial tissue; the velocity and direction of these wavelets depend on the state of recovery of tissue that they encounter. The wavelets can divide, join other waves, or mutually extinguish. The wavelets can travel around anatomic obstacles, such as the pulmonary veins or the vena cava, or around functional areas of block (i.e., a wavelet encountering tissue that is still refractory because of depolarization from another wavelet). The ability to maintain atrial fibrillation appears to depend on tissue mass; atria of small animals such as rats, rabbits, and cats rarely have sustained atrial fibrillation. Since the atria are activated in a random fashion from small wavelets, atrial activity on the ECG is characterized by fine irregular waves. Irregular activation of the AV node leads to irregular ventricular depolarization (i.e., irregular QRS complexes).

Atrial Flutter. In *atrial flutter* a stable reentrant circuit exists (see Fig. 2-38). Most commonly, a region of slow conduction is located at the junction of the coronary sinus, tricuspid valve, and inferior vena cava. This region of relatively slow conduction allows the maintenance of a stable reentrant circuit in the atria (Fig. 2-39). This region is isolated electrically from the rest of the atrium, being formed from the narrow isthmus bounded by the tricuspid annulus and inferior vena cava. Atrial activation normally occurs in a counterclockwise direction at a stable rate of 300 times per minute. The left atrium and septum are activated from inferior to superior, which leads to negative "flutter" waves in the inferior leads (leads II, III, aVF) of the surface ECG (see Fig. 2-38). The AV node allows acti-

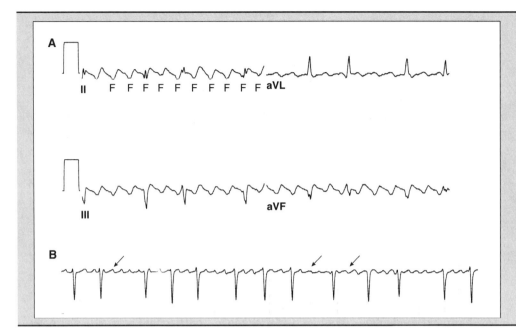

FIG. 2-38

(A) ATRIAL FLUTTER. The atria are activated in regular fashion at 300 beats/min (F). In this case every second or third atrial flutter beat is conducted to the ventricles, which leads to QRS complexes occurring at a rate of 100–150 beats/min.

(B) ATRIAL FIBRILLATION. No definitive P waves can be seen; instead, there are fine baseline irregularities (*arrows*) that are due to fibrillation of the atria. Since the atria are being activated chaotically, the AV node is engaged at random intervals, which leads to a very irregular ventricular activation (QRS complexes).

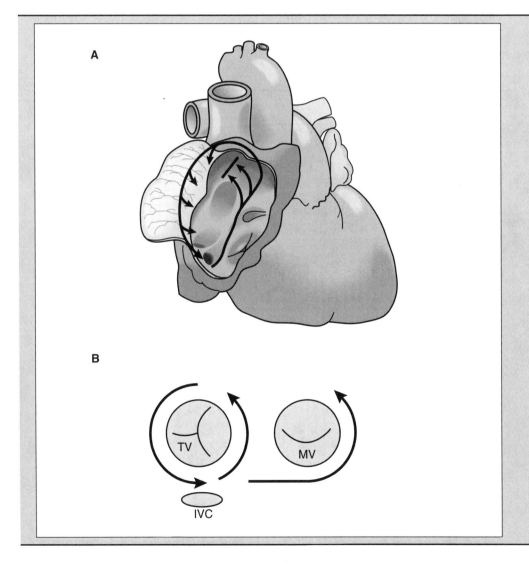

FIG. 2-39

SCHEMATIC OF THE ATRIAL FLUTTER CIRCUIT. Atrial activation proceeds down the lateral wall of the right atrium, through a region of slow conduction bounded by the tricuspid valve, inferior vena cava, and the coronary sinus ostium, and then activates the septum and left atrium in an inferior to superior direction. (A) Anterior right atrium removed. (B) Schematic of the atrial flutter circuit in relationship to the tricuspid valve and mitral valve.

vation of every other or every third atrial beat, which leads to relatively regular ventricular rates of 100–150 beats/min.

The difference between atrial flutter and fibrillation can often be ambiguous, and in some cases, the right atrium can have a stable flutter circuit while the left atrium is activated in a more chaotic fashion, with changing wavefronts suggestive of atrial fibrillation. However, it is important to attempt to make this distinction. Since atrial flutter involves a fixed zone of slow conduction, localized conduction block in this region terminates the arrhythmia. Cauterization of tissues in this region of slow conduction can terminate and potentially cure patients with atrial flutter. However, since atrial fibrillation usually does not involve a fixed area of slow conduction, cauterization of tissue has been less effective for treating this arrhythmia.

AV Node or Junctional Tachycardia. Arrhythmias from junctional tissue can be due to any cellular mechanism. Most commonly, arrhythmias that arise from the junction are due to reentry. The proximal portion of the AV node is an amorphous collection of cells without a distinct beginning. Various regions of atrial tissue provide different inputs to the AV node, often with varying refractory periods and conduction properties. In some patients, electrically distinct pathways can be identified. For example, patients with *AV node reentrant tachycardia* have two electrically separate inputs into the AV node. Most commonly, one input (slow pathway) demonstrates slow conduction properties and a relatively short refractory period, while the other input (fast pathway) has rapid conduction properties and a long refractory period (Fig. 2-40). Normally, atrial activity travels quickly over the fast pathway to engage the AV node; atrial activation that traveled over the slow pathway finds the AV node refractory and is blocked. However, a premature atrial contraction can be blocked in the fast pathway and slowly conduct over the slow pathway. If enough time elapses, the impulse can conduct retrogradely up the fast pathway and start a reentrant circuit.

FIG. 2-40
(A) RHYTHM STRIP SHOWING INITIATION OF ATRIOVENTRICULAR NODE REENTRANT TACHYCARDIA. The first beat is a sinus beat; an atrial premature beat occurs (*arrow*), is followed by a long PR interval, and tachycardia is initiated. The lead shown is V_1. Can you identify how the ventricles are being activated? (This is right bundle branch block.)

(B) SCHEMATIC OF THE EVENTS. *Left:* The first sinus beat is shown. There are two inputs to the atrioventricular node. Activation occurs over the fast pathway. *Center:* With an atrial premature beat the fast pathway is blocked (refractory), and conduction instead travels via the slow pathway (long PR interval). *Right:* The fast pathway has recovered and accepts the impulse in retrograde fashion, and tachycardia begins.

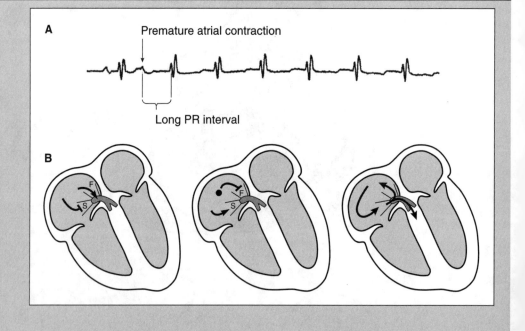

A
Premature atrial contraction
Long PR interval

B

Junctional tachycardia can also arise from triggered activity. For example, toxic concentrations of digitalis, which blocks the $Na^+–K^+$-ATPase, can cause intracellular Ca^{2+} concentrations to increase in junctional tissue, which can lead to the formation of DADs and triggered activity. Junctional tachycardia can also arise from increased automaticity (Fig. 2-41). This mechanism for junctional tachycardia is sometimes observed in newborns and can lead to catastrophic circumstances if not recognized.

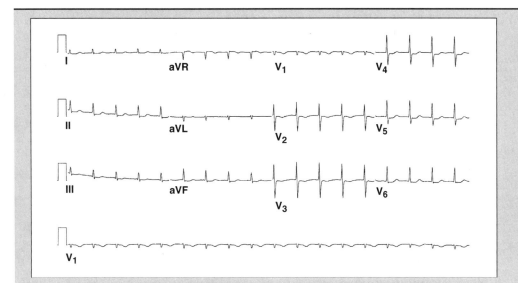

FIG. 2-41
THE TACHYCARDIA RESULTING FROM AN AUTOMATIC FOCUS FROM THE ATRIOVENTRICULAR NODE. Notice that P waves are not seen because of simultaneous activation of the atria and ventricles.

On ECG, junctional tachycardia from any cause most commonly shows QRS complexes that are not preceded by P waves. Since activation of junctional tissue is rapid, this region becomes the dominant pacemaker for the heart rather than the sinus node. Often the junctional tachycardia will not only activate the ventricles but will also activate the atria in retrograde fashion. In this case, the atria and ventricles are activated simultaneously, and the P wave is obscured by the larger QRS complex (Figs. 2-39 and 2-40).

Junctional tachycardias can arise from any mechanism, but re-entry is the most commonly observed cause.

Ventricular Tachycardia. Analogous to the situation with atrial tissues, it is common for a ventricular ectopic focus to cause occasional premature activation of the ventricles. Premature ventricular contractions (commonly referred to as PVCs) can be due to triggered activity, increased automaticity, or a single reentrant beat (Fig. 2-42). In people with normal hearts, PVCs are a benign finding. More than three PVCs in a row are called ventricular tachycardia. By convention, ventricular tachycardia is termed nonsustained if its duration is less than 30 seconds and sustained if the arrhythmia lasts longer than 30 seconds.

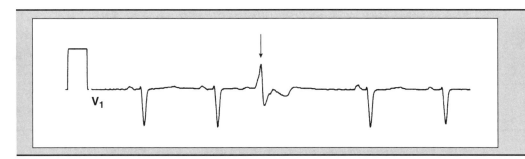

FIG. 2-42
RHYTHM STRIP OF LEAD V$_1$ SHOWING A PREMATURE VENTRICULAR CONTRACTION (*ARROW*). A focus in the ventricle fires early, which leads to the wide QRS complex (since the specialized His-Purkinje tissue is not being used).

Sustained arrhythmias that arise solely from ventricular tissue can be characterized by morphologic appearance. Ventricular tachycardia most commonly occurs in the setting of coronary artery disease. Occlusion of a coronary artery can lead to myocardial infarction and the formation of a scar. This can create adjacent regions with disparate electrophysiologic properties and form the substrate for reentrant circuits. Slow cell-to-cell conduction occurs in the scar as a result of fibrosis, while normal conduction is present in the border zone. While the individual action potentials of cells in the scar are normal, with a rapid phase 0 upstroke, cell-to-cell conduction is slowed; one reason is reduced density of gap junctions in scarred myocardium. If a reentrant circuit is initiated, ventricular tissue is rapidly and repetitively activated. Since the ventricles are now activated abnormally and the His-Purkinje system is not used, the QRS complexes are relatively wide (QRS interval greater than 0.14 sec). If the reentrant circuit is relatively stable, the ventricles are activated in consistent (albeit abnormal) fashion, and the QRS complexes will look uniform (monomorphic). Fig. 2-43 shows an example of sustained *monomorphic ventricular tachycardia.*

FIG. 2-43
MONOMORPHIC VENTRICULAR TACHYCARDIA. Notice the irregular low amplitude deflections (*arrows*), which are best seen in lead III. These are probably P waves that are not related to ventricular activation. Dissociation of ventricular and atrial activity make ventricular tachycardia the most likely diagnosis.

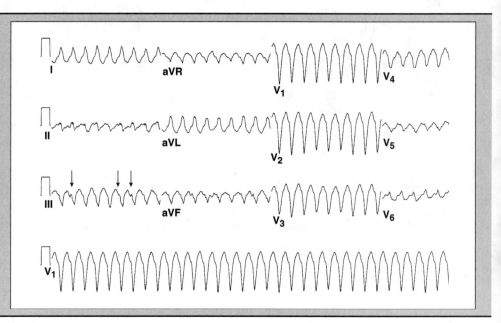

Sustained *polymorphic ventricular* tachycardia can also be observed. In polymorphic ventricular tachycardia, the ventricles are also activated abnormally quickly but are activated differently from beat to beat (Fig. 2-44). This results in QRS complexes on the ECG that have different morphologic characteristics. While coronary artery disease is also the most frequent cause for this arrhythmia, a special form of polymorphic ventricular tachycardia, called torsades de pointes, has been described in a select group of patients with a prolonged QT interval.

FIG. 2-44
POLYMORPHIC VENTRICULAR TACHYCARDIA THAT DETERIORATES TO VENTRICULAR FIBRILLATION.

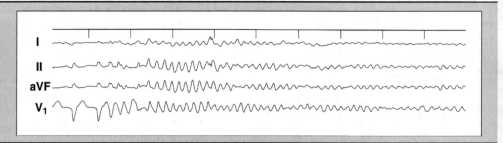

In 1957, Jervell and Lange-Nielsen described a Norwegian family that had congenital deafness and a prolonged QT interval (the interval from the onset of the QRS complex to the end of the T wave). Since then, it has been learned that long QT syndrome can be associated with a variety of genetic mutations. In one family, patients with long QT syndrome had a simple deletion in the amino acid chain between domains III and IV in Na^+ channels, in the region responsible for the inactivation of ion channels.

Deletion of nine amino acids resulted in a subtle change in the behavior of the Na^+ channels' inactivation properties. Experimental data suggested that these abnormal Na^+ channels failed to inactivate properly approximately 3.5% of the time. This resulted in a small maintained inward current, well into the plateau phase, that caused a prolonged action potential. In another family, amino acid substitutions in a gene that may be responsible for the I_K were observed. The actual mechanisms are less well understood, but it is possible that reduced functionality of the I_K causes prolongation of the action potential.

Prolongation of the plateau phase of ventricular myocytes leads to prolongation of the QT interval, which is shown in Fig. 2-45. Prolongation of the action potential can lead to EADs and triggered activity. Triggered activity in ventricular tissue can cause very rapid and disorganized activation of the ventricles. Patients with a prolonged QT interval can display a ventricular arrhythmia in which the QRS complexes undulate, or "twist," from positive to negative. The reason for this ECG appearance is unknown. In fact, while it appears that the tachycardia is initiated by triggered activity, it is unclear whether the arrhythmia continues because of continued triggered activity or because of reentry in the ventricular tissues.

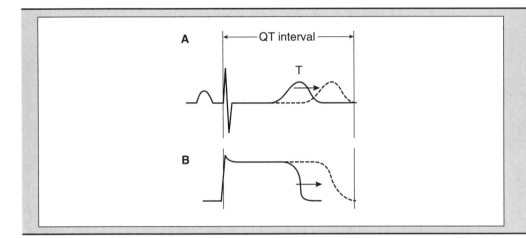

FIG. 2-45
THE BASELINE ELECTROCAR-DIOGRAM IN A PATIENT WITH LONG QT INTERVAL OF APPROXI-MATELY 500 msec. (A) In addition notice that in V_5 and V_6 the T waves are inverted when the predominant QRS forces are positive. (B) The long QT interval is due to prolongation of the plateau phase of the action potential of ventricular cells.

Both monomorphic and polymorphic ventricular tachycardia can deteriorate to *ventricular fibrillation*. As with atrial fibrillation, in ventricular fibrillation, the ventricles are activated chaotically by wandering wavelets of electrical activation. On ECG, very rapid, low-amplitude deflections are observed. The distinction between polymorphic ventricular tachycardia and ventricular fibrillation is rather arbitrary. In polymorphic ventricular tachycardia, some regularization of ventricular activation is present so that some QRS complexes are of normal amplitude. In ventricular fibrillation, the wandering wavelets of ventricular action are manifested by very rapid, low-amplitude QRS complexes on the ECG (see Fig. 2-44).

Accessory Pathway–Mediated Tachycardia. In some people, incomplete formation of the fibrous annulus can lead to thin bands of tissue separating the atria and ventricles, which allow alternative conduction for the cardiac impulse. Accessory pathways occur in approximately 1 in 1000 people, and in 1930, Wolff, Parkinson, and White described 11 patients with accessory pathways associated with episodes of rapid heart rate (i.e., the Wolff-Parkinson-White syndrome).

In patients with accessory pathways, conduction of the atrial impulse occurs over both the accessory pathway and the AV node. Usually, the accessory pathway is formed from normal atrial or ventricular tissue with rapid conduction properties, which causes the ventricle to be "preexcited." On the ECG, the PR interval is shortened, since the ventricles are now partially activated by the accessory pathway (Fig. 2-46). In addition, the region of the ventricle that is activated by the accessory pathway does not use the His-Purkinje system, which leads to a relatively wide QRS complex. The initial portion of the QRS (which mainly represents activation of the ventricles over the accessory pathway) is slurred and is termed a delta wave.

The accessory pathway itself does not cause arrhythmias. In fact, most patients with accessory pathways are asymptomatic. However, in some patients, an atrial premature beat can block in the accessory pathway because the tissue is in its effective refractory period, resulting in conduction solely over the AV node. If, after the ventricles are activated, the accessory pathway has recovered, the atria can be reactivated via retrograde conduction over the accessory pathway. Tachycardia can occur if a sustained reentrant circuit is formed. Since the ventricular activation is now occurring solely over the His-Purkinje system, the QRS complex during tachycardia is narrow. The ventricles

FIG. 2-46
(A) In patients with accessory pathways, activation of the ventricles occurs via both the atrioventricular (AV) node and the accessory pathway. Since the accessory pathway has rapid conduction properties, the PR interval is shortened. Because the ventricular activity from the accessory pathway does not use the His-Purkinje system, the QRS complex is wide. The QRS complex is termed a fusion beat since the ventricles are being simultaneously activated from two separate sites, the AV node and the accessory pathway. (B) A premature atrial contraction can sometimes cause block in the accessory pathway, and the ventricles can be activated solely by the AV node. (C) If enough time has elapsed so that the accessory pathway has recovered, the impulse can travel retrogradely through the accessory pathway, and a reentrant circuit may be initiated.

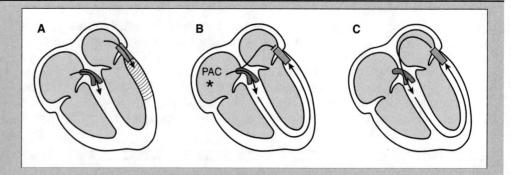

Tachycardias That Involve Accessory Pathways

- Orthodromic AVRT
- Antidromic AVRT
- Atrial tachycardia with rapid conduction down the accessory pathway.

and atria are activated sequentially, and the P wave is inscribed after the QRS complex. The accessory pathway conducts relatively rapidly when compared to AV node conduction so that the P wave is located closer to the preceding QRS than to the QRS following the P wave. Since the atrial insertion point of the accessory pathway is located somewhere on the fibrous annulus, the atria are often activated in a "low-to-high" direction. Retrograde activation of the atria often leads to an inverted P wave in the inferior leads. This type of tachycardia is usually termed *orthodromic* atrioventricular reentrant tachycardia (AVRT) because activation over the AV node is occurring in the normal direction.

Alternatively, activation can occur in a reentrant circuit by traveling down the accessory pathway to activate the ventricles and retrogradely activate the atria via the AV node (see Fig. 2-35). Since activation of the AV node is now occurring opposite to the normal direction, this rarer type of tachycardia is called *antidromic AVRT*. In this situation, the ventricles are repetitively activated solely by the accessory pathway, which leads to a regular tachycardia with wide QRS complexes (the QRS complexes are wide because the ventricles are not activated using the specialized His-Purkinje system).

Finally, patients with accessory pathways can develop atrial tachycardias, particularly atrial fibrillation. Since the accessory pathway does not demonstrate slow conduction properties like the AV node, the ventricles can be activated very rapidly (often at rates greater than 300 beats/min). This rapid activation of the ventricles can in some instances lead to sudden cardiac death. Since activation is occurring rapidly and irregularly over the accessory pathway, the QRS complexes are very wide, very closely spaced, and irregular (Fig. 2-47).

ELECTROCARDIOGRAPHIC CLASSIFICATION

Tachycardias are classified electrocardiographically as wide- or narrow-complex. Regardless of mechanism, if the QRS complex is narrow (< 0.12 sec or < 3 mm wide), the ventricles are being activated normally over the His-Purkinje system. On the other hand, if the QRS complex is wide (> 0.12 sec or > 3 mm wide), the tachycardia is arising from ventricular tissue or from abnormally activated ventricles (i.e., resulting from blocked conduction in the left or right bundle or from activation via an accessory pathway). The

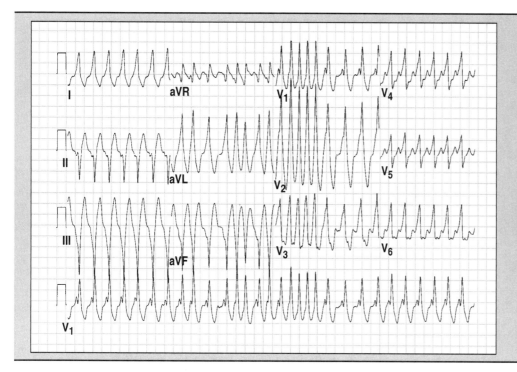

FIG. 2-47
In this 12-lead electrocardiogram, notice that the QRS complexes are very wide, irregular, and at times closely spaced. The interval between the third and fourth QRS complexes is approximately 5 mm or 240 msec (5 × 0.04 sec) apart. This translates to a heart rate of approximately 240 beats/min. This combination of wide, irregular, and very rapid tachycardia is strong evidence for atrial fibrillation with activation of the ventricles via an accessory pathway. Since accessory pathway tissue can conduct very rapidly, rapid rates are possible. In terms of teleology, the student can see that the slow conduction properties of the AV node are useful for preventing ventricular activation from occurring too rapidly.

distinction is clinically important; wide-complex tachycardia resulting from ventricular tachycardia or atrial tachycardia in the presence of an accessory pathway can often lead to catastrophic clinical outcomes.

Narrow-Complex Tachycardia. If the QRS complex is narrow, it follows that the ventricles are being activated in the normal fashion. This finding essentially rules out ventricular tachycardia. (In very rare circumstances, if the ventricular tachycardia focus or exit site from a reentrant circuit is located very near the His bundle where it penetrates the fibrous annulus, the QRS complex can appear normal, since most of the ventricle is activated "normally" over the His-Purkinje system.) However, any atrial tachycardia, junctional tachycardia, or accessory pathway–mediated orthodromic tachycardia can lead to a narrow-complex tachycardia (Fig. 2-48). This group of tachycardias is collectively referred to as supraventricular tachycardias (SVT), since the arrhythmia involves the AV node or atrial tissue (i.e., tissue that is superior to the ventricles).

In atrial tachycardia from a single focus, regular atrial activity is observed preceding the QRS complex. The duration of the PR interval depends on the conduction properties of the AV node in that patient. The shape of the P wave depends on the site of the atrial focus. If the focus is located near the sinus node, the P waves are upright in lead II and negative in aVR. If the focus is from the left atrium—for example, from the orifice of the left upper pulmonary vein—the P wave is negative in aVL. In multifocal atrial tachycardia, several different P waves are seen. Multifocal atrial tachycardia is usually fairly irregular, since each of the atrial foci have different rates of depolarization.

In atrial fibrillation, because the atria are activated via wandering wavelets, the AV node is bombarded by electrical activation at a random and very rapid rate. Fortunately, since the AV node exhibits slow conduction properties, the ventricular rate is much slower than the atrial fibrillation rate. However, the QRS complexes occur quite randomly. Between the QRS complexes, no distinct P waves are observed. Instead rapid and irregular low-amplitude deflections from chaotic activation of the atria are observed. The amplitude of the deflections is determined by the degree of organization of atrial activity. Disorganized atrial activity from many wavelets is manifested by very fine, low-amplitude signals on the ECG. However, if there are relatively few wavelets (6–10), atrial activity may appear more regular and with higher amplitude.

In atrial flutter, the AV node and ventricles are activated in regular fashion (approximately 300 beats/min), but because of slow conduction properties in the AV node, not

FIG. 2-48
ELECTROCARDIOGRAPHIC DIF-FERENTIAL DIAGNOSIS OF SU-PRAVENTRICULAR TACHYCAR-DIA. In atrial tachycardia the P waves are usually located prior to the QRS with a normal AV interval. However, if the patient has first-degree AV block, the PR interval may be prolonged. The shape of the P wave will depend on the atrial tachycardia focus. If the focus is near the sinus node, the P waves will be upright in lead II. If the focus is in the lower portion of the atria, the P waves will appear inverted in lead II. In atrial fibrillation, consistent atrial activity is not observed. Instead atrial fibrillation leads to fine irregular fibrillatory waves (*arrows*). In atrial flutter, the atria are activated in regular fashion at 300 beats/min, and the "flutter waves" are normally negative in the inferior leads (II, III, and aVF), since the atria are activated in counterclockwise fashion and the left atrium is more prominent electrocardiographically. In junctional tachycardias, the atria and ventricles are often activated simultaneously so that the P wave is obscured in the QRS or in the terminal portion of the QRS. In accessory pathway–mediated orthodromic tachycardia, the atria and ventricles are activated sequentially, and the P wave is just after the QRS complex in the ST segment.

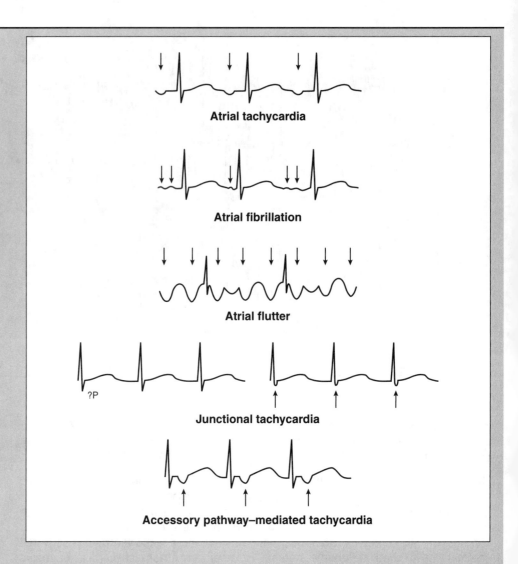

Atrial tachycardia

Atrial fibrillation

Atrial flutter

Junctional tachycardia

Accessory pathway–mediated tachycardia

every impulse is transmitted to the ventricles. For this reason, a regular flutter wave is observed, and QRS complexes occur at a regular rate. Typically, electrical activation travels from lateral to septal in the isthmus formed by the tricuspid valve and inferior vena cava. Electrical activation emerges from this region of slow conduction to activate the septum and left atrium in an inferior-to-superior direction. Since the ECG predominantly measures left atrial activation, the "flutter waves" of atrial activation are usually negative in the inferior leads (i.e., II, III, aVF).

In junctional tachycardias, the electrical impulse often travels both in the retrograde and anterograde directions. The atria are activated by the retrograde impulse, and the ventricles are activated by the anterograde impulse. Since the atria and ventricles are activated simultaneously, the P wave is obscured or barely visible in the terminal portion of the QRS complex.

In narrow-complex tachycardias that use an accessory pathway (orthodromic AVRT), the ventricles are activated via the AV node, and the atria are then activated via retrograde conduction from the accessory pathway. Since the atria and ventricles are activated in sequential fashion, the P wave is often observed in the ST segment. The P wave is usually located closer to the preceding QRS complex because the accessory pathway has rapid conduction properties like atrial or ventricular tissue, and the AV node continues to conduct with relatively slow velocities.

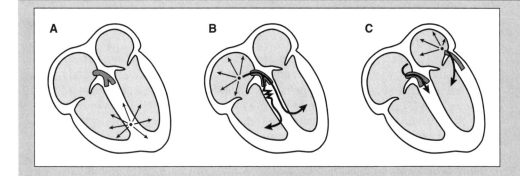

FIG. 2-49
DIFFERENTIAL DIAGNOSIS OF WIDE-COMPLEX TACHYCARDIA. (A) In ventricular tachycardia the ventricles are repetitively activated from a reentrant circuit or abnormal focus. Since His-Purkinje tissue is not used, the QRS complex is wide. (B) Any supraventricular tachycardia can be associated with wide-complex tachycardia by electrocardiogram (ECG) if there is aberrant conduction down the right or left bundle. (C) If the ventricles are activated primarily over an accessory pathway, a wide-complex tachycardia will be observed on the ECG.

In Ms. Eswine's case, while the baseline QRS is widened, the tachycardia actually has a narrow-complex QRS, suggesting that the ventricles were activated utilizing the normal His-Purkinje system. Can you identify atrial activity?

Case Study:
Continued

Wide-Complex Tachycardias. In wide-complex tachycardia, the QRS complex is greater than 0.12 sec (3 mm), and the ventricles are not normally activated over the specialized His-Purkinje system. Wide-complex tachycardia can arise from: (1) ventricular tachycardia, (2) any SVT that is associated with aberrant conduction over the His-Purkinje system, or (3) atrial tachycardia with activation over an accessory pathway or antidromic tachycardia (Fig. 2-49).

In ventricular tachycardia, a focus in the ventricles rapidly activates the heart. Atrial and ventricular activity are usually not associated in a one-to-one fashion. The sinus node continues to fire and activate the atria even as the ventricular focus is repetitively firing. For this reason, the P waves (atrial activity) occur independently from the QRS complexes (ventricular activity). Occasionally, an atrial impulse that originated from the sinus node activates the AV node and activates part or most of the ventricular tissue. If part of the ventricle is activated via the AV node, a fusion beat will be observed, in which the QRS complex has some intermediate form between a normal QRS and the wide QRS as a result of the ventricular tachycardia focus. If most of the ventricle is activated via the AV node, a normal-appearing QRS complex, or "capture beat," will be observed for one beat. Any time fusion or capture beats are observed or atrial and ventricular activity appear to be independent of one another, ventricular tachycardia must be strongly considered.

■ SUMMARY

Abnormal heart rhythms can be classified as either too slow (bradycardias) or too fast (tachycardias). Bradycardias can be due to abnormal impulse formation or blocked conduction. Since the AV node is normally the only connection between the atria and the ventricles, it is the most common site for blocked conduction. A block in the bundle branches leads to sequential activation of the ventricles, which will lead to a wide QRS complex on the ECG. Bradycardias can be used to reduce automaticity or AV block.

Tachycardias can be considered from electrophysiologic, anatomic, and ECG standpoints. Electrophysiologically, tachycardias can be classified by their origin—resulting from increased automaticity, triggered activity, or most commonly, through the formation of reentrant circuits. Anatomically, tachycardias can be classified as atrial, junctional, ventricular, or accessory pathway—mediated. Finally, tachycardias are classified on ECG as either narrow-complex (supraventricular) or wide-complex.

KEY POINTS

- Cyclical changes in membrane permeability to various ions are responsible for the action potential of cardiac cells.
- Cardiac cells can be classified on the basis of their action potential shapes. Slow-response cells (sinus node and AV node) do not have fast Na^+ channels and have a gradual upstroke. Fast-response cells (atria, His-Purkinje tissue, ventricles) have a sharp phase 0 upstroke, resulting from the presence of fast Na^+ channels.
- The ECG can be considered the sum of all the cardiac action potentials; the P wave represents atrial depolarization, the QRS complex ventricular depolarization, and the T-wave ventricular repolarization.
- Tachycardias can be classified by basic mechanism (increased automaticity, triggered activity, reentry), anatomically (atrial tachycardias, junctional tachycardias, ventricular tachycardias, accessory pathway–mediated tachycardias), or electrocardiographically (narrow QRS complex versus wide QRS complex).

Case Study:
Resolution

Examination of the ECG at baseline for Ms. Eswine (see Fig. 2-1A) shows that the QRS complex is relatively wide. This implies that part of the ventricles were activated abnormally, not using the His-Purkinje system. Second, the interval between the P wave and the QRS is normally 120–160 msec in duration, but Ms. Eswine's PR interval is almost nonexistant.

Ms. Eswine not only had normal atrial activation (normal P-wave morphologic characteristics that were positive in lead II and negative in lead aVR) but also had an accessory pathway that preexcited the ventricle and bypassed the slow conduction in the AV node. Her ventricles were actually fusion complexes, since part of the ventricle was activated by the accessory pathway and part of the ventricle was activated via the AV node. Activation via the accessory pathway leads to a short PR interval. In addition, since the accessory pathway inserts into normal ventricular myocardium but not specialized Purkinje tissue, conduction occurred relatively slowly and led to the wide, bizarre-appearing QRS complex.

Examination of the initiation of Ms. Eswine's fast heart rhythm shows that the first two beats were conducted over both the accessory pathway and the AV node; consequently the QRS is wide and bizarre-appearing (left arrows, Fig. 2-1C). There was a PAC, which blocked in the accessory pathway, perhaps occurring in the refractory period of this tissue. The electrical impulse then proceeded solely down the AV node. Because of slow conduction properties in the AV node, the PR interval was lengthened. The ventricles were activated, and the QRS was narrow and normal-appearing because the ventricles were activated solely using the His-Purkinje tissue. The ventricular impulse then reached the distal portion of the accessory pathway, which had by this time recovered its excitable properties, and traveled retrogradely through the accessory pathway to activate the atria. Since the atria were being activated from "low" to "high," the P wave is inverted (right arrows). The cycle repeated as the cardiac impulse again engaged the AV node, and the patient developed persistent supraventricular tachycardia with a narrow QRS complex.

This is an example of a tachycardia utilizing a reentrant mechanism. The two electrically distinct pathways are the AV node and the accessory pathway. Ms. Eswine's sensation of "fluttering" probably correlated with a PAC, and her "racing heart" was due to supraventricular tachycardia. Since Ms. Eswine was otherwise healthy, when her heart rate was 180–200 beats/min, she felt uncomfortable but still maintained perfusion to her brain and so did not lose consciousness.

The site of this accessory pathway can be found and cauterized using special techniques that can cure the patient of this congenital abnormality. A special electrode-tipped catheter is placed at the site of the accessory pathway, and radiofrequency energy cauterizes the tissue (Fig. 2-50). The ECG in Fig. 2-51 is from Ms. Eswine after this procedure was performed. Notice that the PR interval is normal, and the QRS complex now has a normal appearance.

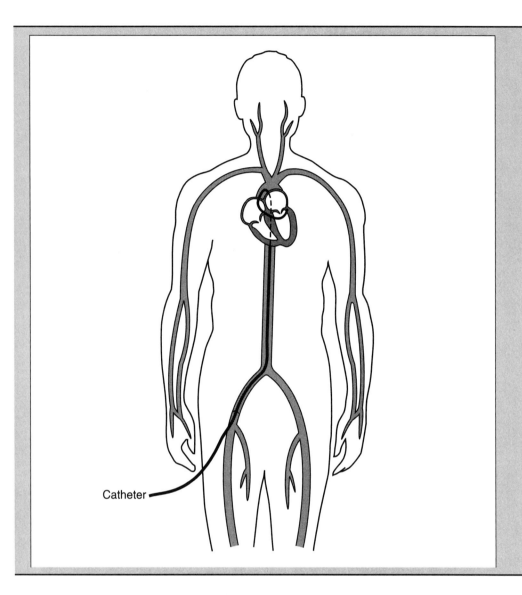

FIG. 2-50
**SCHEMATIC SHOWING THE RA-
DIOFREQUENCY CATHETER AB-
LATION PROCEDURE.** A long
catheter with a special tip is inserted through the femoral artery to the site of the accessory
pathway under fluoroscopy. The
accessory pathway tissue is
cauterized, and abnormal conduction over the accessory
pathway is abolished.

Catheter

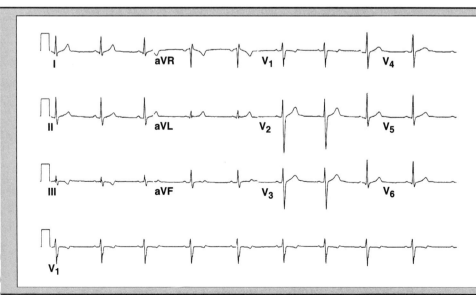

FIG. 2-51
Ms. Eswine underwent a procedure called ablation where a
catheter was placed in the
heart and the accessory pathway was cauterized using radiofrequency energy. Compare this
electrocardiogram to Fig. 2-1.
Notice that the QRS complex
and the PR interval are now normal.

■ REVIEW QUESTIONS

Directions: For each of the following questions, choose the **one best** answer.

Questions 1–2

1. Mr. Wynn Muse is a 57-year-old man who had rheumatic fever as a child. This has caused his mitral valve (the valve that separates the left atrium and ventricles) to become significantly narrowed (mitral stenosis). His baseline electrocardiogram (ECG) is shown below. What is Mr. Muse's arrhythmia?

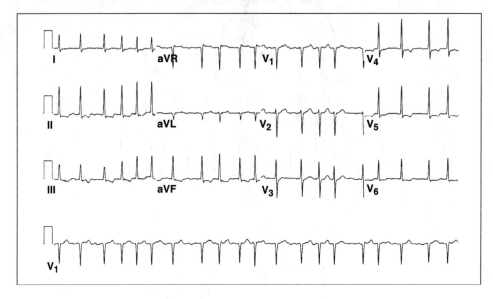

   (A) Atrial fibrillation
   (B) Atrial flutter
   (C) Ventricular tachycardia
   (D) Orthodromic atrioventricular (AV) reentry

2. Mr. Muse is treated with the drug quinidine, which blocks both the sodium (Na^+) channel and the delayed rectifier potassium current (I_K). How will this drug affect the form and structure of his ventricular myocyte action potential?

   (A) Extend the plateau phase
   (B) Shorten the plateau phase
   (C) Slow phase 0 and extend the plateau phase
   (D) Slow phase 0 and shorten the plateau phase

3. Jacob Kwasman is a 67-year-old man who presents with the ECG shown below. He is slightly weak but feels relatively well. He has a history of a myocardial infarction approximately 10 years ago. What arrhythmia is present?

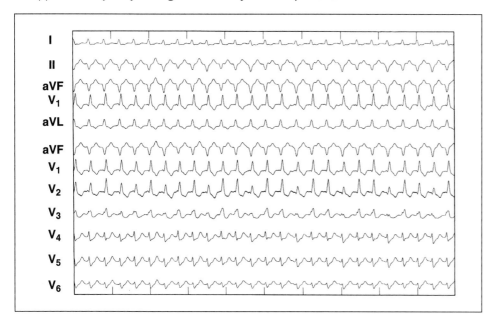

(A) Atrial flutter
(B) Atrial fibrillation
(C) Orthodromic atrioventricular (AV) reentry
(D) Ventricular tachycardia
(E) Ventricular fibrillation

4. Tracy Ung is a healthy 33-year-old woman who has noticed episodes of tiredness. Her ECG is shown below. What are the abnormalities?

(A) Abnormal automaticity
(B) Blocked conduction
(C) Both abnormal automaticity and blocked conduction

■ ANSWERS AND EXPLANATIONS

1. The answer is A. In mitral stenosis the mitral valve is narrowed, which leads to an abnormal pressure gradient between the left atrium and left ventricle. Left atrial pressure increases and causes left atrial enlargement. Left atrial enlargement often is associated with atrial fibrillation. Notice the ventricles (QRS complexes) are activated in an irregular fashion because of the wandering wavelets in the atria, which engage the AV node at irregular intervals. No discrete P waves are observed on the ECG since the atria are activated irregularly. In ventricular tachycardia, the QRS complexes would have been wide (abnormal ventricular activation). In atrial flutter and orthodromic atrioventricular reentrant tachycardia (AVRT), a repeating reentrant circuit exists so that the ventricles are activated in a regular fashion.

2. The answer is C. Atrial fibrillation is commonly treated with quinidine, which blocks Na+ and K+ channels. This changes the action potential as shown in the figure below. Block of Na+ channels causes the phase 0 upstroke to be less steep. Blocking the I_K results in prolongation of the plateau phase. Prolongation of the action potential by blocking the K+ channel may make atrial tissue more refractory and less likely to allow propagation of the wandering wavelets in atrial fibrillation. However, quinidine will also prolong the action potential in ventricular tissue and may lead to the formation of early afterdepolarizations. If these afterdepolarizations lead to triggered activity, life-threatening ventricular fibrillation can occur. Patients on quinidine are at risk for developing torsades de pointes, just like patients with congenital long QT syndrome.

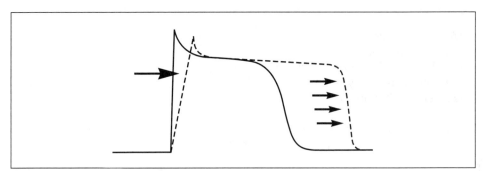

3. The answer is D. The QRS complex is wide and rapid. This suggests either a ventricular origin of the tachycardia or a supraventricular origin with the ventricles aberrantly activated. Notice that P waves can be sporadically observed and are not associated with the ventricular activity. In addition, every third QRS complex is different (see figure below);

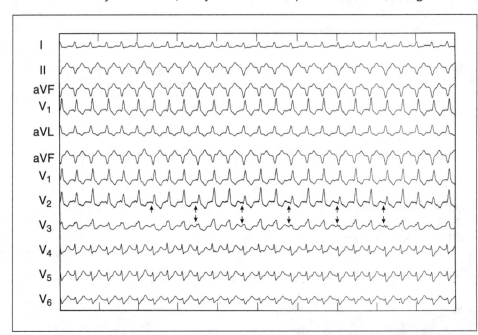

this is due to partial activation of the ventricles via the AV node ("fusion" beat). These findings make ventricular tachycardia most likely.

Even with aberrant activation of the ventricles, atrial fibrillation would be associated with irregular QRS complexes. The presence of the "fusion" beat rules out atrial flutter or orthodromic AV reentry.

Ventricular tachycardia is often poorly tolerated. Patients frequently have associated poor left ventricular function at baseline, and since ventricular and atrial activity are not associated, there is no atrial contribution to cardiac output. In the presence of hemo-dynamic collapse, patients with ventricular tachycardia are treated with a 200- to 360-J shock delivered from external paddles (see figure below). Electrical shock may depolarize enough of the ventricle to terminate the tachycardia. The electrical shock causes simultaneous depolarization of the ventricle, which breaks the reentrant circuit causing tachycardia. While the reentrant circuit is abolished, the substrate for reentry still remains. If patients are relatively stable, antiarrhythmic drugs can be used. Lidocaine and procainamide, which block Na^+ channels, are most commonly used.

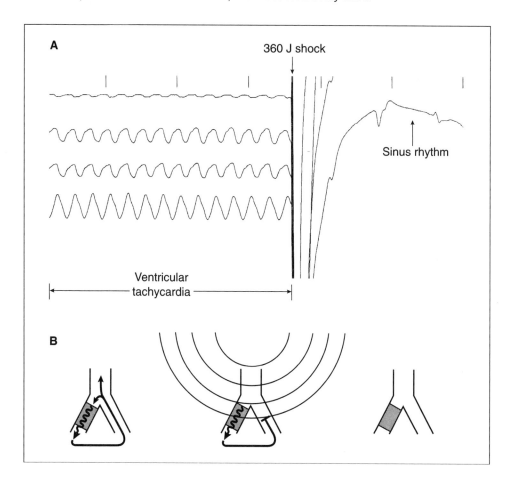

4. The answer is C. Both abnormal automaticity and blocked conduction are present. The first thing that the student should notice is the very slow heart rate of approximately 40 beats/min. Slow heart rates are due to reduced automaticity or conduction block. In this case, notice that the P waves have no relation to the QRS complexes. There is complete block (third-degree AV block) between the atria and ventricles. Next, notice that the P wave is inverted in leads II, III, and aVF and positive in leads aVR and aVL. This suggests that the atria are being depolarized from a focus located in the low septal portion of the atria instead of from the sinus node. Finally, notice that the QRS complex has a right bundle branch block morphology. This implies that the right ventricle is being activated later than the left ventricle. Since conduction is blocked in the AV node, this morphology is not due to right bundle branch block but is due to a subsidiary pacemaker from the left bundle that has now become the primary pacemaker for the heart. Since the left bundle is now the primary pacemaker, it suggests that the block in AV conduction is occurring at the level of the bundle of His. If the block were in the compact AV node, the escape complex is usually narrow since the ventricles are still activated simultaneously from a focus in the His bundle (see figure below).

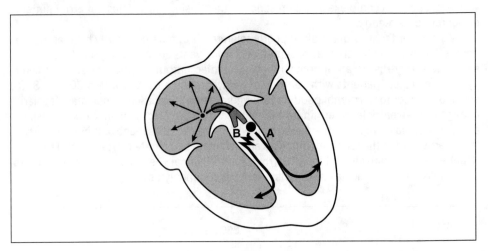

This is a situation where there is both abnormal impulse formation and conduction block. However, the slow rate is due to the block in AV conduction. If activation from the ectopic atrial focus were followed by one-to-one AV conduction, the heart rate would be about 100 beats/min.

■ REFERENCES

Rardon DP, Pressler ML: Cardiac resting and action potentials: current concepts. In *Cardiac Electrophysiology and Arrhythmias*. Edited by Fisch C, Surawicz B. New York NY: Elsevier Science, 1991, pp 3–12.

Chapter 3

CORONARY ARTERY DISEASE

Sreenivas Gudimetla, M.D., and Fred M. Kusumoto, M.D.

■ CHAPTER OUTLINE

Case Study:
Introduction

Mr. Rick Hendrickson was a 50-year-old heavy smoker with a history of type II diabetes mellitus (type II DM) [formerly known as non–insulin-dependent diabetes mellitus] for 7 years, hypertension, and hyperlipidemia, who, while driving home after a stressful day, developed severe midsternal chest pressure that radiated to his jaw and left arm. The chest pain was associated with profound shortness of breath, nausea, and diaphoresis. When the pain continued to worsen over the next 2 minutes, Mr. Hendrickson became concerned and went to a nearby emergency room. Prior to this episode, for the previous several years, Mr. Hendrickson had experienced similar but less severe midsternal chest pain with exertion that would resolve after 3–5 minutes of rest. Over the previous week, however, the pain had become more frequent, and one episode occurred at rest.

Case Study:
Continued

In the emergency room, Mr. Hendrickson's blood pressure was 130/80 mm Hg, and his pulse was 90 beats/min. His cardiac examination was unremarkable.

A previous electrocardiogram (ECG) and his admission ECG are shown in Figs. 3-1 and 3-2, respectively. The emergency room physician gave Mr. Hendrickson a sublingual nitroglycerin pill. What pathophysiologic process was occurring in Mr. Hendrickson? Why was the emergency room physician treating Mr. Hendrickson with sublingual nitroglycerin?

FIG. 3-1
MR. HENDRICKSON'S ELECTRO-CARDIOGRAM FROM 20 YEARS PREVIOUSLY.

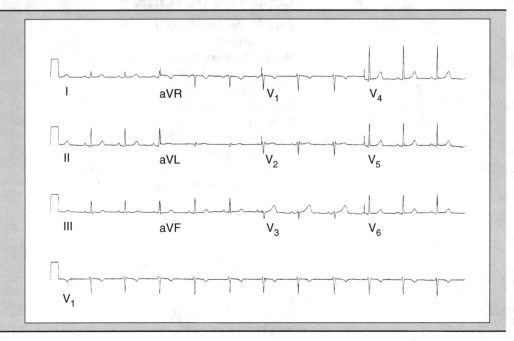

FIG. 3-2
MR. HENDRICKSON'S ELECTRO-CARDIOGRAM IN THE EMERGENCY ROOM.

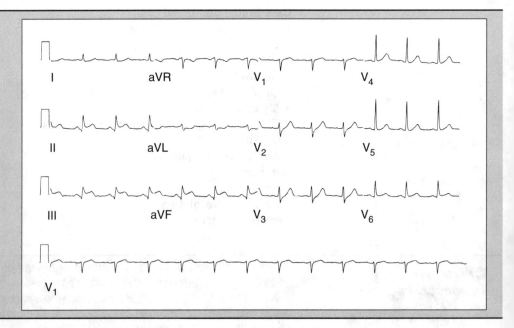

■ INTRODUCTION

The coronary arteries provide blood to the heart. Interestingly, it was not appreciated until the late 1800s that pathophysiologic processes involving the coronary arteries were associated with heart disease. Today it has become apparent that disease of the coronary arteries is very common; the World Health Organization (WHO) predicts that by the year 2000, coronary artery disease will be the leading cause of death in the Western world. Atherosclerosis is the most common form of coronary artery disease. Almost every physician and health care provider encounters atherosclerotic coronary artery disease in his or her practice. Recent data suggest that atherosclerotic lesions are due to an excessive inflammatory and proliferative response in reaction to repeated injury to the vessel wall. The major objective of this chapter is to provide a detailed but concise framework of the multiple, complex processes leading to atherosclerosis and to describe how atherosclerotic lesions give rise to clinical problems.

This chapter is divided into five parts. First, we discuss *normal arterial structure* and functions of the specialized tissues in the arterial wall. Second, we discuss the pathophysiologic basis of the *atherosclerotic process* and the role of hypercholesterolemia and other factors in atherogenesis. Third, the process of *thrombosis* is explored. Fourth, possible pathophysiologic mechanisms for *risk factors* of coronary artery disease are discussed. We conclude with a discussion of the clinical manifestations of coronary artery disease, the *coronary ischemic syndromes*, such as angina pectoris and myocardial infarction; the discussion includes proposed mechanisms, ECG manifestations, and the pathophysiologic basis of some current medical therapies. Throughout the chapter the reader should keep in mind the complex interplay that exists between atherosclerosis and thrombosis; it is the interaction between these two processes that leads to coronary ischemic syndromes.

■ NORMAL CORONARY ARTERY STRUCTURE

The normal coronary artery consists of three layers (Fig. 3-3). The innermost, thin layer consisting of endothelial cells is called the *intima*. With age the intimal layer gradually thickens as small amounts of smooth muscle accumulate in the extracellular matrix

Smooth muscle cells and **endothelial cells** are important for normal vessel physiology.

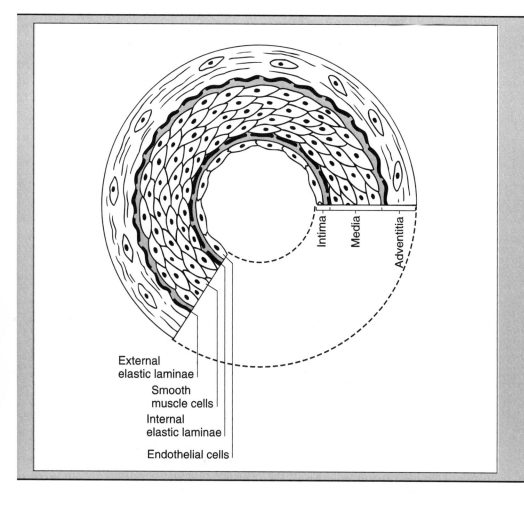

FIG. 3-3
NORMAL LAYERS OF THE ARTERIAL WALL. Intima: endothelial cells. Media: smooth muscle cells. Adventitia: collagenous tissue, connective tissues, vasa vasorum, lymphatics.

External elastic laminae
Smooth muscle cells
Internal elastic laminae
Endothelial cells

Intima
Media
Adventitia

separating the endothelial layer from the internal elastic laminae. The next layer is the *media*, which is demarcated by the internal and external elastic laminae and is made up of smooth muscle cells and an extracellular matrix composed of bundles of collagen fibers and elastic fibrils. The outermost layer of the artery is the *adventitia*, which consists of dense fibroelastic tissue, nutrient vessels, nerves, and lymphatics. Two cell types in the arterial wall, smooth muscle cells and endothelial cells, are particularly important for the normal function of the coronary artery.

SMOOTH MUSCLE CELLS

Smooth muscle cells are spindle-shaped cells that contain three types of filaments: myosin (thick), actin (thin), and intermediate types (Fig. 3-4). Intermediate filaments have diameters between those of actin and myosin and form a cytoskeletal network. Intermediate filaments are composed of polymers of a protein called desmin. Smooth muscle has a higher actin content and a lower myosin content than skeletal muscle. In addition, instead of being arranged in organized sarcomeres with obvious striations (Z bands), the filaments of smooth muscle are arranged in an interlacing network. Thick filaments are complex structures composed of a group of 300–400 myosin molecules (Fig. 3-5). Each myosin protein is composed of two large subunits (each with an approximate molecular weight of 200 kD) and four smaller light-chain subunits, two with molecular weights of 17 kD (LC 17) and the others with molecular weights of 20 kD (LC 20). Thin filaments are composed of two actin molecules, each with a molecular weight of 43 kD, that are arranged in a double α helix.

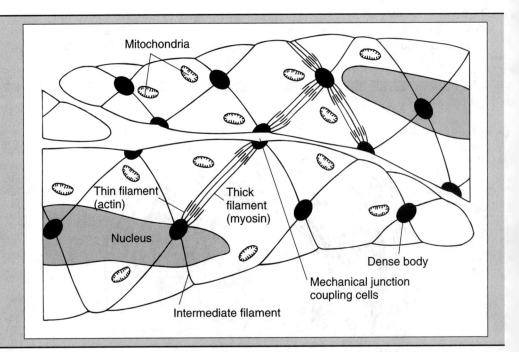

FIG. 3-4
CYTOSKELETAL NETWORK OF SMOOTH MUSCLE. This consists of thick filaments (myosin) and thin filaments (actin), which make up the sarcomere; intermediate filaments link the contractile apparatus via dense bodies.

Smooth muscle contraction is modulated by many vasoactive substances and is calcium-dependent. Most substances that cause smooth muscle contraction (i.e., vasoconstriction of the arteries) do so by increasing intracellular calcium ion (Ca^{2+}) levels. Conversely, smooth muscle relaxation (i.e., vasodilation of the arteries) is mediated by a decrease in intracellular Ca^{2+}.

Unlike skeletal and cardiac muscle cells, smooth muscle cells do not have troponin, a major Ca^{2+}-binding protein involved in regulation of muscle contraction. Instead, a cytosolic protein, *calmodulin*, which has structural and functional similarity to troponin-C, modulates Ca^{2+}-dependent contraction and relaxation of smooth muscle. As illustrated in Fig. 3-6, four intracellular Ca^{2+} bind to calmodulin, and this complex activates myosin light-chain kinase (MLCK). In the presence of adenosine triphosphate (ATP),

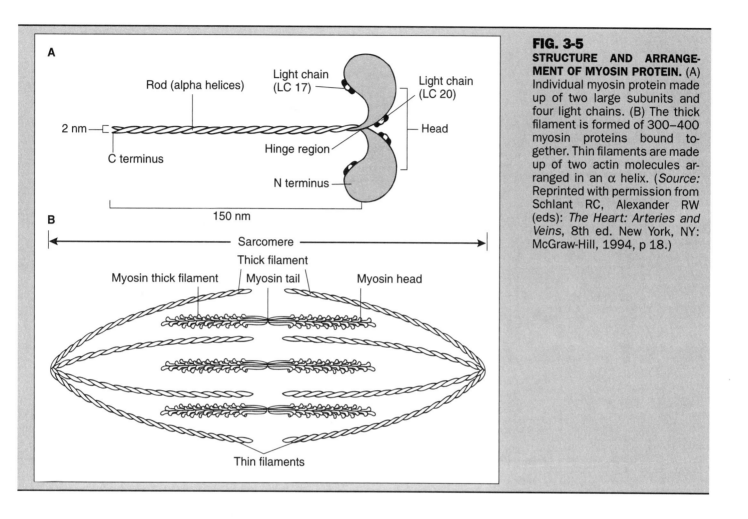

FIG. 3-5
STRUCTURE AND ARRANGE-MENT OF MYOSIN PROTEIN. (A) Individual myosin protein made up of two large subunits and four light chains. (B) The thick filament is formed of 300–400 myosin proteins bound together. Thin filaments are made up of two actin molecules arranged in an α helix. (*Source:* Reprinted with permission from Schlant RC, Alexander RW (eds): *The Heart: Arteries and Veins*, 8th ed. New York, NY: McGraw-Hill, 1994, p 18.)

MLCK mediates phosphorylation of a specialized regulatory site on the 20-kD light chain (LC 20) attached to the myosin head, which results in cross-bridging of the myosin head with the actin filament and smooth muscle contraction. Myosin phosphatase removes the high-energy phosphate from LC 20, which results in detachment of the myosin head from the actin filament. Myosin phosphatase activity causes inhibition or slowing of smooth muscle contraction.

Smooth muscle cells normally function in maintenance of vascular tone, maintenance of structural integrity, and in lipid metabolism. Smooth muscle can contract or relax in response to mediators of vascular tone. Smooth muscle cells can synthesize connective tissue constituents such as collagen, elastin, proteoglycan, and various growth factors and can proliferate in response to growth factors. Smooth muscle cells have numerous surface receptors including low-density lipoprotein (LDL) cholesterol receptors. Understanding smooth muscle physiology is important, since smooth muscle cells may function differently in atherosclerotic lesions. Smooth muscle cells from atherosclerotic lesions respond differently to various growth factors, have different contractile responses, and can accumulate lipids (forming foam cells).

ENDOTHELIAL CELLS

The elliptical endothelial cells form a monolayer that lines the entire vasculature. Endothelial cells occupy a key physiologic position, separating the blood from the smooth muscle in the vessel wall. It is now clear that endothelial cells have multiple functions that include: (1) secretory control of smooth muscle vascular tone; (2) antithrombotic and anticoagulant surface; (3) barrier function; and (4) metabolic tissue. Like smooth muscle cells, endothelial cells associated with atherosclerotic lesions function differently from normal endothelium. These differences are outlined below and in the following section on atherosclerosis.

FIG. 3-6
PROCESS OF MYOSIN CONTRACTIONS. Activation of myosin light-chain kinase (MLCK) by the Ca^{2+}–calmodulin complex results in phosphorylation of the myosin head and cross-bridging of actin and myosin. Myosin phosphatase (MP) removes the high-energy phosphate (P) from the light chain of myosin (LC 20), which prevents cross-bridging (inhibiting muscle contraction) or causes slower detachment of cross-bridging (slowing muscle contraction). ADP = adenosine diphosphate; ATP = adenosine triphosphate; CAM = calmodulin; PO_4 = phosphate.

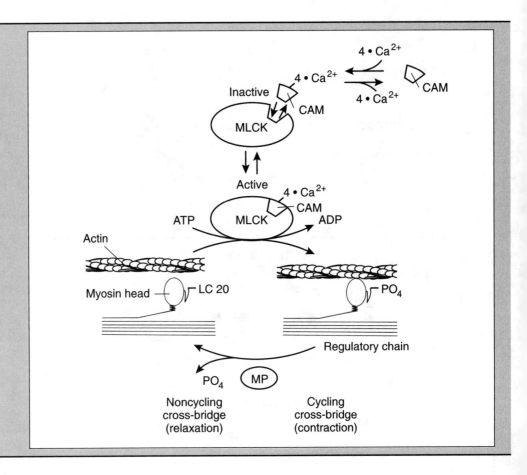

Endothelial Control of Smooth Muscle Vascular Tone.
Vascular endothelium functions as a *paracrine* organ that both secretes many locally acting substances into the intercellular space and metabolizes many vasoactive factors, growth regulatory molecules, and cytokines. Factors secreted by normal endothelium that cause local smooth muscle *vasodilation* include nitric oxide (originally called endothelial-derived relaxation factor or EDRF) and prostacyclin (PGI_2). Factors produced by endothelium that cause local *vasoconstriction* include endothelin I, thromboxane A_2 (TXA_2), prostaglandin H_2 (PGH_2), angiotensin II, and oxygen radicals. Fig. 3-7 summarizes the major mediators produced by endothelium and their effects on vascular tone.

Vasodilatory factors. The most important vasodilatory factor secreted by vascular endothelium is nitric oxide (NO). Less than 20 years ago, Furchgott and Zawadzki discovered that while aortic rings from rabbits normally dilated in response to acetylcholine (ACh), aortic rings denuded of endothelium actually contracted. They postulated that an endothelium-derived vasodilatory factor, which they named EDRF, is the major mediator in this process. EDRF is now known to be the NO molecule.

NO is synthesized and released from endothelial cells. Its major functions include endogenous vasodilation, inhibition of platelet aggregation, and platelet adhesion. Interestingly, NO is also produced by platelets and probably functions as a mediator in the negative feedback to platelet activation. Other important functions of NO include inhibition of leukocyte activation and inhibition of smooth muscle proliferation.

NO is derived from the essential amino acid L-arginine by the action of NO synthase as shown in Fig. 3-8. A variety of stimuli such as ACh, bradykinin, thrombin, adenine nucleotides, TXA_2, histamine, endothelin, and increased shear stress resulting from increased blood flow cause normal endothelium to increase synthesis of NO.

NO produced by endothelial cells diffuses across the internal elastic laminae into the underlying media layer to cause smooth muscle relaxation. The major mechanism of action of NO is activation of guanylate cyclase at the level of the cell membrane, which

Endothelial Factors Controlling Smooth Muscle Tone
Vasodilators
    Nitric oxide (EDRF)
    Prostacyclin (PGI_2)
Vasoconstrictors
    Endothelin I
    Prostaglandin H_2 (PGH_2)
    Thromboxane A_2 (TXA_2)
    Angiotensin II

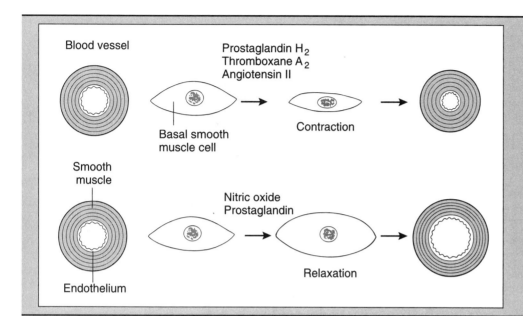

FIG. 3-7
A SUMMARY OF THE MAJOR ME-
DIATORS IN SMOOTH MUSCLE
CONTRACTION AND RELAX-
ATION.

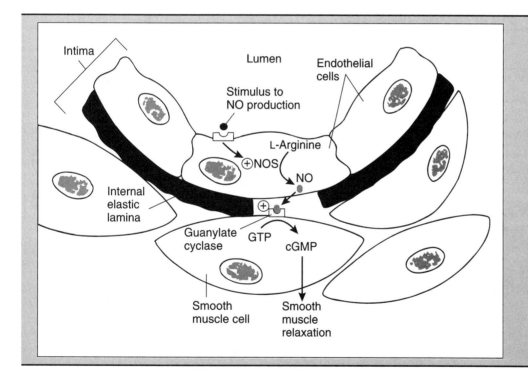

FIG. 3-8
NITRIC OXIDE SYNTHESIS. This
figure shows the activation,
synthesis, and mechanism of
action of nitric oxide (NO). First
of all, stimuli such as acetylcholine, bradykinin, and shear
stress activate NO synthase
(NOS), which increases conversion of L-arginine to NO. NO
then stimulates guanylate cyclase in smooth muscle cells,
which increases cyclic guanosine monophosphate (cGMP)
production, which leads to relaxation. GTP = guanosine triphosphate.

increases conversion of guanosine triphosphate (GTP) to cyclic guanosine monophosphate (cGMP). Increased cGMP activates cGMP-regulated protein kinases. Smooth muscle relaxation then follows by a variety of mechanisms, which all result in reduced
intracellular Ca^{2+}. First, phosphorylation and activation of Ca^{2+}-adenosine triphosphatase (ATPase) reduce intracellular Ca^{2+} levels necessary for calmodulin binding
and MLCK activation. Second, phosphorylation of specific proteins that sequester Ca^{2+}
in the sarcoplasmic reticulum may be a mechanism for reduced intracellular Ca^{2+}. In
addition, some evidence exists that cGMP-mediated decrease of inositol triphosphate
(IP_3), a second messenger that functions to increase cytosolic Ca^{2+} levels, may occur.
Fig. 3-9 demonstrates some of the mechanisms by which NO reduces cytosolic Ca^{2+}.

FIG. 3-9
EFFECTS OF NITRIC OXIDE. Nitric oxide (NO) reduces intracellular calcium (Ca^{2+}) by activating Ca^{2+}-adenosine triphosphatase (ATPase) on the cell membrane and sarcoplasmic reticulum and by reducing inositol triphosphate (IP_3) levels. IP_3 activates Ca^{2+} release from the sarcoplasmic reticulum.

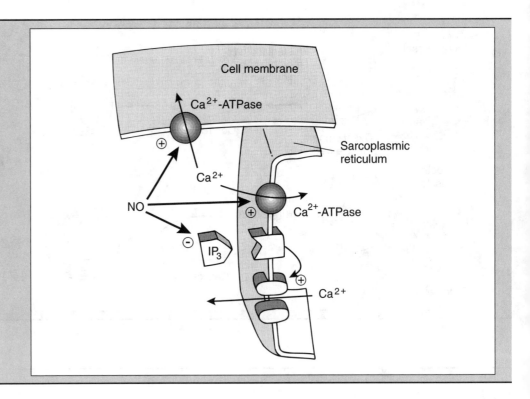

Case Study:
Continued

The emergency room physician was concerned that Mr. Hendrickson's chest pain was due to obstruction of coronary artery blood flow to a portion of his heart. Nitroglycerin, which is rapidly absorbed through the sublingual mucosa, is converted to NO by a sulfhydryl-dependent mechanism and causes vasodilation. Vasodilation of the coronary arteries may help increase blood flow to the heart. Several common conditions decrease PGI_2 production, which can accelerate the atherosclerotic process and increase platelet aggregation. Aging, DM, and nicotine from cigarette smoke can be associated with reduced PGI_2 synthesis. It is possible that Mr. Hendrickson's risk factors (tobacco abuse and DM) reduced PGI_2 synthesis and were contributing to his underlying pathophysiologic process.

Another important vasodilatory factor secreted by endothelium is PGI_2. PGI_2 also inhibits platelet aggregation, decreases the amount of cholesterol that enters into macrophages and smooth muscle cells, and prevents the release of growth factors that cause vascular wall thickening.

PGI_2 is derived from arachidonic acid by the action of cyclooxygenase and PGI_2 synthase. PGI_2 synthesis is stimulated by a variety of factors including thrombin, bradykinin, histamine, high-density lipoprotein (HDL), adenine nucleotides, leukotrienes, TXA_2, platelet-derived growth factor (PDGF), tissue hypoxia, and hemodynamic stress. PGI_2 activates adenylate cyclase, which results in an increase in intracellular cyclic adenosine monophosphate (cAMP).

Vasoconstrictors. Endothelial cells from coronary arteries produce several vasoconstrictors. The most important and most commonly discussed vasoconstrictor is the 21–amino acid peptide, endothelin I. First discovered by Yanagisawa et al. in 1988, endothelin I is one of the most potent vasoconstrictors known and causes prolonged smooth muscle contraction.

Endothelin I is enzymatically produced from prepropeptides in endothelium. Stimulators of its release include thrombin, epinephrine, and hypoxia. Endothelin I binds to a specific membrane receptor, which activates phospholipase C and results in a release of intracellular inositol phosphates and diacylglycerol (DAG). IP_3 binds to a receptor on the sarcoplasmic reticulum, which increases release of Ca^{2+} into the cytoplasm. Increased cytosolic Ca^{2+} levels lead to increased smooth muscle contraction. Fig. 3-10 illustrates the phospholipase C pathway.

Plasma endothelin I levels are known to be two times higher in patients with acute myocardial infarction. Increased binding of endothelin I to cardiac receptors has been demonstrated to occur during prolonged ischemia (> 30 min) and reoxygenation in an animal model. Endothelial binding may improve myocardial contractility but may be deleterious by increasing myocardial oxygen demand and decreasing diastolic relaxation.

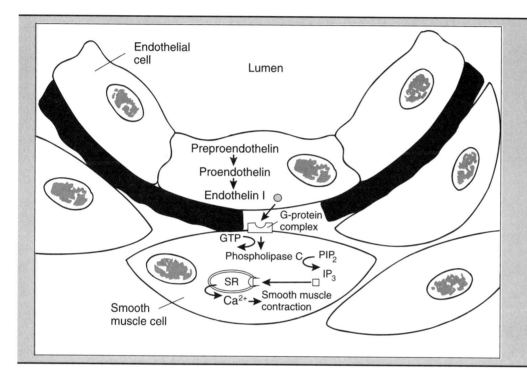

FIG. 3-10
PHOSPHOLIPASE C PATHWAY. A mediator such as endothelin I binds to a membrane receptor, resulting in an α-subunit of a G-protein complex binding to the receptor that requires guanosine triphosphate (GTP). In vascular smooth muscle, the G-protein–receptor complex activates phospholipase C, which in turn converts phosphatidylinositol bisphosphate (PIP$_2$) to diacylglycerol and 1,4,5-inositol triphosphate (IP$_3$). IP$_3$ then binds to a receptor within the sarcoplasmic reticulum, causing release of Ca^{2+} into the cytoplasm and activation of smooth muscle contraction and many other processes.

Endothelium as an Antithrombotic-Anticoagulant Surface. It has been well established that the endothelial layer has antithrombotic properties. The negative charge on the surface of the endothelial cell may account for its antithrombotic effect; negative charges on both platelets and endothelial cells may cause mutual repulsion. Many antithrombotic and anticoagulant substances are produced by the endothelial cell; they include: PGI$_2$, NO, heparin-like molecules, thrombomodulin (an activator of protein C), tissue plasminogen activator (t-PA), and urokinase.

However, in atherosclerosis or states of vascular injury, endothelium may have prothrombotic effects. Cytokines and other inflammatory mediators may stimulate the production and release of prothrombotic factors from the endothelium. In response to injury and inflammation, endothelial cells have been demonstrated to increase the surface expression of tissue factor, leukocyte adhesion molecules, and von Willebrand's factor. Injured endothelial cells associated with atherosclerotic lesions also can bind tissue factor, which leads to the activation of the extrinsic pathway of coagulation. In contrast to the normal state, endothelial injury can also reduce the expression of thrombomodulin. Plasminogen activator inhibitor I is also produced by endothelial cells and can induce a prothrombotic state in lesions of atherosclerosis. Fig. 3-11 lists the various thrombotic and antithrombotic molecules produced by endothelial cells.

Endothelium as a Barrier. Endothelial cells are tightly connected to each other by tight junctional complexes. This arrangement allows the endothelium to regulate the molecules that can enter the underlying smooth muscle layer. The endothelial layer can be crossed by three highly regulated routes. First, some molecules can enter the smooth muscle layer via the tight junctions between endothelial cells. Second, molecules can be

FIG. 3-11
ENDOTHELIAL CELLS CAN SYN-
THESIZE AND SECRETE BOTH
THROMBOTIC AND ANTITHROM-
BOTIC SUBSTANCES.

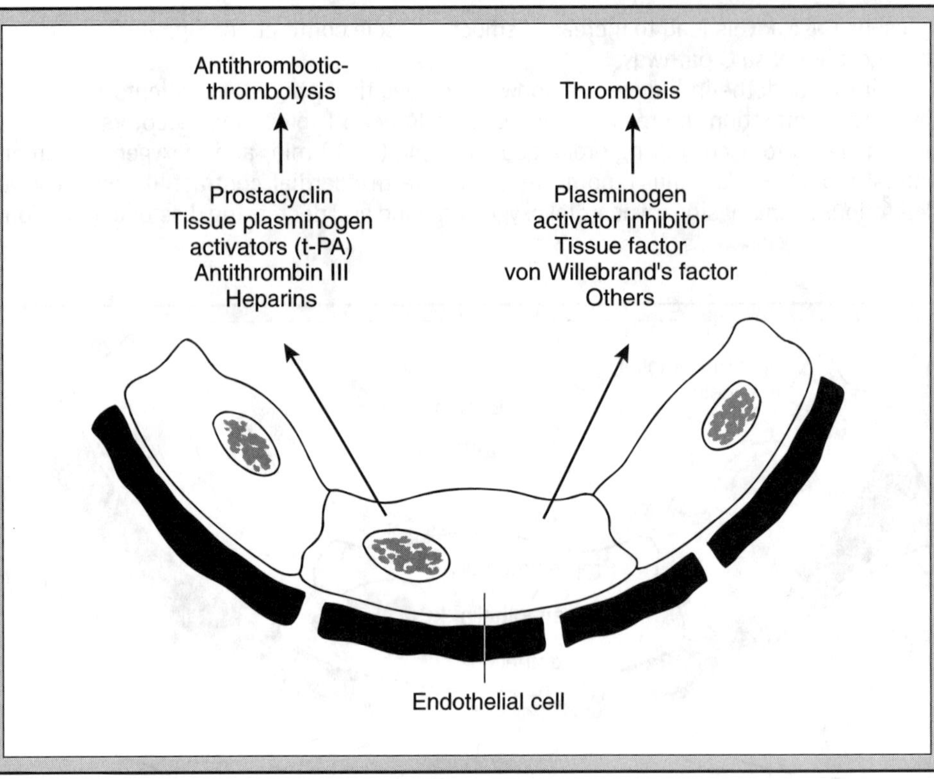

Antithrombotic-
thrombolysis

Thrombosis

Prostacyclin
Tissue plasminogen
activators (t-PA)
Antithrombin III
Heparins

Plasminogen
activator inhibitor
Tissue factor
von Willebrand's factor
Others

Endothelial cell

transported across the endothelial cells via vesicles. Finally, lipid-soluble molecules can travel within the lipid bilayer from the luminal surface to the subintimal space.

Endothelium as a Metabolic Tissue. In addition to mediating smooth muscle vascular tone, endothelial cells produce a variety of growth factors and chemotactic agents and are an important part of lipid metabolism.

Growth factors. Endothelial cells produce both inhibitors and stimulators of smooth muscle growth. When covered by an intact endothelium, underlying smooth muscle is relatively quiescent. Experimentally, removal of the endothelial layer leads to smooth muscle proliferation, which can be inhibited by regrowth of a normal endothelial layer. As mentioned earlier, the endothelium serves as an effective barrier for preventing smooth muscle exposure to various blood growth factors. In addition, it is clear that endothelial cells produce molecules that have an inhibitory effect, including: NO, various glycosaminoglycans (heparin and heparan sulfate), and transforming growth factor–β (TGF-β).

Endothelial cells also produce several growth factors that stimulate smooth muscle proliferation. It may be that endothelial-cell–derived growth factors (EDGFs) are responsible for the smooth muscle cell proliferation that is observed in the atherosclerotic lesion. Endothelial cells can produce PDGF (so named because it was first isolated in platelets), which is a 30-kD dimer of two polypeptide chains. PDGF is an extremely potent mitogen that induces DNA synthesis and cell division. Other growth stimulators produced by the endothelial cell include: fibroblast growth factor (FGF), endothelin, insulin-like growth factor (IGF), and others.

Chemotactic agents. Endothelial cells produce a variety of factors that are important for recruiting white blood cells (WBCs) to areas of intravascular injury. Endothelial cells produce the chemotactic molecule, monocyte chemotactic protein (MCP-1), which attracts monocytes. Endothelial cells also produce adhesion molecules that interact with surface receptors on WBCs: intercellular adhesion molecules (ICAM-1 and ICAM-2) bind to a receptor on B lymphocytes, and vascular cellular adhesion molecule-1 (VCAM-1) binds to surface receptors on T lymphocytes and monocytes.

Lipid metabolism. Cholesterol and triglycerides are transported through the arterial system via a number of different particles called lipoproteins, which are composed of varying amounts of lipids, phospholipids, and proteins. While the details of cholesterol transport are discussed in greater detail in the next section, it is important now to point out that the endothelial cell is an integral part of lipid metabolism. First, endothelial cells can interact with two lipid particles (chylomicrons and very low-density lipoproteins [VLDLs]) via the enzyme lipoprotein lipase (LpL). LpL, which converts triglycerides to free fatty acids, is bound to the endothelial surface by heparan sulfates. Liberated free fatty acids can then enter the subendothelial space to provide an energy source to underlying smooth muscle and other cells. Second, receptors for another particle, LDL, are present in endothelial cells.

> **Endothelial cells** produce a number of molecules with important functions:
>
> Vasomotor control of smooth muscle
> Inhibition and activation of platelets and the coagulation system
> Cell growth and energy metabolism

■ ATHEROSCLEROSIS

The term atherosclerosis is derived from the work of Aschoff, who recognized that differences in intimal lipid deposits exist between children and adults. These differences are the result of progression of one disease process. The Greek term *athero* means "gruel" or "porridge." Thus, atherosis or atheromatosis is defined as lipid deposited in the intima from infancy and thereafter. The Greek term *sclerosis* means "hardening" and hence *atherosclerosis* is defined as the presence of fibrosis (formation of collagen or smooth muscle) in addition to lipid deposits in the intimal layer. Atherosclerosis appears to arise from an excessive amount of the normal inflammatory and proliferative response to vessel wall injury.

RESPONSE-TO-INJURY HYPOTHESIS

While several hypotheses exist to explain the pathophysiologic processes that underlie atherosclerosis, the response-to-injury hypothesis has the largest amount of scientific support and is the basis of our discussion. Virchow, in the mid 1800s, was the first to suggest that injury to the arterial wall, which initiates an inflammatory response, was the underlying mechanism for atherosclerosis. The response-to-injury hypothesis for atherosclerosis was formally proposed in 1973 by Ross and Glomset, who suggested that atherosclerotic lesions develop in response to factors released from platelets at a site of endothelial "injury" induced by hypercholesterolemia. The current form of the hypothesis takes into account newly understood cellular and molecular mechanisms as well as the interplay of risk factors such as hyperlipidemia, hypertension, and cigarette smoking. The current form of the hypothesis is as follows (Fig. 3-12):

1. At baseline, normal endothelium retards development of atherosclerosis by the various mechanisms described (barrier function, antithrombotic function, release of platelet inhibitors such as NO or PGI_2 and release of inhibitors of smooth muscle proliferation such as NO).
2. Some form of injury occurs to the endothelium (oxidized LDL, homocysteine, toxins, infections, mechanical) that results in endothelial dysfunction, the extent of which is dependent on associated risk factors (smoking, DM, and hypertension).
3. Injured endothelial cells become atherogenic and thrombogenic. Monocytes and T lymphocytes from the circulating blood are attracted to the injured area. Monocytes become macrophages. Macrophages and T lymphocytes in the subintimal space and injured endothelial cells secrete molecules that recruit additional macrophages and smooth muscle cells to the area. As this process continues, an atherosclerotic lesion develops.

The initial injury to the endothelial cell can arise from multiple sources. *Oxidized LDL* particles are probably the most common cause of injury in the Western world. The proposed mechanism of injury by oxidized LDL is discussed below. Another possible source of injury includes *infectious agents* such as *Chlamydia* and herpesvirus. While these organisms have been isolated from some atherosclerotic lesions, a causal nature in the atherosclerotic process has not been established. Atherosclerotic lesions can occur at branch points in the coronary arteries. It is possible that increased *mechanical stress* at these sites is the initial form of endothelial cell injury. Patients with elevated levels of

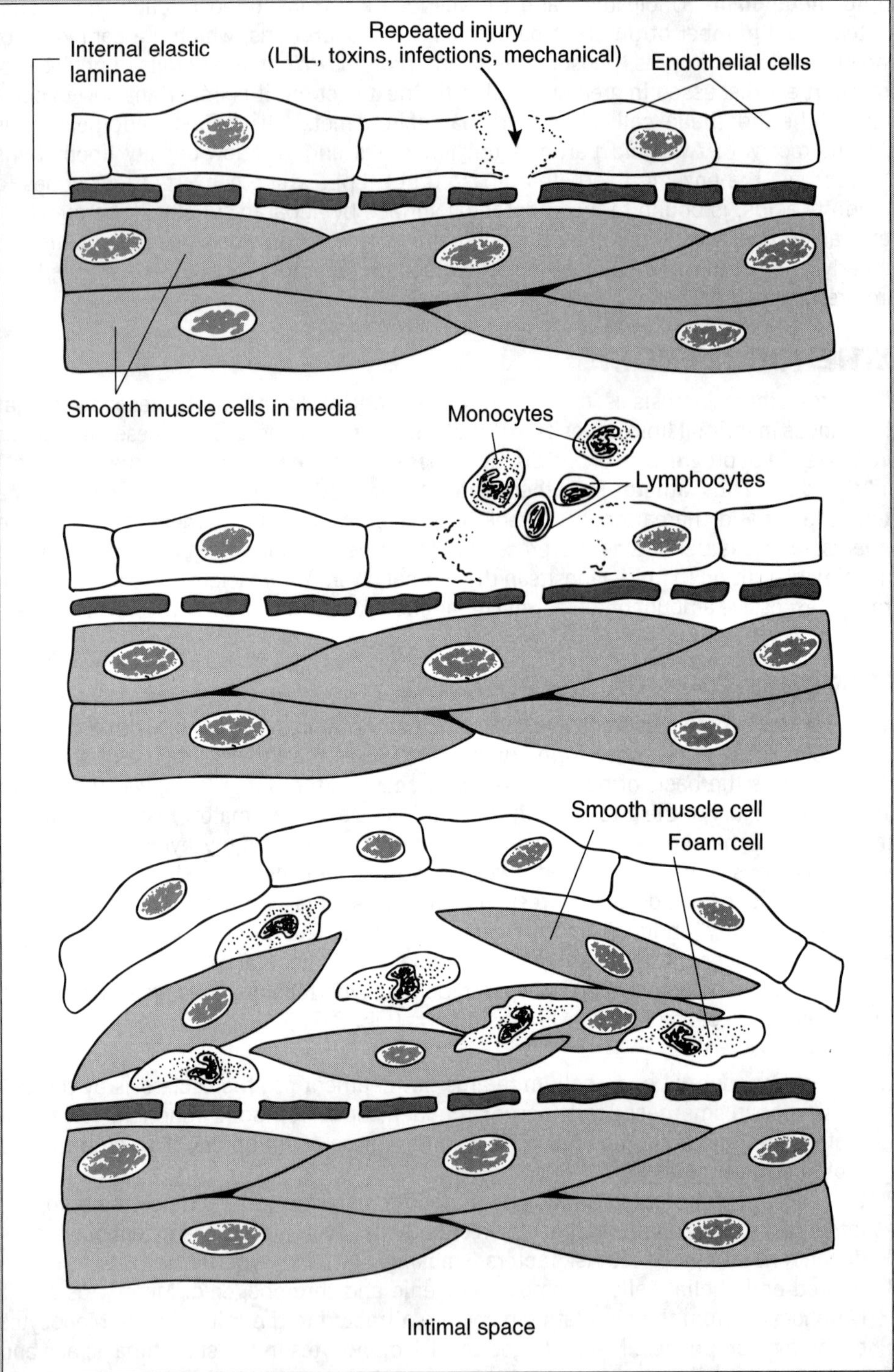

FIG. 3-12
RESPONSE-TO-INJURY HYPOTHESIS. First, endothelial cells are repeatedly injured (oxidized low-density lipoprotein [LDL] particles, infectious agents, toxins, mechanical stresses). Second, circulating monocytes and T lymphocytes are attracted to the injured area. Third, smooth muscle cells and macrophage foam cells accumulate in the subintimal space to form an atherosclerotic lesion.

homocysteine are more likely to have atherosclerosis; experimental studies have found that homocysteine may act as a direct *toxin* to endothelial cells. Toxic effects of chemical irritants in tobacco smoke and glycosylated end products are thought to be possible mechanisms for endothelial cell injury for smoking and DM, respectively.

After initial injury, there are several explanations for the increased atherogenicity and thrombogenicity of endothelial cells. In injured endothelial cells, the barrier function is compromised, which results in increased permeability and exposure of smooth muscle to various growth factors and other molecules. Also, injured endothelial cells produce less

PGI_2 and NO, which results in increased thrombogenicity. Injured endothelial cells produce increased PDGF and endothelin I, which along with decreased NO levels cause smooth muscle migration and proliferation. Secretion of MCP-1 and upregulation of monocyte-binding cell surface receptors on endothelial cells cause macrophage recruitment.

ROLE OF HYPERCHOLESTEROLEMIA

Cholesterol has a central role in the process of atherogenesis. Numerous studies have reported on the causal relationship between cholesterol levels and atherosclerotic coronary artery disease. In a large multicountry study (Fig. 3-13), the prevalence of coronary artery disease and overall mortality was lower in countries associated with low–saturated-fat diets and low serum cholesterol (Japan) and higher in countries where the traditional diet is high in saturated fat with an accompanying increase in serum cholesterol (United States, Finland, Denmark). Before we begin a detailed discussion of the process of atherogenesis, it is appropriate to review briefly cholesterol biosynthesis and discuss the mechanisms by which cholesterol increases atherogenesis.

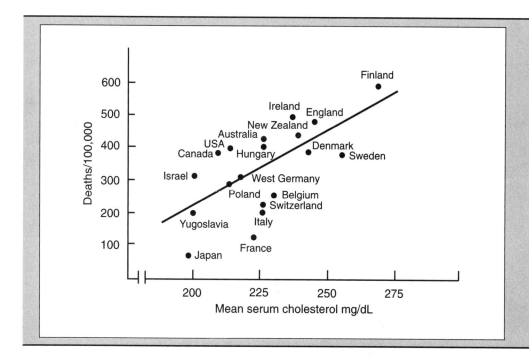

FIG. 3-13
THE RELATIONSHIP BETWEEN DEATHS RESULTING FROM CORONARY ARTERY DISEASE AND SERUM CHOLESTEROL LEVELS IN NUMEROUS COUNTRIES. (*Source:* Reprinted with permission from Simons LA: Interrelations of lipids and lipoprotein with coronary artery disease mortality in 19 countries. *Am J Cardiol* 57:56, 1986.)

The current models of lipoprotein metabolism and cholesterol biosynthesis involve two major pathways: the *exogenous* and *endogenous* pathways (Fig. 3-14). Both pathways transport cholesterol and triglycerides in large particles called lipoproteins, which have a hydrophobic lipid core of triglycerides and cholesterol, covered by a polar monolayer of phospholipids and protein. Fig. 3-15 summarizes the different lipoprotein particles found in the body.

The *exogenous* pathway processes dietary lipids that are absorbed from the intestine. Free fatty acids and cholesterol are absorbed by the enterocytes of the small intestine. Free fatty acids are converted into triglycerides, which are incorporated, along with absorbed cholesterol, into large particles called chylomicrons. The chylomicrons then undergo a two-step process of metabolism. First, the chylomicrons enter the bloodstream and within 5 minutes interact with the enzyme LpL, which is present on the endothelial cells of muscle and adipose tissue capillaries. LpL hydrolyzes chylomicron triglycerides into free fatty acids, monoglycerides, and diglycerides. The liberated free fatty acids enter the cells, where they either are oxidized for energy or reform triglycerides. In the second step of chylomicron processing, the triglyceride-depleted chylomicron "remnants" return to the circulatory system and are taken up by the liver.

Lipid Metabolism
Exogenous and endogenous pathways
Lipids transported in particles called lipoproteins

FIG. 3-14
EXOGENOUS AND ENDOGENOUS PATHWAYS OF CHOLESTEROL METABOLISM. FFA = free fatty acids; HDL = high-density lipoprotein; IDL = intermediate-density lipoprotein; LCAT = lecithin–cholesterol acyltransferase; LDL = low-density lipoprotein; VLDL = very low-density lipoprotein.

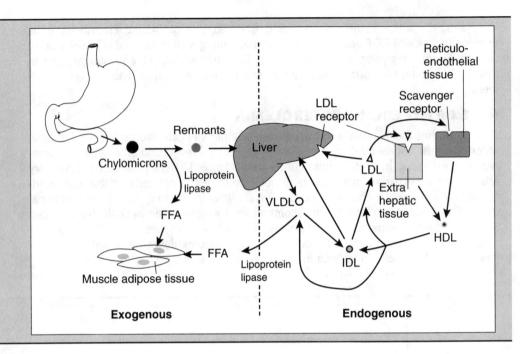

FIG. 3-15
LIPOPROTEIN PARTICLES IN THE BODY. Each particle has a lipid core of varying amounts of cholesterol (C) and triglycerides (TG). The surface of the lipoprotein particles is covered by phospholipids and proteins that are particle-specific. Chylomicrons and very low-density lipoproteins (VLDLs) have a lipid core that is composed predominantly of triglycerides with relatively little cholesterol. In contrast, low-density lipoprotein (LDL), lipoprotein (a) [Lp(a)], and high-density lipoprotein (HDL) particles have cores that are made up of only cholesterol. Intermediate-density lipoproteins (IDL) have roughly equal amounts of triglycerides and cholesterol. ■ = apoprotein.

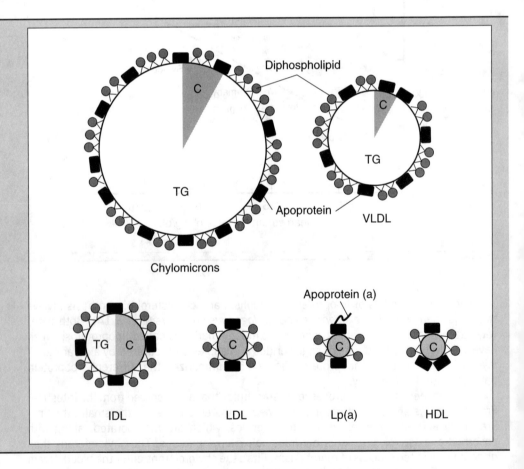

As illustrated in Fig. 3-14, the *endogenous* pathway transports lipids that are synthesized within the body to provide tissues with a stable source of cholesterol and triglycerides despite dietary fluctuations. The liver incorporates triglycerides and cholesterol along with protein into a moderately large particle called a VLDL. The triglyceride-rich VLDL enters the bloodstream and, like chylomicrons, interacts with LpL. LpL hydrolyzes the triglycerides of the VLDL, and a triglyceride-depleted intermediate-density lipoprotein (IDL) particle is formed. Some of the IDL particles are taken up by the liver, while the remainder of the IDL particles continue to have triglyceride removed and are converted into the cholesterol-rich LDL particles.

The physiologic role of LDL particles is to transport cholesterol, which is necessary for the synthesis of cell membranes and steroid hormones, to the extrahepatic tissues. LDL particles bind to LDL receptors that are present on many tissue types, including endothelial cells. LDL-receptor numbers and activity are highest early in life and diminish with age. LDL particles bind to LDL receptors and are internalized by endocytosis. Approximately 70% of the LDL particles are taken up by this receptor system. The remainder of the LDL particles are metabolized via a "scavenger receptor" by reticulo-endothelial cells.

HDL particles, which exert a protective effect against the development of atherosclerosis, are synthesized in the liver and intestine. HDL metabolism is quite complex. For the purposes of this discussion, it is important to know that HDL particles are important for the process of "reverse cholesterol transport"; HDL particles exchange cholesterol with LDL, VLDL, and IDL particles, and ultimately cholesterol is transported back to the liver.

LDL particles are particularly atherogenic. Foam cells, which are macrophages or smooth muscle cells filled with vacuoles of fat, are the first cell types found in the precursor lesion of atherosclerosis. Early studies by Brown and Goldstein demonstrated that macrophages incubated with high concentrations of native unmodified LDL cholesterol did *not* convert into foam cells. It was subsequently discovered that LDL particles which are "modified" by acetylation, acetoacetylation, or conjugation with malondialdehyde is rapidly taken up by macrophages, and these latter become foam cells in culture. Macrophages have a "scavenger receptor" that can only recognize "modified" LDL particles. These observations led to the finding that LDL particles undergo peroxidation by endothelial cells, smooth muscle, and macrophages, which allows the LDL particle to be recognized by the "scavenger receptor" on macrophages. Oxidized LDL particles can cause direct endothelial cell damage, stimulate endothelial cells to produce MCP-1, and inhibit motility of resident macrophages. The concept of LDL oxidation forms the basis of antioxidant therapy with vitamin E, which in one study recently has been shown to reduce cardiovascular mortality.

Oxidized LDL
Cytotoxic for cells
Attracts circulating monocytes and inhibits macrophage motility
Stimulates endothelial cells to produce chemotactic molecules

LDL particles are the principle lipoprotein associated with atherosclerosis. However, other lipoproteins such as IDL and chylomicron remnants have atherogenic potential. In addition, another particle, lipoprotein (a), or Lp(a), has significant atherogenic potential. Lp(a) particles are formed when an unusual protein, apoprotein (a) [apo(a)], is linked to the normal protein component of a LDL particle. People with high concentrations of Lp(a) are at particular risk for the development of atherosclerosis and for clinical coronary syndromes (angina pectoris and myocardial infarctions). The apo(a) protein has close structural homology to plasminogen; it is possible that apo(a) functions as a competitive inhibitor of plasminogen binding and promotes thrombosis. Thrombosis is the final pathophysiologic process that makes the atherosclerotic lesion cause angina pectoris and myocardial infarction.

CLASSIFICATION OF ATHEROSCLEROTIC LESIONS

Recently, atherosclerotic lesions have been formally classified into a histologic schema that is summarized in Fig. 3-16. Atherosclerotic lesions are classified by the amount and location of cholesterol, the amount of accompanying fibrous tissues and smooth muscle, and the presence or absence of associated thrombus or bleeding. Type I lesions contain scattered isolated macrophages with *intracellular* lipid droplets (macrophage foam cells) in the intimal layer. Type I lesions are not evident from surface examination of the arterial wall. Type II lesions consist of large numbers of macrophage foam cells and lipid-laden smooth muscle cells that are arranged in layers in the intima. Type III lesions, called intermediate lesions, are characterized by scattered collections of *extracellular* lipid droplets and particles within the layers of intimal smooth muscle cells. When the extracellular lipid droplets coalesce and become larger to form a lipid core, a type IV lesion, or atheroma, is formed. Type V lesions are characterized by thick layers of fibrous connective tissue. Finally, in type VI lesions, the atherosclerotic lesion has a disrupted surface associated with adherent thrombus or has fissured and is associated with blood and thrombus within the atherosclerotic lesion (hematoma). It is important to note that considerable overlap is present within this classification scheme, and single lesions can fall within several categories. In addition, while the schema is ordered from least to most complex, it is important to remember that lesions are quite dynamic. For example, a type IV lesion could suddenly rupture and become a type VI lesion, and conversely, healing and scar formation could transform a type VI lesion to a type V lesion. Despite these shortcomings, this classification is helpful for the discussion of the pathogenesis of atherosclerosis.

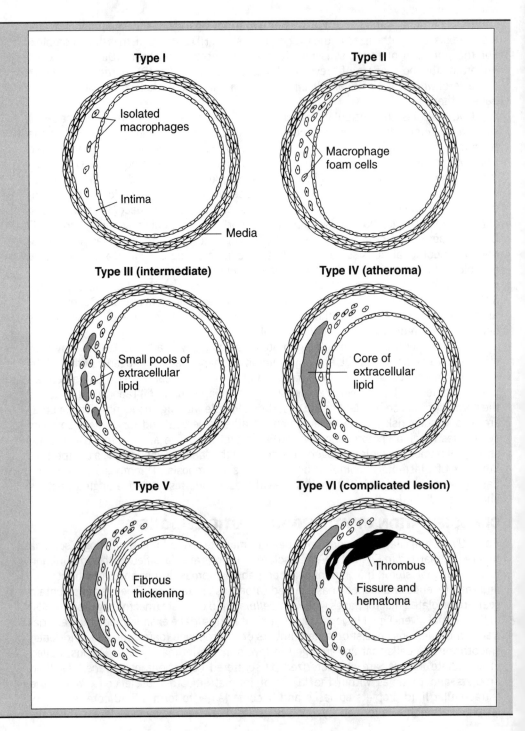

FIG. 3-16
ATHEROSCLEROTIC LESION CLASSIFICATION. (*Source:* Reprinted with permission from Fuster V, Ross R, Topol EJ (eds): *Atherosclerosis and Coronary Artery Disease.* Philadelphia, PA: Lippincott-Raven, 1995, Fig. 4.)

PATHOLOGY AND HISTOLOGY OF ATHEROSCLEROSIS

Fatty Streaks. The fatty streak corresponds to type II and type III lesions and is the earliest recognizable lesion in atherosclerosis. Fatty streaks grossly appear as longitudinally oriented, slightly raised, narrow yellow areas that occur throughout the arterial tree but are most common at branches and bifurcations.

It appears that fatty streaks form when endothelial injury causes monocytes and T lymphocytes to migrate to the subintimal space just below the injured endothelial region. It appears that oxidized LDL particles may be the initial stimulus for attracting leukocytes to the area. Upon entering the vessel wall, monocytes (now referred to as macrophages) can become foam cells as they accumulate oxidized LDL, via scavenger receptors, in intracellular vacuoles. Continued endothelial cell damage attracts platelets that, along with endothelial cells and macrophages, produce PDGF and other growth-stimulating factors. These growth factors stimulate migration and proliferation of smooth muscle cells from the media. Smooth muscle proliferation marks the transition of a type I lesion to a type II lesion. Smooth muscle cells can also take up lipid and function as foam cells. Some of the lipid-laden macrophages rupture, and other cell types die, which results in extracellular deposition of lipid, and the lesion progresses to a type III lesion.

Fatty streaks are known to form throughout life (fatty streaks have been reported as early as 3 years) and develop in areas both susceptible and unsusceptible to developing clinical lesions later in life. In coronary arteries, fatty streaks occur in the same anatomic sites that are prone to plaque formation later in life, especially in predisposed individuals. However, fatty streaks in the aorta may not progress or may spontaneously disappear. Thus, fatty streaks can undergo three courses. They can progress through atherogenesis and form fibrous plaques, remain unchanged throughout life, or regress.

Atheromas. Fatty streaks can progress to form atheromas, or type IV lesions. Continued migration of LDL particles into the subintimal space and confluence of small extracellular collections of lipid leads to the formation of a large extracellular "lipid core." This lipid core is usually large enough to be seen by the naked eye; the core has the consistency of toothpaste. In general, the lesion is still covered by the original endothelial cells, but the space between the endothelium and the lipid core has large numbers of macrophages, T lymphocytes, and foam cells. Atheromas may be particularly susceptible to rupturing because the large amounts of fibrous tissue that define the type V lesion have not yet formed.

Atheromas grossly appear as rounded, raised lesions that are whitish in color and approximately 4 cm in diameter. They usually do not significantly reduce the lumen diameter of the coronary artery.

Fibrous Plaques. Atheromas can progress to form fibrous plaques, which correspond to type V and VI lesions, the fundamental lesions in atherosclerosis. Several important changes are associated with fibrous plaque formation. Foam cells begin to protrude between endothelial cells and enter the lumen as a result of disruption in the endothelial cell junction. Foam cells can act as thrombogenic sites, with formation of platelet microthrombi on their exposed surfaces. In addition, numerous smooth muscle cells migrate and proliferate in all regions of the atherosclerotic lesion. A fibrous cap forms as a result. It consists of smooth muscle cells surrounded by and intermixed with collagen, proteoglycan, elastic components, macrophages, and T lymphocytes.

Some fibrous plaques are composed mostly of fibrous tissue and have very little extracellular lipid. Other fibrous plaques are characterized by large amounts of lipid. As is discussed later, the lipid content may be one factor in determining the susceptibility of rupture of a fibrous plaque. In addition, fibrous plaques can contain varying amounts of calcium. The mechanism for calcium deposition in some atherosclerotic lesions is not known.

Fibrous plaques can develop surface defects that can range from a small area of focal loss of endothelial cells to deep fissuring that can expose the underlying smooth muscle cells, macrophages, and extracellular lipid to the blood. Adherent blood clots on the surface or intraplaque bleeding (hematoma) mark the progression of the type V lesion to the complicated type VI lesion. It is rupture of type IV and type V lesions, with the rapid formation of a type VI lesion, that is responsible for the majority of acute clinical

---

Fatty Streak Formation
Chronic endothelial injury
Increased endothelial permeability to lipids and attraction of macrophages to form foam cells
Smooth muscle cell proliferation

syndromes associated with coronary artery disease. Fibrous plaques can lead to symptoms when coronary blood flow is compromised. Compromise in coronary blood flow can occur gradually (slow increase in fibrous tissue) or rapidly (deep plaque fissure that leads to the formation of an occlusive thrombus).

CELL BIOLOGY OF ATHEROSCLEROSIS

Atherosclerotic lesions are due to the interaction among three circulating blood cells (monocytes, lymphocytes, platelets) and two vessel wall components (endothelial cells, smooth muscle cells). Fig. 3-17 illustrates the functions for each cell type under normal conditions and during the atherosclerotic process.

Atherosclerosis results from abnormal interactions among monocytes, lymphocytes, platelets, endothelial cells, and smooth muscle cells.

FIG. 3-17
NORMAL AND ABNORMAL FUNCTIONS FOR EACH CELL TYPE.

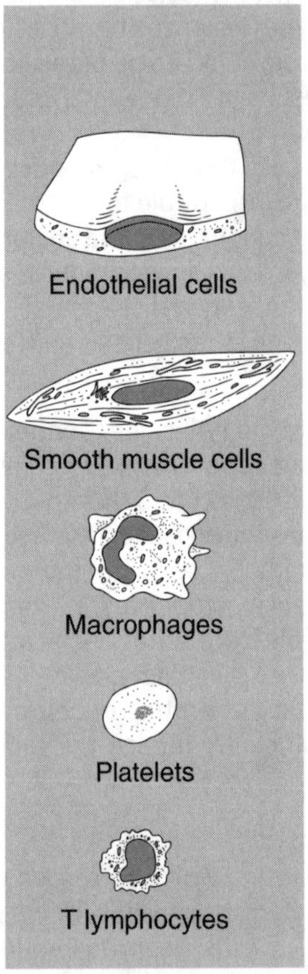

	Normal	Atherosclerosis
Endothelial cells	• Vasodilation of smooth muscle cells • Antithrombogenic • Barrier • Synthesize inhibiting growth factors • Smooth muscle growth inhibitor	• Increased vasoconstriction of smooth muscle cells • Thrombogenic • Increased permeability • Synthesize large amounts of stimulating growth factors
Smooth muscle cells	• Contractile phenotype • Myofibrils • Respond to vasoactive substances	• Synthetic phenotype • Golgi bodies • Secrete growth factors • Secrete connective tissue matrix
Macrophages	• Not present or present in very small numbers in the subintimal space	• Take up lipid to form foam cells • Chemotactic factors • Growth factors • Proteases
Platelets	• Not present	• If activated, recruit more platelets • Chemotactic factors • Growth factors
T lymphocytes	• Not present	• Activate macrophages • Chemotactic factors • Growth factors • Interleukin-2

Endothelial Cells. Endothelial cell dysfunction is an important part of the atherosclerotic process. In the initial stages, endothelial cells produce several glycoprotein molecules (ICAM-1, VCAM-1) that are responsible for the initial recruitment of monocytes and T lymphocytes. In addition, endothelial cells allow increased permeability of LDL particles. Endothelial cells are capable of producing oxidized LDL particles, which are particularly atherogenic.

As the atherosclerotic process progresses, the endothelial cells continue to be involved. Endothelial-cell–dependent relaxation is abnormal in atherosclerotic lesions. The mechanism for this is unclear, although some investigators have reported reductions in functional NO associated with atherosclerosis. Endothelial cell secretion of various growth factors (such as PDGF) may be responsible for stimulation of smooth muscle cells and macrophages in the subintimal space. It is possible that endothelial cells produce more procoagulant materials during the atherosclerotic process, thus increasing the risk of thrombosis. Finally, once the endothelial cell surface is denuded, unlike smooth muscle cells and fibroblasts, endothelial cells are unable to crawl over one another to repair the injured site. Once the endothelial layer is lost, the injured vessel wall becomes particularly thrombogenic as underlying smooth muscle cells, foam cells, and other tissue types become directly exposed to blood.

Smooth Muscle. Smooth muscle cell proliferation within the intima is a critical event in the progression of atherosclerosis. An important function of smooth muscle cells is the synthesis of the bulk of the connective tissue matrix. In addition, smooth muscle cells can accumulate lipid and function in some cases as a foam cell. Two major phenotypes of smooth muscle cells exist: the contractile phenotype and synthetic phenotype. Fig. 3-18 diagrammatically illustrates these two phenotypes. The phenotypic differences may be relevant because of the effect on the capacity of each type to respond to various mediators involved in atherosclerosis.

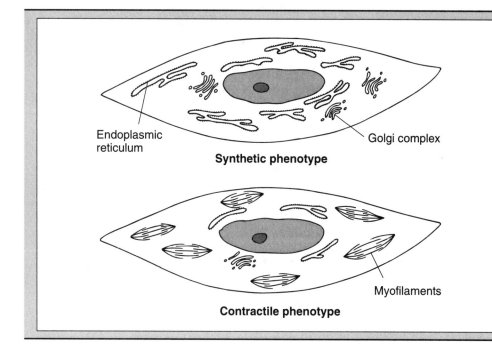

Endoplasmic reticulum

Golgi complex

Synthetic phenotype

Myofilaments

Contractile phenotype

FIG. 3-18
COMPARISON OF THE CONTRACTILE AND SYNTHETIC PHENOTYPE IN SMOOTH MUSCLE CELLS. It is believed that in atherosclerotic lesions, the synthetic phenotype is predominantly expressed, resulting in proliferation and synthesis or secretion of extracellular matrix components.

The contractile phenotype is myofilament-rich and is very responsive to vasoconstrictors or vasodilators. The predominant type in adults, the contractile phenotype responds to various agents including endothelin I, catecholamines, angiotensin II, prostaglandin E (PGE), PGI_2, neuropeptides, leukotrienes, and NO.

In contrast, the synthetic phenotype is myofilament-poor and relatively rich in rough endoplasmic reticulum (RER) and Golgi complex. It is found in normal intima of the embryo and the young growing organism. The synthetic phenotype is capable of gene expression for several growth-regulatory molecules and cytokines. The synthetic phenotype can also respond to growth factors such as PDGF via cell surface receptors and synthesize extracellular matrix. Several investigators have reported that smooth muscle cells in atherosclerotic lesions change from the contractile phenotype to the synthetic phenotype.

Monocytes or Macrophages. As mentioned previously, foam cells in a fatty streak are predominantly macrophages. Macrophages have several important functions in the development of atherosclerosis. Macrophages can take up oxidized LDL via the "scavenger receptor" and become foam cells. In addition, by peroxidation of free fatty acids, macrophages can generate oxidized LDL. Macrophages can produce several growth-regulatory molecules and cytokines, including: PDGF, interleukin-1 (IL-1), tumor necrosis factor–α (TNF-α), and MCP-1. In this way macrophages play an important role in the proliferative responses associated with atherosclerosis. They also can stimulate matrix production by smooth muscle.

Lymphocytes. Lymphocytes also contribute to atherosclerosis, which suggests an immune component to the atherosclerotic process. Interleukin-2 (IL-2), produced by macrophages, may stimulate lymphocyte proliferation in the atherosclerotic lesion. Lymphocytes can produce various growth factors and cytokines that may be important for macrophage activation in the atherosclerotic lesion.

In patients who undergo cardiac transplant, the coronary arteries of the transplanted heart often are associated with a unique concentric atherosclerotic lesion. In these lesions, large numbers of T lymphocytes are present, which suggests an immune-mediated response in this specialized form of atherosclerosis.

Platelets. Platelets are small, anucleate, disk-shaped structures that are formed from bone marrow megakaryocytes. Platelets are important for the process of hemostasis at regions of vessel injury. However, inappropriate activation of platelets at sites of intravascular injury can also be important for the process of atherosclerosis. Thrombi that contain adherent and aggregated platelets are present in regions associated with injured endothelium, particularly if deep fissuring of the atherosclerotic plaque has occurred. While platelets are capable of very little protein synthesis, they contain granules that are filled with a number of potent growth factors. Platelets appear to be a source of various growth-stimulatory molecules such as PDGF, transforming growth factor-α (TGF-α), and others in some atherosclerotic lesions. Several effective therapies for the treatment of coronary artery disease are directed specifically at platelets (aspirin).

❚ THROMBOSIS

In certain clinical syndromes, such as unstable angina pectoris and myocardial infarction, symptoms occur when the atherosclerotic lesion becomes disrupted and associated with intraluminal thrombus. The process of thrombosis is similar to the physiologic response to rupture of an artery; however, when an atherosclerotic plaque ruptures, intraluminal activation of this physiologic response can lead to severe problems. If thrombus formation is extensive, blood flow through the coronary artery can be severely reduced or even stopped completely. Lack of blood to the heart (myocardial ischemia) supplied by that particular vessel will cause the chest pain and other symptoms associated with coronary artery disease.

DISRUPTION OF ATHEROSCLEROTIC LESIONS

"Vulnerable" Lesions
Large lipid core
Less fibrous tissue
Large numbers of macrophages
Mild-to-moderate luminal narrowing

Identifying characteristics of atherosclerotic lesions that are prone to rupture has been the subject of intense research. Identification of "vulnerable" lesions could spur the development of pathophysiologically based preventative therapies that would be a major advance in the treatment of coronary artery disease.

There are several histologic characteristics of atherosclerotic lesions that have been associated with plaque rupture (Fig. 3-19). First, plaques associated with large lipid cores appear to be more prone to rupture. It is likely that larger lipid cores reduce the structural strength of the atherosclerotic lesion. When the lipid core of an atherosclerotic lesion involves more than 40%–50% of the vessel circumference, plaque rupture becomes much more likely. Second, pathologic studies have found higher numbers of macrophages in plaques that have ruptured. Protease release and release of toxic substances (oxidized LDL) may be the reason that lesions with high numbers of macrophages tend to be unstable. Third, atherosclerotic lesions with thinner fibrous caps covering the lipid core are more likely to rupture.

In addition to histologic characteristics, it is also clear that atherosclerotic lesion geometry plays an important role in the likelihood of plaque disruption. Stress in the atherosclerotic plaque can be estimated by applying Laplace's law, which states that wall stress is related to pressure and vessel geometry in the following manner:

$$\text{Wall stress} = \frac{\text{arterial pressure} \times \text{radius}}{\text{cap thickness}}$$

Hence, higher arterial blood pressures, larger luminal diameters (radius), and thinner fibrous caps increase wall stress or tension on the vessel wall. For this reason, atherosclerotic plaques associated with only mild or moderate stenosis actually bear more

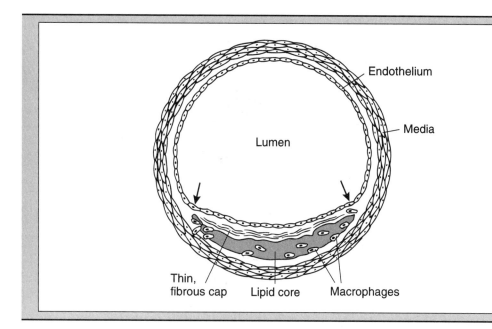

FIG. 3-19
**CROSS SECTION OF A CORO-
NARY ARTERY SHOWING CHAR-
ACTERISTICS OF A PLAQUE
"VULNERABLE" TO RUPTURE.**
Present are large lipid core,
thin fibrous cap, increased
number of macrophages, and
high stress (relatively mild stenosis). Rupture normally occurs at the "shoulder" of the
plaque (*arrows*).

tension and wall stress than plaques associated with severe stenosis. Retrospective data support this observation with the demonstration that 60%–70% of acute coronary syndromes actually occur in areas of mild (< 50% diameter) or moderate (50%–70% diameter) narrowing of the coronary artery lumen. Thus, mildly stenotic plaques can be more prone to rupture than severely stenotic plaques.

To summarize, plaque rupture most commonly occurs at the "shoulder," or lateral edge, of lipid-rich atherosclerotic lesions associated with mild-to-moderate narrowing of the coronary artery. The lateral edge is particularly vulnerable to rupture. In this region the fibrous cap is thinnest, tensile support from the underlying lipid core is low, and macrophage concentration is relatively high.

THROMBOTIC PROCESS

Once an atherosclerotic plaque is disrupted, the thrombotic process is initiated when cells and extracellular materials in the subintimal space are exposed to blood. Thrombosis within the coronary arteries is due to closely intertwined activation of *platelets*, which leads to a platelet plug, and of the *coagulation system*, which produces a fibrin clot.

The process of **thrombosis** involves the synergistic action of platelets and the coagulation system.

Platelet Adhesion and Aggregation. In the first step of thrombosis, platelets adhere to exposed collagen and other extracellular and cellular ligands (Fig. 3-20). Platelet adherence is mediated by von Willebrand's factor (vWF), which is a complex glycosylated protein produced by endothelial cells and secreted into the subendothelial space. The platelets spread out over the injured area to form a monolayer. After binding, the platelets become activated and release the contents of their storage granules (adenosine diphosphate [ADP], serotonin, and TXA_2), which recruit more platelets to the injured region. In addition to release of storage granule contents, platelet activation induces two platelet surface glycoproteins, Gp IIb and Gp IIIa, to assemble. The Gp IIb-IIIa complex is a functional receptor for fibrinogen, which is a molecule that is commonly found in plasma.

Additional platelets can now bind to each other via the Gp IIb-IIIa receptor fibrinogen complex, and an aggregate of platelets, or platelet plug, is formed. The platelet plug continues to form, as platelets are activated and in turn express the Gp IIb-IIIa receptor, until the platelet plug is affected by antiaggregatory molecules. Propagation of the platelet plug is limited by adjacent uninjured endothelial cells that produce NO and PGI_2. However, if the atherosclerotic plaque is deeply ruptured and endothelial injury is extensive, the platelet plug continues to propagate, and a large occlusive thrombus may form.

Coagulation System Activation. The coagulation system is traditionally divided into an *intrinsic* pathway, which uses circulating coagulation factors to activate thrombin, and an *extrinsic* pathway, which requires tissue factor, a surface coenzyme

FIG. 3-20
(A) Endothelial cells are denuded, exposing collagen and subintimal cells to circulating blood. (B) Von Willebrand's factor (vWF) in the subendothelial space initiates binding of a spreading platelet monolayer. Activated platelets release their storage granule contents, which attract more platelets and initiate assembly of the glycoprotein (Gp) IIb–IIIa receptor. The Gp IIb–IIIa receptor then allows fibrinogen to cross-link platelets, forming a large platelet aggregate. The activated platelet also acts as a surface for promoting thrombin production. Platelet aggregation is inhibited by molecules secreted by neighboring, normal endothelial cells (nitric oxide, prostacyclin [PGI_2]).

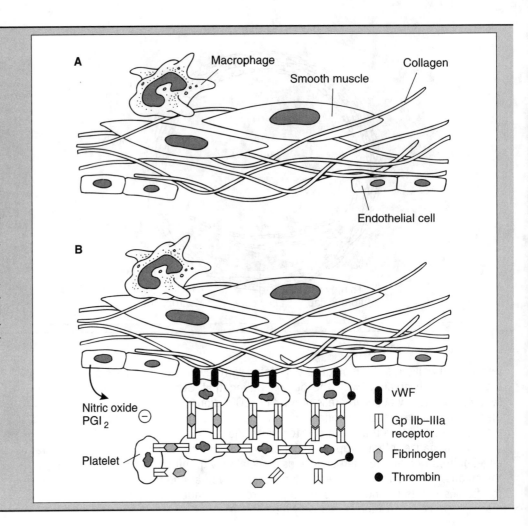

produced by cells. In general, coagulation in the setting of atherosclerotic lesion rupture involves activation of the extrinsic system (Fig. 3-21). When subendothelial cells are exposed by plaque rupture, tissue factor on the surface of macrophages, smooth muscle cells, fibroblasts, and injured endothelial cells forms complexes with and activates circulating factor VII. The tissue factor–activated factor VII complex preferentially assembles on the surface of activated platelets and activates factor IX, which catalyzes the proteolysis of factor X to Xa.

If factor Xa production is sufficient, thrombin can be produced. Thrombin is the final product of both the extrinsic pathway and intrinsic pathway. Thrombin occupies the central role in the coagulation system. Since it can generate itself via potent positive feedback mechanisms, production of thrombin is tightly controlled. Thrombin catalyzes the cleavage of fibrinogen to fibrin. Fibrin molecules can form dense polymers, which can cross-link to form a tight mesh that traps leukocytes and red blood cells (RBCs) and stabilizes the platelet plug.

Once formed, fibrin polymers can be degraded by a highly regulated, complex fibrinolytic system. Briefly, circulating plasminogen molecules can bind to the fibrin polymers. Tissue plasminogen activator (t-PA), which is produced by neighboring uninjured endothelial cells, catalyzes the hydrolysis of a single peptide bond, which converts plasminogen to plasmin (Fig. 3-22). Plasmin causes lysis of the fibrin polymers and the formation of fibrin degradation products.

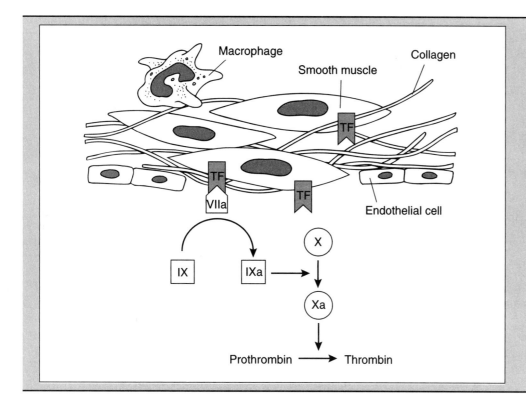

FIG. 3-21
EXTRINSIC COAGULATION SYSTEM. Denudation of endothelial cells exposes blood to the subintimal space. Tissue factor (TF) can interact with factor VIIa, which can lead to the production of thrombin, via activation of factor IX and X. If thrombin production is large enough, thrombin will self-amplify in a positive feedback loop, which leads to the formation of a fibrin mesh.

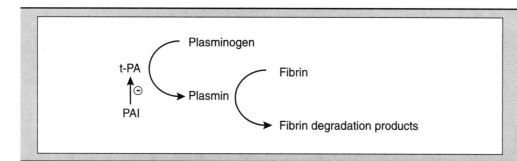

FIG. 3-22
FIBRINOLYSIS. Tissue plasminogen activator (t-PA) generates plasmin from plasminogen. Plasmin degrades fibrin polymers. The action of t-PA is inhibited by plasminogen activator inhibitor (PAI).

■ RISK FACTORS FOR CORONARY ARTERY DISEASE

Large epidemiologic studies have identified several risk factors that are associated with the development of coronary artery disease. The possible pathophysiologic bases for these risk factors are explored below.

CIGARETTE SMOKING

Cigarette smoking is an important cause of coronary artery disease and is the leading preventable cause of death in the United States, where approximately 25% of people over 18 years of age smoke; cigarette smoking increases the risk of cardiovascular mortality by 20%–30% in both men and women.

Cigarette smoking has a number of effects that increase the risk for symptomatic coronary artery disease. First, it appears that cigarette smoking is associated with reduced HDL concentrations. Although the reductions are modest (5%–10%), reduced cholesterol removal from extrahepatic sites leads to an increased incidence of atherosclerotic lesions. Second, nicotine may cause direct endothelial cell injury. Third, cigarette smoking is associated with increased coagulability. Cigarette smoking is associated with increased platelet reactivity and elevated fibrinogen and factor VII levels.

Risk Factors for Coronary Artery Disease
Cigarette smoking
Hypercholesterolemia
Diabetes mellitus
Hypertension
Age
Male gender
Family history

Finally, nicotine can directly cause ischemia by increasing metabolic demand of myocardial cells and vasoconstriction of coronary arteries.

HYPERCHOLESTEROLEMIA

Hypercholesterolemia, particularly if LDL levels are elevated, is associated with increased risk for coronary artery disease. As outlined above, LDL and oxidized LDL appear to play an important part in the process of atherogenesis.

DIABETES MELLITUS (DM)

Accelerated atherosclerosis is a well-known consequence of DM, especially type I diabetes mellitus (type I DM) [formerly known as insulin-dependent diabetes mellitus], but also type II DM. Both type I and II DM are associated with significant lipid abnormalities, characterized by elevation of triglycerides and LDL cholesterol and reduction in HDL cholesterol. Other abnormalities may occur as a consequence of DM, such as hypertension from diabetic nephropathy. DM can predispose to increases in platelet reactivity and coagulation factors that lead to atherosclerosis and thrombosis. DM is also associated with elevations in plasminogen activator inhibitor I (PAI-I), which decreases fibrinolysis. Fig. 3-22 shows the fibrinolytic process and the level at which PAI-I acts to inhibit fibrinolysis. Insulin and glycosylated proteins may stimulate smooth muscle proliferation. Poorly controlled diabetics have a higher risk of myocardial infarction and microvascular disease. Increasing concentrations of glucose reduce endothelial cell production of NO and increase endothelial cell production of TXA_2. The neuropathy associated with DM may lead to a decreased perception of cardiac chest pain symptoms and an increased incidence of silent ischemia.

HYPERTENSION

Numerous studies demonstrate a direct relationship between systolic and diastolic arterial pressure elevations and cardiovascular risk. Hypertension can cause left ventricular hypertrophy and endothelial dysfunction. In hypertensive vessels, endothelial cells enlarge and bulge into the lumen. Endothelial cell production of NO is reduced and PGH_2 (vasoconstrictor) production is increased. Elevated blood pressure increases the stress on atherosclerotic plaques and increases the potential for plaque rupture. Blood pressure reduction has been shown to decrease the development of cardiovascular disease, and in some studies, improvement in endothelial function has been reported.

AGE, GENDER, AND FAMILY HISTORY

These risk factors are also called nonmodifiable risk factors, unlike hypertension, hyperlipidemia, DM, and cigarette smoking, all of which are modifiable risks. In terms of age and gender, men below 55 years of age have a three to four times increased incidence of coronary artery disease compared to women. Estrogens have several salutary effects. First, estrogen increases HDL levels by 15% and reduces LDL by 15%. Second, estrogen is associated with coronary artery vasodilation. The exact mechanism of arterial vasodilation is unknown and is probably multifactorial. After the age of 55 years, the incidence of coronary artery disease equalizes between men and women. If postmenopausal women are given estrogen replacement, a 50% reduction in the rate of cardiovascular mortality has been reported. Several age-related effects on endothelial cell function have been reported. With increasing age, there is decreased production of NO. Regenerated endothelial cells appear to produce less NO in response to platelet-derived serotonin.

Coronary artery disease has an important genetic component. After correcting for other risk factors (hypertension, DM, smoking, age), people with relatives who have coronary artery disease are two to four times as likely to develop coronary artery disease when compared to people without relatives with coronary artery disease. A histologic study found that subintimal muscle cell accumulation was more common in people with a family history of coronary artery disease.

Case Study:
Continued

Mr. Hendrickson had a significant number of risk factors for the development of coronary artery disease. It is very helpful to identify the presence or absence of risk factors in a given patient that will increase or decrease the suspicion that the patient's symptoms are due to coronary artery disease.

■ CORONARY ISCHEMIC SYNDROMES

Atherosclerotic heart disease is the most common cause for mortality in the United States, where it is estimated that 1.5 million myocardial infarctions occur annually.

Coronary artery ischemic syndromes can be classified by the duration of symptoms and precipitating causes. Chest pain is the most common symptom of coronary artery ischemia. If pain occurs only in the setting of increased myocardial demand (usually exercise) and has been stable over a period of time, it is termed *stable angina*. If the pain occurs at rest, it is called *unstable angina*. Finally, regardless of precipitating causes, if the chest pain continues and is associated with irreversible myocardial cell damage, a *myocardial infarction* has occurred. Before discussing each of these clinical syndromes, a brief review of coronary artery anatomy is necessary.

CORONARY ANATOMY

The left main coronary artery arises from the ascending aorta just distal to the aortic valve cusps, as seen in Fig. 3-23. It has a somewhat posterior takeoff from the ascending aorta and is a relatively short vessel of less than 10 mm in length. The left main coronary artery bifurcates into the left anterior descending (LAD) coronary artery and the circumflex coronary artery systems. Fig. 3-24 illustrates the left main, LAD, and the circumflex coronary arteries.

The LAD coronary artery courses anteriorly and extends to the apex. It gives rise to one or several diagonal branches, which follow an anterolateral and apical course. Septal perforators, which branch downward into the interventricular septum, also arise from the LAD and supply the anterior two-thirds of the interventricular septum. Thus, stenosis or occlusion of the LAD causes ischemia to the anteroseptal wall and can extend to the apex.

The circumflex coronary artery courses down the left atrioventricular (AV) groove and gives rise to one or several obtuse marginal branches. Usually, stenosis or occlusion of the circumflex system results in ischemia to the lateral wall of the left ventricle.

The right coronary artery arises from the ascending aorta at the level of the right coronary sinus. It has a lower and more anterior takeoff than the left main coronary artery

Ischemia is derived from the Greek words *ischo*, "to hold back," and *haima*, "blood."

Coronary Ischemic Syndromes
Stable angina
Unstable angina
Myocardial infarction

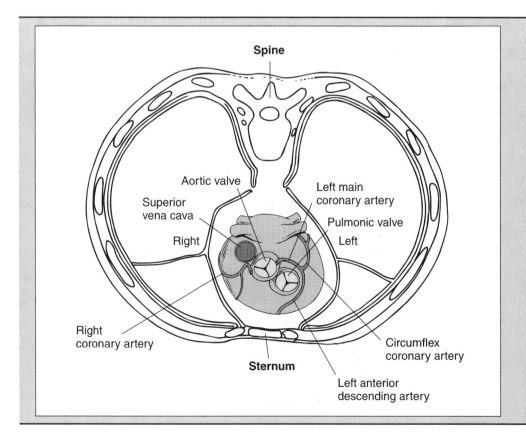

FIG. 3-23
SUPERIOR VIEW OF THE HEART, SHOWING THE ORIGIN OF LEFT AND RIGHT CORONARY ARTERIES FROM ASCENDING AORTA. Note that the right coronary artery originates more anteriorly compared to the left main coronary artery. The left main coronary artery courses around the pulmonic valve and divides into the left anterior descending and circumflex coronary arteries.

FIG. 3-24
ANTERIOR VIEW OF THE ANATOMY OF THE CORONARY CIRCULATION. The left main coronary artery divides into the left anterior descending (LAD) and circumflex coronary arteries. The LAD courses anteriorly, between the right and left ventricles to the apex, and gives rise to septal perforators and diagonal branches. The circumflex artery courses laterally down the left atrioventricular (AV) groove and gives rise to obtuse marginal branches. The right coronary artery travels around the right AV groove and gives rise to atrial and acute marginal branches. At the inferior portion of the interventricular septum, the posterior descending artery travels to the apex between the left and right ventricles.

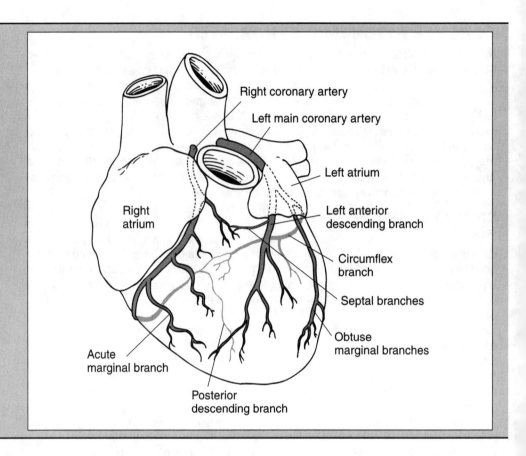

as seen in Figs. 3-25 and 3-26. The right coronary artery courses in the right AV groove. The sinoatrial (SA) nodal branch of the right coronary artery arises from the proximal vessel and courses posteriorly and superiorly to the right atrium, interatrial septum, and superior vena cava. The SA nodal branch supplies blood to the SA node and both atria. Right ventricular (also called acute marginal) branches arise from the mid-portion of the right coronary artery and supply the right ventricular wall. A posterior descending artery (PDA) arises from the distal right coronary artery and supplies the inferior and posterior interventricular septum as well as the diaphragmatic portion of the left ventricle. The right coronary artery often continues and gives rise to one or two posterolateral branches that supply blood to the posterior region of the left ventricle. The AV nodal artery usually branches off in the same area as the PDA branches. Fig. 3-25 illustrates normal anatomy of the right coronary artery. Ischemia of infarction in the right coronary artery system involves the inferior and basal septal walls. Since the SA and AV nodal branches supply blood to the sinus and AV nodes respectively, occlusion of the right coronary artery may be associated with transient sinus node dysfunction (sinus bradycardia) and AV node dysfunction (AV block).

There is great heterogeneity in the actual location and configuration of individual coronary arteries. The configuration of a coronary artery system is traditionally classified by the term *dominance*. A dominant vessel in the context of epicardial coronary anatomy is defined as that which supplies the inferior-posterior aspect of the interventricular septum and the diaphragmatic portion of the left ventricle. In approximately 85% of individuals, the right coronary artery supplies this territory by giving rise to the PDA, as demonstrated in Figs. 3-24 and 3-25. Therefore, these individuals are said to have a right dominant system. Around 8% of people have a left dominant system, in which this territory is actually supplied by the terminal portion of the circumflex coronary artery. The right coronary artery in this setting is usually small with very few branches. The remaining approximately 7% of individuals have a co-dominant system. Fig. 3-26 illustrates right, left, and co-dominant coronary artery systems.

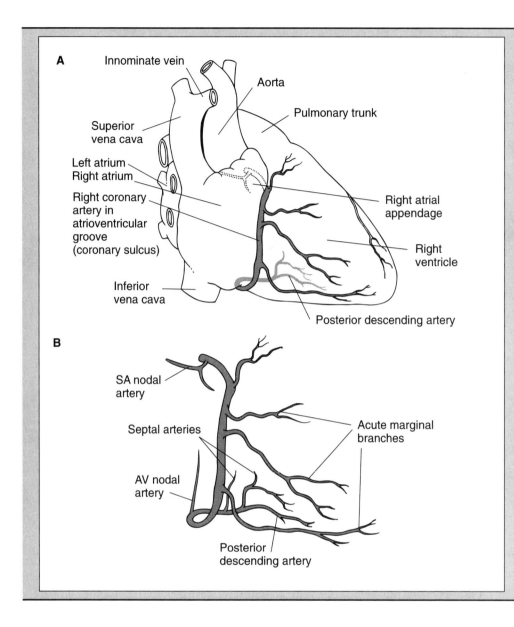

FIG. 3-25
ANATOMY OF THE RIGHT CORO-NARY CIRCULATION. (A) The *top* illustration shows the relation-ship of the right coronary artery and the heart. (B) The *bottom* illustration shows only the right coronary artery and its branches. The right coronary ar-tery courses down the right atri-oventricular (AV) groove and gives rise to branches to the sinoatrial (SA) node and acute marginal branches. At the dia-phragmatic portion of the heart, the right coronary artery gives off a large branch called the posterior descending artery (PDA), which travels toward the apex in the interventricular groove. The PDA divides into septal branches that supply the bottom third of the inter-ventricular septum. The AV no-dal artery, which supplies blood to the AV node, branches up-ward at the junction of the right coronary artery and the PDA.

STABLE ANGINA

Angina pectoris is derived from the Latin words *angere*, which means "to choke," and *pectus*, "breast." Angina is usually described as a dull, substernal chest pain that may radiate to the jaw or arm and can be associated with shortness of breath, nausea, or vomiting. Phrases that patients may use to explain angina include "strangling," "tighten-ing," "burning," and "squeezing."

Pathophysiology. Angina pectoris occurs as a response to inadequate oxygen supply for meeting the metabolic need of cardiac myocytes. The pathophysiologic pro-cesses that cause angina pectoris can be classified by whether they affect oxygen *supply* or oxygen *demand*. Oxygen supply by the coronary arteries can be estimated as the product of *oxygen-carrying capacity* and *blood flow*. Reduced arterial oxygen content (anemia, carbon monoxide poisoning, and hypoxia) can cause angina pectoris if flow cannot be increased to compensate for the reduced oxygen. For this reason, reduced oxygen content usually precipitates angina in the presence of a flow-limiting lesion. Reduced blood flow resulting from a narrowing of the coronary artery lumen is the most common cause of angina. Coronary artery narrowing can be due to fixed obstruction from an atherosclerotic plaque, vasospasm of the coronary artery, or vasospasm at the site of an atherosclerotic plaque. Unlike all other organs of the body, in the coronary arteries blood flow is greatest during diastole.

Angina pectoris is the result of a reduced supply or increased de-mand for oxygen.

Oxygen Supply
Oxygen-carrying capacity
Flow

Oxygen Demand
Heart rate
Contractility
Wall tension

FIG. 3-26
CLASSIFICATION OF CORONARY ARTERY CONFIGURATIONS IN DIFFERENT PEOPLE. Schematics of the main coronary arteries are shown. Most people have a right dominant system in which the posterior descending coronary artery (PDA) is formed from the right coronary artery. In a left dominant system, the PDA branches off the circumflex coronary artery. In a co-dominant system, the diaphragmatic aspect of the left ventricle is supplied by small branches of the circumflex coronary artery and the right coronary arteries.

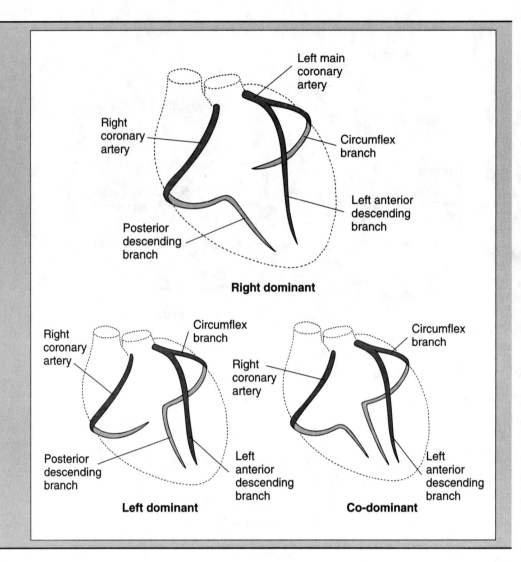

Right dominant

Left dominant

Co-dominant

Coronary artery blood flow is greatest during diastole. During systole as the velocity through the aorta increases, artery pressure drops in the coronary artery, which is known as the **Venturi effect**.

During systole, rapid blood flow through the aortic valve past the ostia of the coronary arteries causes a Venturi effect, reducing the systolic pressure in the coronary arteries themselves. In addition, during systole, contraction of the left ventricle causes external compression on the coronary artery arterioles within the ventricular wall, which further reduces delivery of blood to the cardiac myocytes. Myocytes in the ventricular subendocardium (the myocytes that line the ventricular cavity) are particularly susceptible to ischemia; they are exposed to high intracavitary pressures during systole, which further reduces the systolic pressure gradient in capillaries that supply these cells.

Oxygen demand of cardiac myocytes is dependent on three factors: heart rate (HR), wall tension, and contractility. Oxygen demand is directly proportional to the HR. With increased HR, the absolute increase in the rate of ventricular contractions means more myosin–actin interactions and a proportional increase in ATP requirements. The second important factor determining oxygen demand is wall tension. Wall tension in the left ventricle is the force exerted on cardiac myocytes in response to the intracavitary pressure resulting from ventricular contraction. Wall tension is related to intracavitary pressure and volume by Laplace's law:

$$\sigma = \frac{p \times r}{2h}$$

where σ is ventricular wall tension, p is left ventricular intracavitary pressure, r is the radius of the left ventricle, and h is wall thickness. Increased cavitary pressure and increased ventricular size both increase the oxygen demand of the heart. Finally, increased contractility from catecholamines or other causes increases the amount of ATP consumed by the myocardial cells.

Stable angina pectoris is characterized by symptoms that occur in the setting of higher metabolic demand. Most commonly, patients complain of chest pain that occurs when they exercise, then resolves when they stop to rest. Stable angina is defined as a chest pain pattern that does not change in severity, duration, threshold, or inciting factors over at least a 6- to 8-week period.

Stable angina can be observed when a patient has a stable atherosclerotic plaque that has become large enough to occlude blood flow partially (Fig. 3-27). Normally, the main coronary arteries (left main, LAD, circumflex, right coronary artery) do not offer significant resistance to flow. For this reason the arterial lumen must be reduced by 90% to produce cellular ischemia at rest. With exercise and the accompanying increase in metabolic demand, ischemia can occur with a 50% reduction in the intra-arterial lumen.

In addition to precipitation of ischemia by fixed obstruction to flow by an atherosclerotic lesion, it is now becoming more evident that dynamic obstruction resulting from vasospasm is an important precipitant of myocardial ischemia. Endothelial cells

Reduced coronary artery blood flow can result from fixed obstruction or focal spasm.

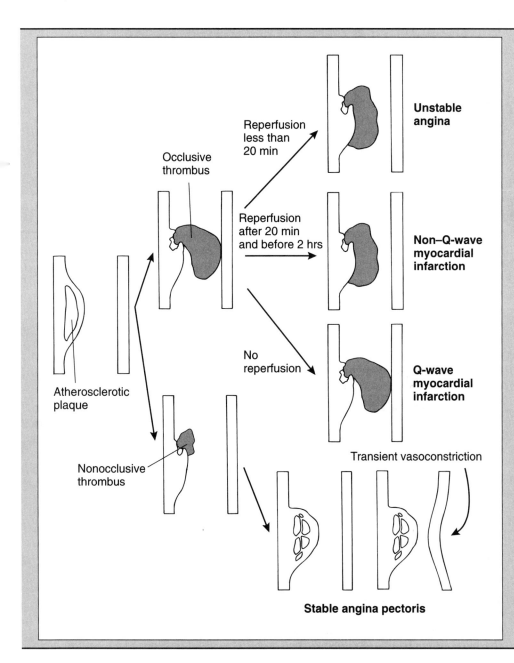

FIG. 3-27
PROPOSED PATHOPHYSIOLOGY OF VARIOUS CLINICAL SYNDROMES. In *stable angina*, small surface disruptions lead to nonocclusive thrombi, which cause the atherosclerotic lesion to increase in size slowly and ultimately limit blood flow in the presence of high metabolic demand. In addition, flow may be limited by some component of vasospasm. In the other clinical syndromes, a larger intimal surface disruption leads to formation of an occlusive thrombus that causes chest pain at rest. If the thrombus resolves quickly (less thrombus load as a result of a smaller surface disruption) the symptoms resolve after a few minutes, and the patient is classified as having *unstable angina*. If the thrombus is more persistent but still resolves within several hours, the patient will present with a *non–Q-wave myocardial infarction*. If the occlusive thrombus is permanent, the patient will develop a *Q-wave myocardial infarction*.

associated with atherosclerotic lesions have abnormal function. In particular, they tend to secrete relatively less NO and more vasoconstrictors (such as endothelin I). Coronary artery vasospasm can also occur without accompanying atherosclerotic lesions in some cases. In 1959, Printzmetal described a syndrome of ischemic chest pain that occurs at rest. It is now known that *Printzmetal's* or *variant angina* is due to focal spasm in relatively normal coronary arteries. Several possible pathophysiologic mechanisms exist, including abnormal endothelial cell function and abnormalities in smooth muscle cell responsiveness. Interestingly, the focal spasm in Printzmetal's angina is often associated with a very minor atherosclerotic lesion.

The mechanism of chest pain resulting from cardiac ischemia is not well understood. Stimulation of free nerve ends in the myocardium causes impulses to travel via afferent fibers to the first five thoracic ganglia. In the spinal cord, impulses from the heart converge with other impulses from the neck, arm, and back, which is probably responsible, in part, for the pain in these regions that may accompany cardiac ischemia. The actual trigger for nerve stimulation may be adenosine. Interestingly, adenosine infused into the coronary arteries produces chest pain with similar qualities to angina pectoris, without actual ischemia.

Treatment. Stable angina can be treated with a number of medications. Most commonly, sublingual nitroglycerin is used. As mentioned, nitroglycerin metabolism yields NO, which is a potent vasodilator. Drugs that block the β-adrenergic receptor (β-blockers) are also used for the treatment of angina. Many of the conditions that precipitate angina (e.g., exercise) are associated with increased sympathetic activity. β-Blockers antagonize sympathetic activity, which results in reduced HR, decreased contractility, and reduced blood pressure. Another class of drugs used to treat angina are the calcium channel blockers. The mechanism of action of calcium channel blockers for the treatment of angina is complex; it is in part mediated by reduced blood pressure, reduced HR, and negative inotropic effects. Finally, aspirin reduces platelet aggregation, which is probably important for reducing the chance that a stable atherosclerotic lesion will become unstable. Daily aspirin has been associated with a 70%–80% reduction in the risk of future myocardial infarction in patients with stable angina.

Treatment of Stable Angina
Nitrates
β-Blockers
Calcium channel blockers
Aspirin

Case Study: *Continued*

Mr. Hendrickson's original symptoms were probably stable angina from an atherosclerotic plaque that obstructed the arterial lumen by more than 50% but less than 90%.

UNSTABLE ANGINA

Just as the name implies, in unstable angina, patients complain of chest pain or angina, but now the pattern of pain has accelerated or occurs at rest. An unstable pattern can be characterized by increased frequency of pain, pain occurring at lower levels of exercise, or pain that is less responsive to medication (such as sublingual nitroglycerin).

Pathophysiology. In unstable angina the chronic stable atherosclerotic lesion becomes unstable (Fig. 3-27). Often the atherosclerotic plaque develops a small fissure or surface disruption, which initiates the process of thrombosis. Symptoms occur as the lumen is transiently occluded by thrombus (usually 10–20 min) and improve when spontaneous lysis of the thrombus (via plasmin production) reestablishes partial blood flow. It also appears that in addition to thrombosis, local vasoconstriction produced by platelet-mediated release of TXA_2 and other molecules occurs. The exact mechanism that causes initial plaque instability is unknown; several studies have suggested that disrupted atherosclerotic plaques are associated with increased numbers of macrophages and monocytes. It is possible that macrophage degradation of collagen is the initiating cause of plaque disruption.

Treatment. Unstable angina can be treated with a number of medicines. Intravenous nitroglycerin is commonly used. As mentioned above, increased NO production from nitroglycerin may allow coronary artery vasodilation. In addition, intravenous heparin is frequently used. Heparin is a naturally occurring molecule composed of repeating disaccharide units containing glucosamine and uronic acid. Heparin binds to the antithrombin

Treatment of Unstable Angina
Intravenous nitroglycerin
Intravenous heparin
β-Blockers
Aspirin

III molecule; the heparin–antithrombin III complex has a high affinity for thrombin, thus limiting the coagulation cascade (Fig. 3-28). Beta-blockade, by reducing myocardial oxygen demand, is also useful for the treatment of unstable angina.

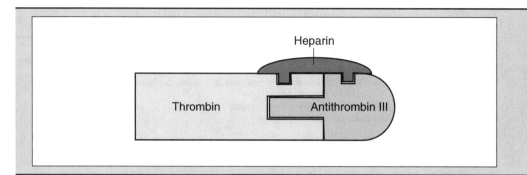

Heparin

Thrombin   Antithrombin III

FIG. 3-28
HEPARIN BINDS TO ANTITHROMBIN III. The heparin–antithrombin III complex has a high affinity for thrombin, which limits the coagulation cascade.

The development of pain at rest over the previous week suggests that Mr. Hendrickson's atherosclerotic plaque had become unstable and was now associated with intermittent thrombosis.

Case Study:
Continued

MYOCARDIAL INFARCTION

In myocardial infarction, deep fissuring of an atherosclerotic plaque leads to the formation of an occlusive thrombus. Unlike unstable angina, in myocardial infarction the thrombus does not resolve quickly and irreversible myocardial damage occurs as blood flow is completely stopped. Myocardial infarctions are clinically classified by the presence or absence of *Q waves*. In patients with non–Q-wave myocardial infarctions, thrombotic occlusion of the artery lasts approximately 1 hour (20 min–2 hr), and in Q-wave myocardial infarctions thrombotic occlusion is persistent and lasts for more than several hours and is sometimes permanent unless treated aggressively.

Pathophysiology. Abrupt sudden occlusion of a coronary artery has several important biochemical consequences that follow from reduced oxygen supply. First, there is a rapid shift to anaerobic metabolism, which results in lactic acid production. High-energy phosphates such as ATP and creatine phosphate (CP) drop within minutes, a drop that is associated with a marked increase in intracellular inorganic phosphate. Second, within 1 minute of coronary artery occlusion, extracellular potassium ion (K+) concentration increases in the ischemic region. Increased extracellular K+ appears to be due to an ATP-modulated K+ channel (I_{KATP}), which opens in response to low ATP levels and, to a lesser extent, because of reduced Na+–K+-ATPase activity. By the Nernst equation, increased extracellular K+ results in depolarization of the cell membrane. Third, Ca2+ concentrations increase. Increased intracellular Ca2+ is due to reduced Na+–K+-ATPase activity, which causes increased intracellular sodium (Na2+), which in turn favors accumulation of intracellular Ca2+ by the Na+–Ca2+-exchanger.

Histologically, the earliest changes observed in myocardial ischemia are cellular and mitochondrial swelling, myofibrillar relaxation, and margination of nuclear chromatin. With prolonged ischemia, mitochondria with calcium phosphate deposits can be observed, myofibrils become hypercontracted and form contraction bands, and the cell membrane becomes disrupted. Cell necrosis begins after 20–30 minutes of ischemia and spreads from endocardium to epicardium. If ischemia persists for 6–8 hours, 70%–80% of the cells supplied by that particular artery will die. Collateral blood flow from other coronary arteries minimizes the ischemia in the peripheral regions of the myocardium that is affected.

Functionally, myocardial cells quickly lose their contractile ability within several minutes. As already mentioned, irreversible necrosis begins after 20–30 minutes. Interestingly, even if blood flow is restored within 15–20 minutes, myocardial contractility

Nernst Equation

$$E_m = \frac{RT}{F} \ln \frac{[K^+]_0}{[K^+]_i}.$$

will sometimes remain abnormal despite the absence of any permanent histologic changes. It appears that reperfusion of the injured area is associated with transient Ca^{2+} overload and generation of oxygen free radicals, which "stun" the myocardium. After several days function in this region slowly normalizes. The effects of myocardial ischemia are summarized in Table 3-1.

Table 3-1
Effects of Myocardial Ischemia

TYPE OF EFFECT	EFFECT
Biochemical	Increased lactic acid and protons
	Decreased adenosine triphosphate and creatine phosphate
	Increased inorganic phosphate
	Increased extracellular potassium
	Increased intracellular calcium
Histologic	Mitochondrial swelling
	Breaks in cytoplasmic membrane
	Cell necrosis
Functional	Loss of contractility (may persist despite reestablishment of blood flow)

Diagnosis of Myocardial Infarction
History
ECG
Enzymes and proteins

Clinical Diagnosis. The clinical diagnosis of myocardial infarction takes into account three important criteria. First and most important is the history obtained from the patient. Persistent chest pain is the most common complaint of patients in the midst of a myocardial infarction. Like angina, the pain can be described as "strangling," "tightening," "burning," and "squeezing." Associated symptoms such as diaphoresis (sweating), nausea, vomiting, and shortness of breath may or may not be present. The diagnosis of myocardial infarction by history requires a significant amount of clinical experience and skill.

The second criterion for myocardial infarction is the ECG. The ECG findings in various ischemic syndromes are described separately below.

The third criterion for the diagnosis of myocardial infarction uses blood measurement of enzymes and proteins. Three enzymes have historically been used for the diagnosis of myocardial infarction: aspartate transaminase (AST), lactate dehydrogenase (LDH), and creatine kinase (CK). Of these enzymes, the CK is most commonly used. CK catalyzes the transfer of phosphate from ATP to creatine and is found in muscle, brain, and heart tissue. CK is made up of two monomers; two types of monomers have been identified and are named B and M. CK with two B monomers (BB-CK) is found predominantly in the brain, and CK with two M monomers (MM-CK) is most commonly found in muscle. MB-CK, which is composed of one M and one B monomer, is found in relatively high concentrations in the heart. With myocardial injury, MB-CK is released into the blood. An elevated blood CK, particularly if it has a high concentration of the MB form, should arouse suspicion of myocardial damage.

Recently, measurement of cardiac-specific troponins has become available. Remember that the troponin complex consists of three subunits: troponin-C, which binds calcium, troponin-I, which binds to actin and inhibits actin–myosin interaction, and troponin-T, which binds to tropomyosin. Antibodies for the troponins found in the heart (troponin-T and troponin-I) have been developed and are now commercially available in quantitative assays. The clinical use of the cardiac-specific troponins is still under clinical study.

Treatment of Myocardial Infarction

Pharmacologic therapies
Thrombolytic: t-PA, streptokinase, urokinase
Platelet-directed: Gp IIb-IIIa receptor blockers, aspirin
Heparin
β-Blockade

Mechanical therapy
Angioplasty

Treatment. Treatment for myocardial infarction is evolving quickly. All therapies are directed toward reestablishing blood flow in the coronary artery in a timely fashion. Currently, pharmacologic and mechanical interventions are used for the acute treatment of myocardial infarction. Since an occlusive thrombus is usually responsible for a myocardial infarction, pharmacologic agents (thrombolytics) that are directed toward dissolving or "lysing" the thrombus are commonly used. For example, several molecules that activate plasminogen have been developed: streptokinase, urokinase, t-PA, and others. While the structures of these molecules differ, all of them cleave plasminogen to produce plasmin, which breaks up the fibrin network of the occlusive thrombus. In addition to agents targeting the fibrin polymers, several agents that reduce platelet aggregation have been developed. Several agents that block the platelet Gp IIb-IIIa receptor have been developed; these can significantly reduce platelet aggregation, and preliminary data suggest that they may be useful in the treatment of acute myocardial infarction. Instead of pharmacologic methods, mechanical methods can be used to break up thrombus by performing angioplasty, where a specialized balloon is dilated in the region of the ruptured atherosclerotic lesion and thrombus. The remnants of the thrombus flow to the distal vessel where they are metabolized by the normal fibrinolytic system.

Finally, adjunctive treatment of acute myocardial infarction with heparin and β-blockers is usually indicated for the pathophysiologic reasons mentioned earlier.

ELECTROCARDIOGRAM IN ISCHEMIC SYNDROMES

The ECG may be useful for the diagnosis of ischemia, since it measures the electrical activity of the heart. Ischemia can be associated with three different ECG findings: *Q waves, ST-segment changes*, and *T-wave changes*.

Q Waves. To understand the importance of Q waves, the student must remember several important fundamentals of the ECG. First, the QRS complex measures electrical activation or depolarization of the ventricles in the frontal (leads: I, II, III, aVL, aVR, aVF) and precordial (V_1 through V_6) planes. Second, the student must remember how the ventricles are normally activated (Fig. 3-29). In the frontal plane, ventricular activation is directed downward and to the left. In the precordial plane, initial ventricular activation of the septum is from left to right, which is followed by a predominant right to left activation

ECG Changes Associated with Coronary Ischemic Syndromes
Q waves (changes in ventricular depolarization)
ST-segment changes (voltage gradients present during the normally isoelectric ST segment)
T-wave changes (changes in repolarization)

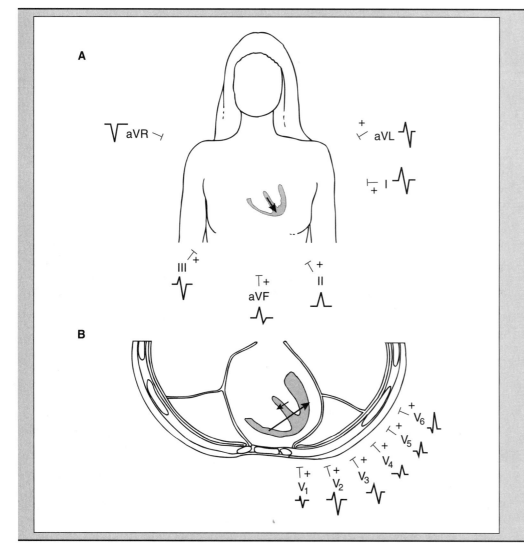

FIG. 3-29
NORMAL ACTIVATION OF THE HEART. (A) In the frontal plane, activation of the ventricles can be approximated by a spreading dipole traveling at approximately 60 degrees. (B) In the precordial plane, activation first occurs in the septum from left to right, and then the left ventricle is activated from right to left.

of the rest of the heart. Third, electrical activation traveling away from the positive electrode of a lead produces a negative deflection. A Q wave is simply defined as an initial negative deflection in the QRS complex, which means that initial depolarization of the ventricles is directed away from the positive electrode of that particular lead.

These fundamentals can first be applied to the normal ECG (see Chap. 2, Fig. 2-28). In the frontal plane, since ventricular activation is normally directed downward and to the left, a Q wave is normally seen in lead aVR. Similarly, depending on variations in body habitus and relative position in the heart, small Q waves can sometimes be observed in any of the "inferior leads" (II, III, aVF), particularly in lead III. In the precordial plane, small Q waves produced by initial septal activation can sometimes be observed in leads V_4 to V_6. In Fig. 2-28, only lead aVR has a Q wave; in the rest of the leads the initial deflection of the QRS complex is positive. Now refer to Fig. 3-30. This also is a normal ECG. Notice the very small initial deflections in leads II, III, aVF, aVL, V_4, V_5, and V_6. These small Q waves are a normal finding.

FIG. 3-30
NORMAL ELECTROCARDIO-GRAM. This is the same one shown in Fig. 3-1. *Arrows* mark the small, insignificant Q waves.

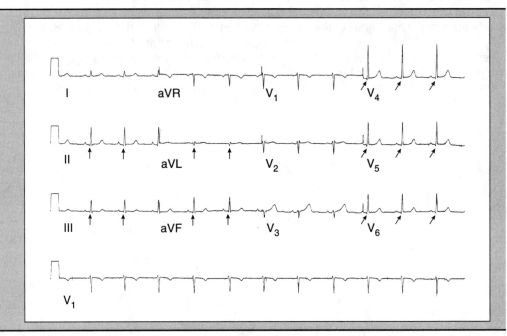

Large Q waves in any lead other than aVR must be evaluated carefully. Q waves resulting from myocardial ischemia are usually wide (> 0.04 msec in duration) and deep (> 3 mm negative). Q waves in the setting of a myocardial infarction are due to inactive myocardial tissue that fails to contribute to normal electrical activity. This leads to relative ventricular activation away from the injured area. For example, occlusion of the right coronary artery leads to ischemia in the inferior wall of the heart. Electrical inactivity of the inferior wall of the heart causes a relative negative activation away from the "inferior leads" (II, III, and aVF) [Figs. 3-31 and 3-32]. Similarly, occlusion of the LAD artery causes ischemia to the anterior portion of the heart, which yields Q waves in the "anterior leads" (V_1, V_2, V_3, and V_4) [Figs. 3-33 and 3-34]. Finally, occlusion in the circumflex coronary artery leads to Q waves in the "lateral" leads (V_5, V_6, aVL, and I). While Q waves signify abnormal electrical activity of a relatively large region of myocardium, it is important to remember that Q waves are not synonymous with myocardial cell death. Q waves can temporarily appear in the setting of acute coronary artery occlusion and then disappear some time later, if blood flow is promptly reestablished.

It is important to remember that Q waves can also be seen in other circumstances, such as left bundle branch block (LBBB), infiltrative diseases of the heart, and accessory pathway activation. The detailed evaluation of Q waves is beyond the scope of this text; for more information the student is referred to texts that are devoted exclusively to electrocardiography.

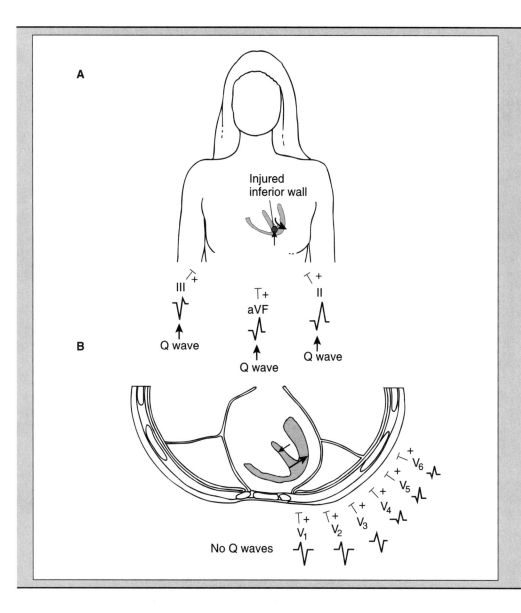

FIG. 3-31
In an inferior myocardial infarction (usually the result of thrombotic occlusion of the right coronary artery), myocardial injury of the inferior wall changes early activation of the ventricle. (A) Since the injured area does not contribute to ventricular activation, there is a relative early force directed away from the inferior leads (*small arrow*) that yields an early negative deflection in the inferior leads (II, III, aVF). (B) This early upwardly directed force is not observed in the precordial leads since the force is well out of the plane subtended by those leads.

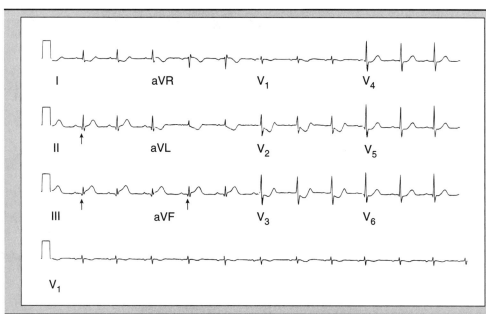

FIG. 3-32
ELECTROCARDIOGRAM FROM A PATIENT IN THE EARLY PART OF AN INFERIOR WALL MYOCARDIAL INFARCTION. (A) Small Q waves in leads II, III, and aVF are denoted by the *arrows*. If blood flow in the coronary artery (the right coronary artery in this case) is not promptly restored, these Q waves will become larger as the area of ischemia and cell necrosis spreads outward (B). Notice also that the ST segment is elevated in leads II, III, and aVF, and depressed in leads V_2 through V_5.

FIG. 3-33
In an anterior myocardial infarction (usually the result of thrombotic occlusion of the left anterior descending coronary artery), myocardial injury of the anterior wall and septum changes early activation of the ventricle. (A) Since the injured area is out of the frontal plane, no Q waves are noted in the frontal leads. (B) However, in the precordial plane, the injured anterior and septal regions do not contribute to ventricular activation; there is a relative early force directed away from the precordial leads V₁ and V₂ (*small arrows*).

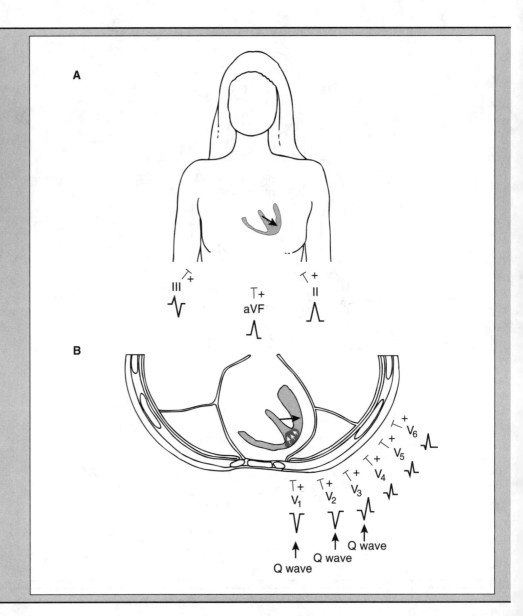

FIG. 3-34
ELECTROCARDIOGRAM FROM A PATIENT IN THE EARLY PART OF AN ANTERIOR WALL MYOCARDIAL INFARCTION. Q waves in leads V₁ and V₂ are denoted by the *arrows*. If blood flow in the coronary artery (the left anterior descending coronary artery in this case) is not promptly restored, these Q waves will become evident in leads V₃ and V₄ as the area of ischemia and cell necrosis spreads outward. Notice also that the ST segment is elevated in leads V₁, V₂, and V₃ (arrowheads).

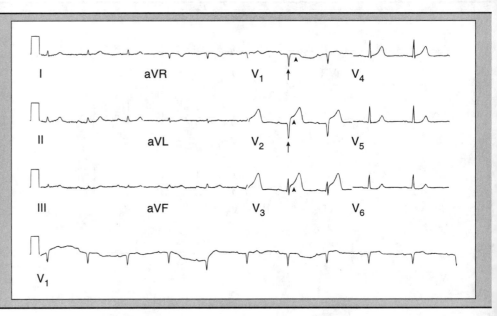

ST Segment. The ST segment correlates with the plateau phase or phase 2 of the ventricular myocytes. Normally all of the ventricular myocytes are simultaneously at the plateau phase at this time, and no voltage gradients exist in the heart, which leads to an isoelectric ST segment. Myocardial ischemia can be associated with both ST-segment elevation and ST-segment depression. Deviations of the ST segment from the baseline suggests that voltage gradients are present and measurable from the surface during the period after ventricular contraction.

ST-Segment Elevation. Myocardial infarction is an important cause of ST-segment elevation. At the present time, the pathophysiology of ST-segment elevation is best explained by two important concepts: the systolic current of injury and the diastolic current of injury (Figs. 3-35 and 3-36) [Review Figure 2-26.]

The systolic current of injury (see Fig. 3-35) suggests that the ischemic heart is electrically identical to the nonischemic heart at rest. However, after ventricular activation, the injured area is unresponsive to depolarization or repolarizes earlier relative to adjacent normal segments. In either case, the exteriors of the myocytes in the injured area are relatively positive compared to the normal regions of the myocardium. This voltage gradient yields a positive deflection in the leads with positive electrodes facing the injured area. For example, if the LAD artery is occluded, the anterior wall of the heart becomes ischemic and does not depolarize or repolarizes earlier than the rest of the heart. A voltage gradient is generated with the cells of the anterior wall having a relatively positive surface charge compared to the rest of the heart (see Fig. 3-34), which leads to an elevated ST segment in some of the precordial leads (in the example, V_1 through V_3). The specific precordial leads that display ST-segment elevation depend on the exact part of the artery that is occluded and the orientation of the heart relative to the surface. Remember that, by convention, a positive deflection is recorded when the positive pole of a dipole faces the positive electrode. This results in ST-segment elevation on the surface ECG in those leads with the positive electrode lying directly over the anterior wall.

The concept of diastolic current of injury was proposed in 1977 by Vincent et al. (see Fig. 3-36). They partially and completely occluded coronary arteries in dogs and recorded ECGs during this process. They noted that the TQ segment (the segment between

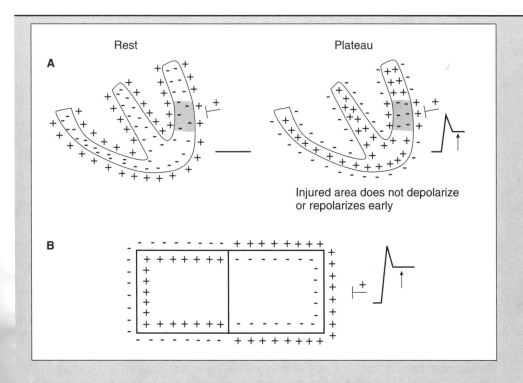

FIG. 3-35
SYSTOLIC CURRENT OF INJURY THEORY FOR ST-SEGMENT ELEVATION. (A) At rest, every myocyte is at a normal resting state (−85 mV), no voltage gradients exist, and the electrocardiogram records 0 mV. With depolarization, the majority of the cells become depolarized (10 mV, surface relatively negative). However, the myocytes in the injured area do not depolarize or repolarize early and are at −85 mV (surface relatively positive). This leads to ST-segment elevation in those leads where the positive electrode lies over the injured area. (B) A model of the systolic current of injury theory. The myocardium can be modeled as a single large cell. At the plateau phase, the right side of the cell remains positive, which yields ST-segment elevation if the positive electrode of a recording system is located on the right of the cell.

Inside figure A:
Rest   Plateau

Injured area does not depolarize or repolarizes early

FIG. 3-36
DIASTOLIC CURRENT OF INJURY THEORY FOR ST-SEGMENT ELEVATION. (A) At rest, uninjured myocytes are at a normal resting state (−85 mV), but myocytes in the injured region are partially depolarized (−70 to 0 mV), which yields a voltage gradient during the TQ segment. Since the injured region has a relatively negative surface charge, the TQ segment of a lead lying over the injured area will show TQ-segment depression. With depolarization, all of the cells become depolarized (10 mV, surface relatively negative). Since the modern electrocardiograph machine calibrates the TQ segment as zero, TQ depression is manifested as ST-segment elevation. (B) A model of the diastolic current of injury theory. The myocardium can be modeled as a single large cell. At rest, the right side of the cell is partially depolarized, which yields TQ-segment depression if the positive electrode of a recording system is located on the right of the cell.

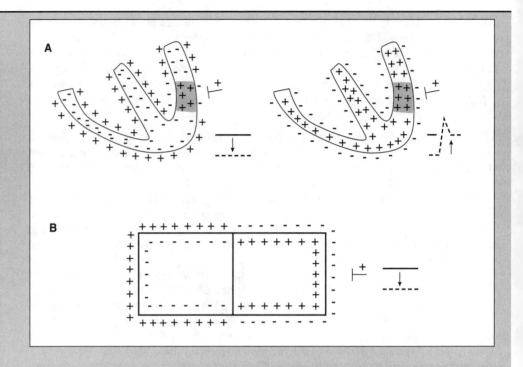

ventricular repolarization and ventricular depolarization of the *next* contraction) became depressed during occlusion of the coronary artery, and the magnitude of depression increased with duration of occlusion. Downward shift of the TQ segment is due to resting depolarization of the ischemic area (see Fig. 3-36). Since the modern ECG machine always defines the TQ segment as "zero," TQ-segment depression is manifested as ST-segment elevation.

It appears that the ST-segment elevation observed during a myocardial infarction is due to a combination of systolic and diastolic effects. However, diastolic effects appear to be predominant. Remember that ischemia causes local extracellular K^+ increase and depolarization of the resting membrane potential.

It is important to remember that ST-segment elevation can be observed in a number of conditions. A discussion of the subtleties of ST-segment elevation is beyond the scope of this text; the reader is referred to Appendix I for a limited list of the causes of ST-segment elevation.

Case Study:
Continued

Mr. Hendrickson had an atherosclerotic plaque in his right coronary artery that progressed slowly at first, limiting blood flow only during periods of increased metabolic need (period of stable angina). The plaque became unstable and probably ruptured, which initially caused intermittent thrombosis (unstable angina) but now was associated with a persistent occlusive thrombus (myocardial infarction).

Evaluation of his ECG showed profound ST-segment elevation in his inferior leads (II, III, and aVF). In this situation, it is mandatory to reestablish flow in the culprit vessel by medications or by mechanical means.

ST-Segment Depression. The astute student will recognize that an ST segment will become depressed if normal myocardial tissue is present between the positive recording electrode and the injured region of myocardium. The pathophysiologic mechanisms are similar to those described for ST-segment elevation. For this reason, ST-segment depression is observed in the "reciprocal leads" where a region of injury is separated by normal tissue. For example, occlusion of the right coronary artery leads to ischemia of the inferior wall, which generates ST-segment elevation in the inferior leads (II, III, and aVF). In the precordial leads, ST-segment depression is noted because the positive electrodes of these leads are separated from the ischemic area by normal myocardium (see Fig. 3-32).

In Mr. Hendrickson's ECG, notice the "reciprocal" ST-segment depression in leads aVL, I, and V_1 through V_4.

Case Study:
Continued

In addition to "reciprocal" ST-segment depression, ST-segment depression can be observed as the only manifestation of myocardial ischemia. ST-segment depression without accompanying ST-segment elevation can be observed if the ischemic region only involves the endocardium (no electrodes are located within the heart chamber!) [Fig. 3-37]. For this reason, a myocardial infarction that is characterized only by ST-segment depression has traditionally been called a "subendocardial" infarction, although the phrase non–Q-wave myocardial infarction is now more commonly used. ST-segment depression can be observed in a number of conditions other than myocardial ischemia. For example, ST-segment depression can be seen in left ventricular hypertrophy.

The **subendocardium** is the region most prone to ischemia. (Remember the relationship between wall stress and myocardial oxygen demand.)

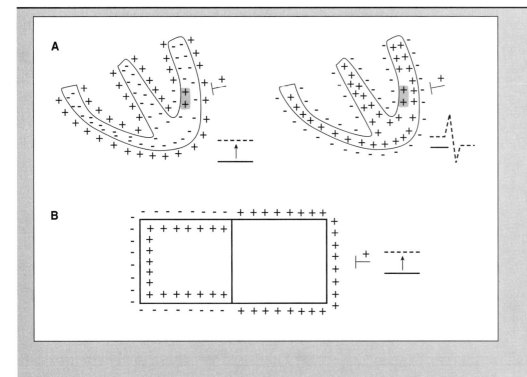

FIG. 3-37
SUBENDOCARDIAL ISCHEMIA IS ASSOCIATED WITH ST-SEGMENT DEPRESSION. Both diastolic and systolic currents of injury theories can explain ST-segment depression. (A) In this figure, only the diastolic current of injury theory is illustrated. At rest, the subendocardial region is partially depolarized as a result of ischemia. This yields TQ-segment elevation, which is manifested as ST-segment depression because the electrocardiograph machine arbitrarily defines the TQ segment as zero. This is shown in a similar schematic form in the bottom panel (B). At rest, a voltage gradient exists with the left side of the cell with a relatively negative surface charge. A lead positioned to the right of the cell will "see" the injured area through a region of normal tissue. Since the positive pole of the dipole faces the positive electrode, TQ-segment elevation is noted.

T-Wave Changes. Myocardial ischemia can be associated with repolarization abnormalities, which are reflected by a variety of T-wave changes. Inverted T waves and other abnormalities can be observed in ischemia but are very nonspecific findings. The T wave generally is in the same direction as the QRS complex (see Chap. 2). For example, leads like II, III, and aVF with positive QRS complexes are associated with upright T waves (see Chap. 2, Fig. 2-28). A T wave that is opposite in direction to the QRS complex should always arouse suspicion, but this can also be a normal finding. Notice that in Fig. 3-30 in leads aVL and V_3 the T wave is upright even though the QRS complex is predominantly negative. These are normal findings. In addition to T-wave inversion, T-wave "peaking" can also be associated with ischemia and myocardial infarction (Fig. 3-38).

FIG. 3-38
(A) A 12-LEAD ELECTROCAR-DIOGRAM IN A HEALTHY 43-YEAR-OLD POLICEMAN EXPERIENCING CHEST PAIN. (B) FIVE MINUTES LATER, AFTER THE PAIN RESOLVED SPONTANE-OUSLY. Notice the prominent T waves in leads V_2 and V_3 during chest pain, which normalize in the second tracing. This subtle finding led to an extensive cardiac evaluation, which found a critical narrowing in the left anterior descending coronary artery.

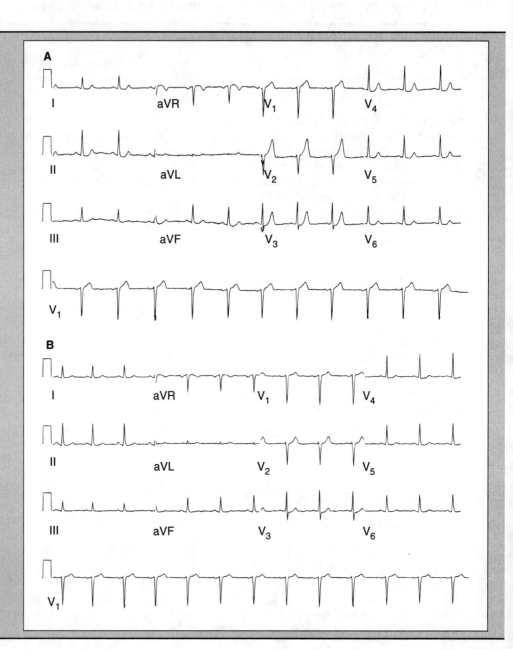

ECG Changes and Ischemic Syndromes. The ECG changes in different ischemic syndromes are summarized in Table 3-2. In both unstable and stable angina, Q waves and ST-segment elevation are normally not observed. In both of these conditions myocardial ischemia is relatively transient and usually involves the subendocardial tissue. For this reason, these conditions are usually characterized by ST-segment depression and T-wave changes when the cells become ischemic, which often resolve when blood flow is restored.

Myocardial infarctions are classified by the presence or absence of Q waves. In non–Q-wave myocardial infarction, while myocyte damage has occurred (usually confirmed by

ELECTROCARDIOGRAM	STABLE ANGINA	UNSTABLE ANGINA	MYOCARDIAL INFARCTION non–Q-wave	MYOCARDIAL INFARCTION Q-wave
Q waves	Not present	Not present	Not present	Present
ST segment	ST-segment depression during pain (ischemia)	ST-segment depression during pain (ischemia)	ST-segment depression or elevation	ST-segment elevation
T waves	T-wave inversion or peaked T waves may be present during pain (ischemia)	T-wave inversion or peaked T waves may be present during pain (ischemia)	T-wave inversion or peaked T waves may be present	T-wave inversion or peaked T waves may be present

Table 3-2
Electrocardiographic Changes in Coronary Ischemic Syndromes

an elevated MB-CK level in the peripheral blood), the damage is not extensive enough to cause abnormal ventricular depolarization patterns to be detected by the surface ECG. For this reason, by definition, no abnormal Q waves are recorded. Non–Q-wave infarctions can be associated with ST-segment elevation, ST-segment depression, T-wave changes, and in some cases, no repolarization abnormalities.

In a Q-wave myocardial infarction, enough myocardium has become ischemic to cause abnormal ventricular depolarization to be detected on the surface ECG. Q-wave myocardial infarctions are almost always associated with ST-segment elevation.

The distinction between Q-wave and non–Q-wave myocardial infarctions is important since they have a number of important clinical differences, which are summarized in Table 3-3. Non–Q-wave myocardial infarctions are generally smaller and have an excellent short-term prognosis. However, non–Q-wave myocardial infarctions are associated with significant residual ischemia, increased risk of reinfarction, and a similar long-term mortality to Q-wave myocardial infarctions. These findings have led some clinicians to call non–Q-wave myocardial infarctions "incomplete" myocardial infarctions.

CHARACTERISTIC	Q-WAVE	NON–Q-WAVE
Prevalence	47%	53%
Incidence of coronary occlusion	80%–90%	15%–25%
ST-segment elevation	80%	25%
ST-segment depression	20%	75%
Postinfarction angina	15%–25%	30%–40%
Incidence of early reinfarction	5%–8%	15%–25%
Mortality at 1 month	10%–15%	3%–5%
Mortality at 2 years	30%	30%
Infarct size	Moderate to large	Usually small
Residual ischemia	10%–20%	40%–50%
Acute complication	Common	Uncommon

Table 3-3
Distinctions between Q-Wave and Non–Q-Wave Myocardial Infarctions

Source: Reprinted with permission from Roberts R, Morris D, Pratt CM, et al: Pathophysiology recognition, and treatment of acute myocardial infarction and its complications. In *Hurst's The Heart*, 8th ed. Edited by Schlant RC, Alexander RW, O'Rourke RA, et al. New York, NY: McGraw-Hill, 1994, p 1113.

■ SUMMARY

Coronary artery disease resulting from the development of atherosclerosis is the most common cause of death in the Western world. Atherosclerotic plaques develop over time as the normal biologic response to repeated injury of the vessel wall. The clinical manifestations of coronary artery disease depend on how acutely the atherosclerotic plaque causes ischemia. If the plaque only increases in size slowly, when the narrowing reaches 70%–90% of the vessel lumen, the patient begins developing stable angina. If the plaque ruptures and intracoronary thrombosis ensues, the patient develops unstable angina (if blood flow is only intermittently stopped) or myocardial infarction (if relatively long-lasting thrombosis develops). Each of these syndromes causes characteristic symptoms and findings on the ECG. Recognition of the clinical coronary syndromes and a clear understanding of the pathophysiology of coronary artery disease is necessary for all physicians.

KEY POINTS

- Atherosclerosis is the most common form of coronary artery disease. The atherosclerotic process appears to be an inflammatory and proliferative response to repeated injury to the vessel wall.
- Atherosclerosis involves the abnormal and complex interaction of three circulating cell types: monocytes, platelets, and lymphocytes, and two vessel wall cells: endothelial cells and smooth muscle cells.
- Rupture of the atherosclerotic plaque initiates the process of thrombosis. Thrombosis involves the interaction between platelets and the coagulation system.
- Coronary ischemic syndromes are due to the interaction between the atherosclerotic process and thrombosis, which can reduce or stop blood flow to a portion of the heart. In *stable angina*, slow progression of the atherosclerotic process limits blood flow when metabolic demand is increased. In *unstable angina*, surface rupture of an atherosclerotic lesion results in transient vessel occlusion as a result of thrombus. In *myocardial infarction*, deep fissuring of the atherosclerotic lesion leads to persistent thrombus formation.
- Clinically, coronary ischemic syndromes can be identified by using the patient history, myocardial enzyme levels, and the ECG.
- All therapies for the treatment of coronary ischemic syndromes are aimed at improving blood flow to the ischemic area or reducing myocardial demand.

Case Study:
Resolution

Mr. Hendrickson was in the midst of an acute inferior myocardial infarction resulting from occlusion of the right coronary artery. He was treated with aspirin, nitroglycerin, heparin, and t-PA. Increased plasmin production by t-PA resulted in lysis of the occlusive thrombus; his pain resolved with reestablishment of flow to myocardial tissue supplied by the right coronary artery. His CK level peaked at 2000 at 12 hours after the initial onset of chest pain. Two days later, the patient began to complain of recurrent chest pain and was promptly taken to the cardiac catherization laboratory. There, injection of dye into his right coronary artery showed obstruction of his right coronary artery. He underwent percutaneous transluminal coronary angioplasty (PTCA) of this lesion, and the final angiogram is seen in Fig. 3-39. In PTCA, a balloon is placed at the site of the lesion; the balloon is inflated, which reduces the amount of narrowing associated with the atherosclerotic lesion (Fig. 3-40). Alternatively, he could have undergone coronary artery bypass graft surgery (CABG) in which arteries and veins from different parts of the body are grafted to the coronary artery distal to the obstruction (Fig. 3-40C). The choice between medicines, angioplasty, and surgery depends on a number of factors including lesion number and severity, presence or absence of myocardial damage, and patient preference.

For the student, the major point of this case is to understand the pathophysiologic mechanisms of different coronary ischemic syndromes and to use this knowledge as a basis for understanding the clinical presentation, diagnosis, and medical therapies for coronary artery disease.

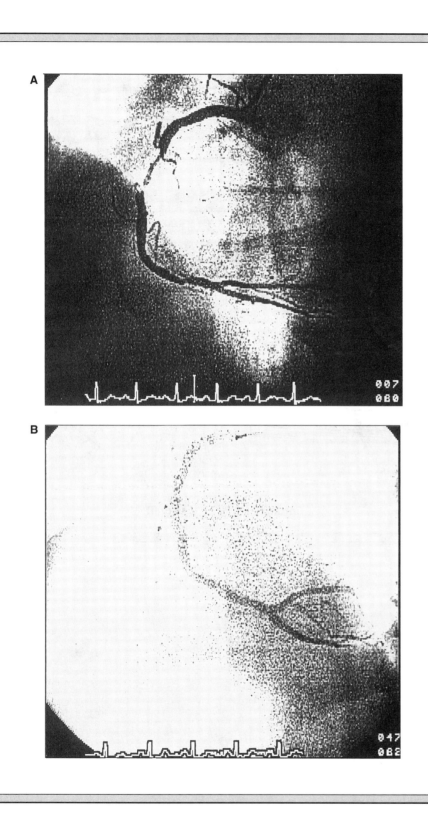

FIG. 3-39
ANGIOGRAM OF MR. HENDRICK-
SON'S RIGHT CORONARY AR-
TERY BEFORE (A) AND AFTER
(B) ANGIOPLASTY.

FIG. 3-40
MECHANICAL METHODS FOR TREATING A FLOW-LIMITING ATHEROSCLEROTIC LESION. (A) In angioplasty a special balloon catheter is placed at the lesion and inflated. This tends to compress and crack the atherosclerotic lesion. Recently an improvement to the angioplasty technique has been developed. (B) A stent is placed on a balloon. After inflation the stent remains in place, reducing recoil of the vessel. (C) Finally, the lesion can be bypassed with a separate conduit by cardiac surgery. The best conduit is the internal mammary artery. The saphenous vein is also commonly used.

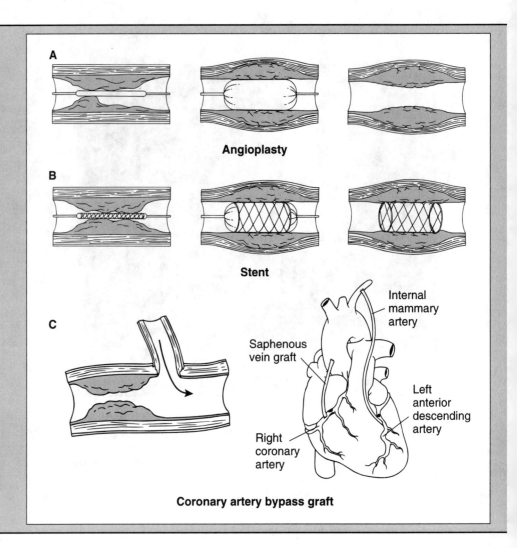

■ REVIEW QUESTIONS

Directions: For each of the following questions, choose the **one best** answer.

1. Which of the following statements is true regarding vascular smooth muscle cells?

   (A) Calcium (Ca^{2+}) binds to troponin-C, which increases actin and myosin cross-bridging.
   (B) Nitric oxide (NO) in normal states increases smooth muscle contraction by a mechanism that results in decreased intracellular Ca^{2+} levels.
   (C) Vasoconstriction by endothelin I is mediated by a mechanism causing an increase in intracellular Ca^{2+} levels.
   (D) Smooth muscle cells do not have synthetic capabilities for various mediators involved in atherosclerosis.

2. Trixie Lunsford, a 49-year-old patient with a long history of hyperlipidemia, diabetes mellitus, hypertension, and tobacco use, presents to the physician's office for a fasting lipid profile. She has the following findings: total cholesterol, 290 mg/dL; triglycerides, 150 mg/dL; high-density lipoprotein (HDL), 20 mg/dL; and low-density lipoprotein (LDL), 240 mg/dL. Which of the following statements is correct regarding the management of this patient?

   (A) The patient would benefit from lipid-lowering therapy.
   (B) The patient will not benefit from antioxidant therapy.
   (C) Dietary therapy alone should be the first step in managing this patient.
   (D) The patient does not have a higher risk for cardiovascular mortality if the hypercholesterolemia is left untreated.
   (E) Lipoprotein (a) [Lp(a)] decreases the risk of thrombus formation by competitively inhibiting plasminogen binding.

3. Which of the following will make the atherosclerotic lesion rupture and accompanying thrombosis more likely?

   (A) High smooth muscle content in a plaque
   (B) Higher concentration of macrophages in a plaque
   (C) Thick fibrous cap
   (D) Increased local nitric oxide
   (E) Decreased platelet aggregability and hypercoagulability

4. Justis Johnson, a 56-year-old man with a history of known hyperlipidemia, obesity, and hypertension, had sudden onset of midsternal chest tightness radiating to his left arm, with shortness of breath and diaphoresis, after his favorite football team was beaten on a last-second touchdown. The pain was constant. On arrival at the emergency room his blood pressure was 95/50, pulse 90, and he appeared very anxious. A 12-lead electrocardiogram (ECG) is shown below. Which of the following statements is true regarding this patient?

   (A) The pattern on ECG is suggestive of subendocardial ischemia.
   (B) Prompt reperfusion therapy is indicated.
   (C) The likely ischemic territory is the inferior wall.
   (D) His endothelium is functioning normally.
   (E) Q waves will not likely develop if this is left untreated.

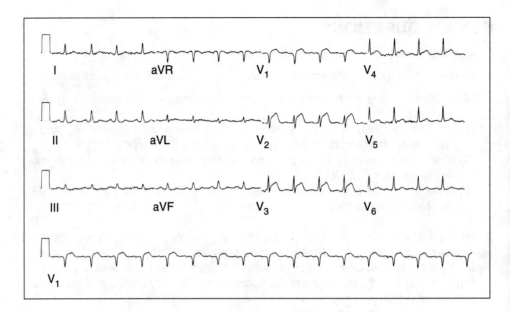

5. Which of the following statements regarding acute myocardial infarctions is true?

   (A) Anterior and anteroseptal myocardial infarctions are almost always due to disease of the left anterior descending (LAD) coronary artery.
   (B) In a left dominant system, the right coronary artery supplies the lateral wall of the left ventricle.
   (C) The sinus node and the atrioventricular (AV) node are normally supplied by the LAD coronary artery.
   (D) ECG findings in a non–Q-wave myocardial infarction are very specific and often make the diagnosis.
   (E) The ECG in acute myocardial infarctions always demonstrates ST-segment elevation.

ANSWERS AND EXPLANATIONS

1. The answer is C. Endothelin I is derived from preproendothelin in endothelial cells. Endothelin I functions by binding to a membrane receptor and activating phospholipase C resulting in inositol triphosphate (IP_3) production. IP_3 releases Ca^{2+} from the sarcoplasmic reticulum into the cytoplasm. This results in vasoconstriction. Choice A is incorrect because troponin-C is not present in smooth muscle. Choice B is incorrect because NO causes smooth muscle relaxation, not contraction. Choice D is incorrect because smooth muscle can synthesize many mediators in atherosclerosis (see text for details).

2. The answer is A. The National Cholesterol Education Program (NCEP) formulated guidelines regarding treatment decisions based on LDL cholesterol levels. In patients without coronary artery disease and two or more risk factors, drug treatment is indicated if the LDL level prior to therapy is $\geq$ 190 mg/dL. Diet therapy should be used in conjunction with drug therapy for this patient. Antioxidant therapy may be beneficial in this patient. Several recent trials have demonstrated an improved long-term mortality from lipid-lowering therapy in patients with hypercholesterolemia.

3. The answer is B. Several histologic characteristics in an atherosclerotic plaque can predispose to disruption. They include a soft atheromatous lipid-rich core, decreased smooth muscle density, and increased macrophage activity and number. NO levels are lower in plaques, and this is perhaps related to a breakdown of NO by superoxide in injured tissue. Hypercoagulability and increased platelet activity are important characteristics in thrombosis.

4. The answer is B. The ECG in the question shows marked ST-segment elevation in the anterior leads. The patient has acute thrombotic occlusion of his left anterior descending coronary artery and is in the midst of an anterior wall myocardial infarction. No ST-segment elevation is observed in the inferior leads, which suggests the inferior wall is being perfused normally. Patients with only subendocardial ischemia usually do not have ST-segment elevation on the ECG. In a patient with this ECG and active chest pain, prompt reperfusion therapy is indicated to preserve viable myocardium. If this is left untreated, transmural myocardial necrosis will follow, and Q waves will be seen in the anterior and possibly lateral leads on the ECG. As described in the text, endothelium is dysfunctional in diseased states.

5. The answer is A. The LAD coronary artery supplies the anterior wall and courses to the apex. Septal perforators arise from the LAD and supply the anterior two-thirds of the interventricular septum. The right coronary artery primarily supplies the inferior and basal septal walls as well as the sinus and AV nodes. In a left dominant system, the right coronary artery is often a very small vessel that supplies the right ventricular free wall only. ST-segment changes in a non–Q-wave myocardial infarction are nonspecific and can be present in other conditions unrelated to coronary artery disease.

REFERENCES

Fuster V: Lewis A. Conner memorial lecture: mechanisms leading to myocardial infarction: insights from studies of vascular biology. *Circulation* 90:2126–2146, 1994.

Hayden MR, Reidy M: Many roads lead to atheroma. *Nat Med* 1:22–31, 1995.

Kleiman NS: Treatment of acute myocardial infarction. *Cardiol Clin* 13:283–470, 1995.

Levine GN, Keaney JF Jr, Vita JF: Cholesterol reduction in cardiovascular disease: clinical benefits and possible mechanisms. *N Engl J Med* 332:512–519, 1995.

Ross R: The pathogenesis of atherosclerosis: a perspective for the 1990s. *Nature* 362:801–808, 1993.

Chapter 4

VALVULAR HEART DISEASE

Andrew U. Chai, M.D., and Fred M. Kusumoto, M.D.

■ CHAPTER OUTLINE

Case Study:
Introduction

A previously healthy 36-year-old woman presented to her physician complaining of a recent increase in shortness of breath and fatigue. She had been in her usual state of good health until 2 months previously when she first noticed that she could not finish her usual evening walk without stopping to rest. Her stamina and breathing had suddenly worsened several days before and now she complained of shortness of breath at rest. She had noticed that her heart rate was irregular and relatively fast even when she was resting. At night she now could have a sudden sensation of breathlessness, which was relieved by sitting up. She often could not sleep lying flat in bed and often fell asleep sitting up in a chair.

Physical examination revealed several significant findings. She was a thin woman who was obviously short of breath. Her pulse was irregularly irregular and was rapid (approximately 120 beats/min) with a blood pressure of 92/58 mm Hg. The lung examination revealed crackles heard over the lower half of both sides. Cardiac examination was significant for an irregularly irregular weak arterial pulse, mild bilateral lower extremity edema, and a right ventricular heave. Cardiac auscultation revealed an irregularly irregular rhythm, an accentuated pulmonic second sound (P_2), an opening snap, and a low-frequency diastolic rumble heard best at the apex. An elevated jugular venous pressure was estimated to be 10 mm Hg. An electrocardiogram (ECG) is shown in Fig. 4-1. What are the underlying reasons for this patient's symptoms? Why did her symptoms suddenly worsen?

FIG. 4-1
THE PATIENT'S ELECTROCARDIOGRAM.

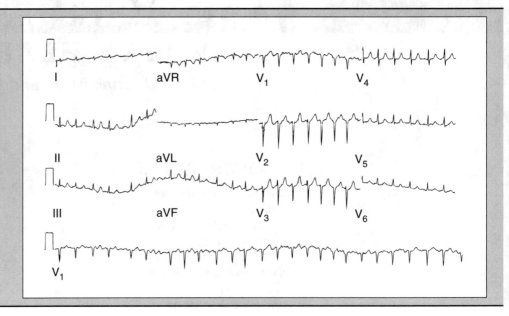

INTRODUCTION

The primary function of the cardiac valves is to allow unidirectional flow of blood through the cardiac chambers. The normal valve performs this function without causing obstruction or reversal of flow, which ensures efficient transformation of energy from myocardial contraction into circulation of blood throughout the body.

The heart contains four valves; two are semilunar and two are atrioventricular. The two semilunar valves, the pulmonic and aortic, are located at the outflow tract of the right and left ventricles, respectively (Fig. 4-2). The two atrioventricular (AV) valves are located between the atria and the ventricles (Fig. 4-3). The tricuspid valve separates the right atrium and right ventricle, and the mitral valve performs the same function for the left chambers. The cardiac valves consist of a central collagenous core covered by a fibroelastic tissue rich in mucopolysaccharides. The "fibrous rings" of the four valves interconnect to form the backbone of the cardiac skeleton (Fig. 4-4).

Malfunction of the cardiac valves results in an obstruction (stenosis) or regurgitation of flow (insufficiency). Although the two conditions often coexist, the pathophysiology is usually dominated by either obstruction or regurgitation, not both. When the valves malfunction, compensatory mechanisms initially allow the heart to function efficiently; however, over time, these mechanisms may become inadequate and the heart eventually fails to meet the metabolic requirements of the body. Signs and symptoms of valvular disease develop, and the patient comes to the physician.

The epidemiology and presentation of valvular disease has changed considerably since the advent and widespread use of effective antibiotics. Rheumatic heart disease is no longer the most common etiology of valvular disease and is uncommon in developed countries. Congenital, degenerative, and infective etiologies are prevalent in patients presenting with valvular disease.

Although rheumatic valvular disease may not be common today, early recognition and diagnosis of valvular disease are more important than ever. This is because major advances in recognition, evaluation, and surgical treatment during the past 2 decades have yielded striking improvements in quality of life and long-term survival for patients with valvular heart disease.

After a brief review of normal cardiac and valvular physiology, the pathophysiology of regurgitant and stenotic lesions is considered individually for each valve.

Semilunar valves are the aortic and pulmonic valves.
Atrioventricular valves are the mitral and tricuspid valves.

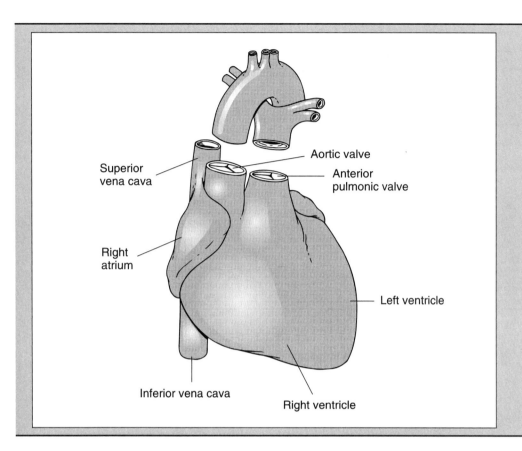

FIG. 4-2
ANTERIOR VIEW OF THE HEART.
The great vessels (aorta, main pulmonary artery) are cut and lifted to expose the anterior pulmonic valve and, just posterior and to the right of the pulmonic valve, the aortic valve.

Aortic valve

Anterior pulmonic valve

Superior vena cava

Right atrium

Left ventricle

Inferior vena cava

Right ventricle

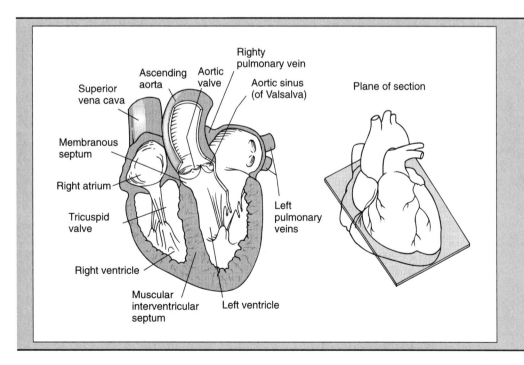

FIG. 4-3
THE HEART CUT IN HALF AND OPENED, EXPOSING THE MITRAL AND TRICUSPID VALVES.

Righty pulmonary vein

Ascending aorta

Aortic valve

Aortic sinus (of Valsalva)

Plane of section

Superior vena cava

Membranous septum

Right atrium

Tricuspid valve

Left pulmonary veins

Right ventricle

Muscular interventricular septum

Left ventricle

FIG. 4-4
FIBROUS SKELETON OF THE HEART. The atria and great vessels are removed so that the relationship of the four valves can be appreciated. The aortic valve is wedged between the mitral and tricuspid valves, and the pulmonic valve is the most anterior.

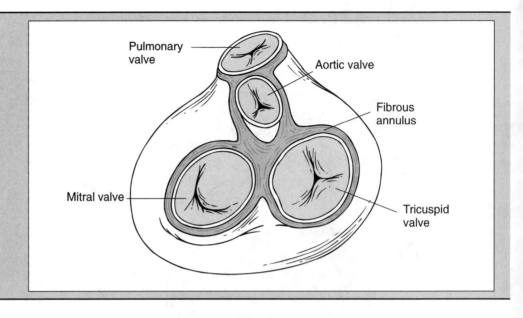

■ NORMAL VALVULAR PHYSIOLOGY

Valvular function can be evaluated by pressure–time analysis or pressure–volume analysis.

Normal physiology of the heart can be examined using *pressure–time (temporal)* or *pressure–volume* analysis. Understanding both methods of analyzing ventricular function allows a clear understanding of the pathophysiologic mechanisms that occur with valvular diseases.

PRESSURE–TIME (TEMPORAL) ANALYSIS

Fig. 4-5 shows the temporal relationship between the surface ECG, heart sounds, left ventricular volume, and aortic, left ventricular, and left atrial pressure. By studying Fig. 4-5 closely, one can get a better understanding of the relationship between the different phases of the cardiac cycle, the ECG, and the heart sounds. Traditionally, the cardiac cycle is divided into ventricular *diastole*, when open mitral and tricuspid valves allow left and right ventricular filling, and ventricular *systole*, when contraction of the left and right ventricles causes ejection of blood through the aortic and pulmonic valves into the systemic and pulmonary circulations, respectively. Parallel events occur in the right and left chambers; this discussion focuses on the left atrium and left ventricle.

Cardiac Cycle
- Diastole: ventricular relaxation and filling
    Isovolumic relaxation
    Rapid (early) filling phase
    Diastasis
    Atrial systole
- Systole: ventricular contraction
    Isovolumic contraction
    Ejection phase

Ventricular Diastole. During ventricular contraction, the mitral valve is closed and blood collects in the atrium. When ventricular contraction is completed, the ventricle begins relaxing. Shortly thereafter, the elevated pressures in the distended large arteries begin to push blood back toward the ventricle, causing the aortic valve to snap closed. Aortic valve closure marks the beginning of diastole. For the next 3–6 msec, the ventricular muscles continue to relax, even though the ventricular volume remains unchanged (mitral and aortic valves are closed), giving rise to the first period of diastole, *isovolumic relaxation*. When ventricular pressure falls to a level lower than atrial pressure, the mitral valve opens, and there ensues rapid filling of the ventricle with the accumulated blood in the left atrium. The *rapid filling phase* lasts approximately the first third of diastole. In the middle third of diastole the ventricular volume changes very little, since there is only passive inflow of blood from the pulmonary venous system. This phase is sometimes referred to as *diastasis*. In the last third of diastole the atrium contracts (*atrial systole*) and accounts for the final portion of ventricular filling (approximately 20%–30%).

Ventricular Systole. Ventricular systole can be divided into two parts, isovolumic contraction and the ejection phase. Immediately following the completion of ventricular filling, ventricular systole begins. Ventricular contraction causes the ventricular pressure to rise rapidly, which closes the mitral valve. Then an additional 2–3 msec are required for the ventricle to build up enough pressure to push the aortic valve open against aortic pressure. Therefore, during this phase the left ventricle is contracting, but both the mitral and aortic valves are closed and there is no change in ventricular volume. This period is called the period of *isovolumic*, or isometric, *contraction* because there is an increase in myocardial muscle tension without change in ventricular volume or shortening of the muscle fibers.

As the ventricular pressure rises above aortic diastolic pressure, the aortic valve opens. Blood immediately begins to flow out of the ventricle with about 70% of the stroke volume (the difference between end-diastolic volume and end-systolic volume) ejected during the first third of the ejection phase and the remaining 30% ejected in the second two-thirds of the ejection phase. Therefore, the first third of systole is sometimes called the phase of rapid ejection and the second two-thirds, the phase of slow ejection. The ventricle begins to relax, and once aortic pressure becomes greater than left ventricular pressure, the aortic valve closes, and the cycle repeats.

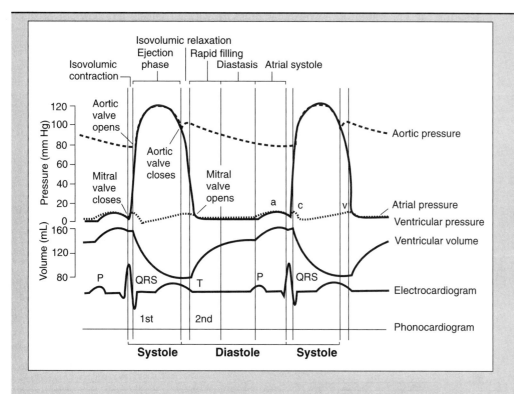

FIG. 4-5
THE RELATIONSHIPS AMONG HEART SOUNDS, ELECTROCARDIOGRAM, LEFT VENTRICULAR VOLUME, AND AORTIC, LEFT VENTRICULAR AND LEFT ATRIAL PRESSURE IN A NORMAL HEART. There are four phases in diastole. First, during the *isovolumic relaxation period*, the ventricle is relaxing, and both the aortic and mitral valves are closed (no volume changes in the ventricle). Second, when ventricular pressure drops below atrial pressure, the mitral valve opens and the *rapid filling phase* begins. During the third period of diastole, *diastasis*, left ventricular volume filling slows. The final period of diastole, *atrial systole*, is responsible for the final portion of ventricular filling. Systole represents ventricular contraction. In the first phase of systole, *isovolumic contraction*, the mitral valve and aortic valve are closed. When the intraventricular pressure becomes greater than aortic pressure, the aortic valve opens, and blood is ejected into the body. This is the second period of systole, called the *ejection period*. (*Source:* Guyton AC: *Textbook of Medical Physiology*, 8th ed. Philadelphia, PA: W. B. Saunders, 1991, p 102.)

PRESSURE–VOLUME ANALYSIS

The different phases of the cardiac cycle described above can also be depicted using pressure–volume analysis. Much can be learned about the functional capabilities of the heart (or any pump for that matter) by studying the relationship between volume and pressure. Although pressure–volume relationships can be examined for any cardiac chamber (right or left atria and right or left ventricles), since the left ventricle is primarily responsible for systemic circulation of blood, pressure–volume analysis of the left ventricle is most commonly used and is reviewed here. Pressure–volume analysis requires an understanding of two curves. First, the *diastolic pressure curve* is generated by progressively filling the ventricle with larger volumes of blood and measuring the intraventricular

Pressure–volume analysis is generated from two curves:

1. Diastolic pressure curve measures "passive" compliance properties of the ventricle.
2. Isovolumic systolic pressure curve measures the "active" ability of the ventricle to generate pressure.

pressure. The diastolic pressure curve measures the compliance of the ventricle (Fig. 4-6). In a normally compliant heart, the diastolic pressure curve remains relatively flat, and the pressure does not rise significantly until the end-diastolic volume reaches 150 mL. Above this volume, the pressure curve becomes steeper and rises more rapidly, because the heart has reached the compliance plateau and cannot tolerate a further increase in volume without a significant increase in pressure. There are two reasons for the compliance plateau: (1) the myofibrils reach their absolute limit and cannot stretch further, and (2) the pericardium, which surrounds the heart, begins to have a constraining effect.

The second important curve for pressure–volume analysis is the *isovolumic systolic pressure curve* (Fig. 4-7). The isovolumic systolic pressure curve is generated by filling the ventricle to a given amount of volume, allowing the ventricle to contract, and then measuring the generated intraventricular pressure without letting any flow out of the ventricle (fixed volume). By the Starling relationship, as the ventricle is filled with more fluid, the pressure generated during contraction is initially higher. However, at high filling volumes the systolic pressure begins to drop as individual sarcomeres stretch and

FIG. 4-6
DIASTOLIC PRESSURE CURVE OF THE LEFT VENTRICLE.

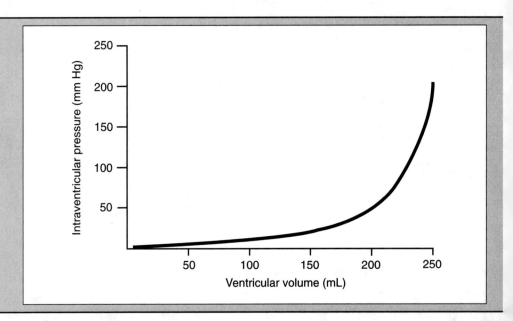

FIG. 4-7
ISOVOLUMIC SYSTOLIC PRESSURE CURVE OF THE LEFT VENTRICLE. The ventricle is filled to varying amounts. The ventricle is allowed to contract but not allowed to expel blood. The pressure generated at different amounts of filling generates the isovolumic systolic pressure curve.

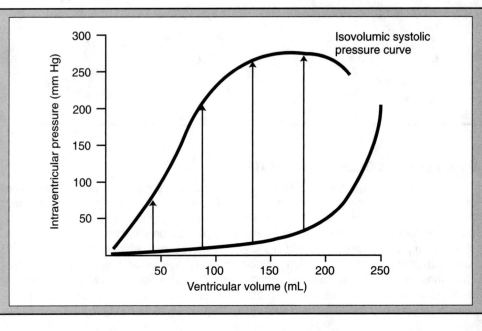

become relatively inefficient. This is because as myofibrils stretch, the interaction between the actin and myosin fibers is no longer optimum and the myocardium cannot generate the same degree of contractile force.

The diastolic pressure curve and the isovolumic systolic pressure curve can be combined to generate a pressure–volume diagram (Fig. 4-8). Point A in Fig. 4-8 represents mitral valve opening and the beginning of ventricular filling (start of the early filling phase). There are approximately 50 mL of blood that remain in the ventricle after the completion of the previous systole; this is referred to as the end-systolic volume. The ventricular pressure at this time is normally close to zero. As the ventricle passively fills, the pressure begins to rise very slowly until it reaches the end of diastole at point B. The ventricular volume at point B is called the end-diastolic volume and is approximately 120 mL. The pressure at this point is referred to as the end-diastolic pressure and is usually about 5 mm Hg. Therefore, the pressure–volume curve in diastole extends from point A to point B and is labeled I, with the volume increasing from 50 mL to 120 mL and the pressure increasing from 0 mm Hg to 5 mm Hg. This portion of the pressure–volume curve corresponds to most of diastole (early filling phase, diastasis, and atrial contraction).

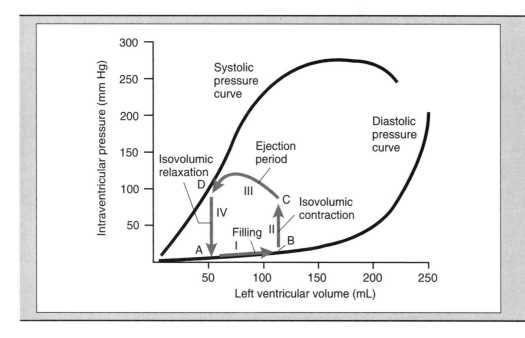

FIG. 4-8
PRESSURE–VOLUME RELATION-SHIP OF THE LEFT VENTRICLE. The diastolic pressure curve and the isovolumic systolic pressure curve are combined here to generate a pressure–volume curve. Ventricular filling begins at point A and continues to point B (end diastole) along the diastolic pressure curve (I). Ventricular systole is composed of isovolumic contraction (II) and the ejection period (III). Diastole begins with isovolumic relaxation (IV).

During the isovolumic contraction phase of systole, the ventricular volume remains the same but the pressure rises sharply and moves the curve from point B to point C and is labeled II. This is the point at which the intraventricular pressure equals the diastolic aortic pressure and the aortic valve opens to start the ejection phase. As soon as the aortic valve opens, the ventricular volume decreases, but ventricular pressure continues to rise as a result of continued myocardial contraction. The ejection phase is labeled III on the curve, and moves the curve from point C to D. At the end of the ejection phase, aortic pressure becomes greater than ventricular pressure, and the valve closes, starting the isovolumic relaxation period, which is labeled IV and marks the beginning of diastole. During isovolumic relaxation, the ventricular volume remains constant but the pressure falls rapidly, moving the pressure volume curve from point D to point A, which completes the cardiac cycle.

Knowledge of the function of the normal left ventricle and how it relates to pressure, volume, heart sounds, and ECG provides the basis for understanding valvular heart diseases and how each valve lesion affects these relationships.

■ DISEASES OF THE AORTIC VALVE

Aortic valve diseases are classified as aortic stenosis or aortic regurgitation.

The normal aortic valve is a symmetric structure with three equal cusps. These have been named the left, right, and noncoronary cusps. This is because the left and right main epicardial coronary arteries arise from the left and right sinuses of Valsalva, respectively, and no coronary arteries arise from the noncoronary sinus of Valsalva. The normal function of the aortic valve is to allow blood to flow from the left ventricle to the body without obstruction or regurgitation. Functionally, aortic valve diseases can be divided into those that cause an obstruction at the aortic valve (aortic valve stenosis) or cause a leaky aortic valve (aortic valve regurgitation).

AORTIC STENOSIS

Obstruction at the valvular, subvalvular, or supravalvular level may cause obstruction of blood flow from the left ventricle to the aorta. Discussion here is limited to valvular aortic stenosis. Subvalvular obstruction resulting from septal hypertrophy is discussed in Chap. 1. Discussion of supravalvular obstruction is beyond the scope of this chapter. The pathophysiologic effects of supravalvular obstruction are similar to valvular obstruction.

Etiology. The causes of aortic stenosis can be divided into congenital and acquired forms (Table 4-1). In congenital aortic stenosis, the valve can be unicuspid, bicuspid, or tricuspid with fused commissures. Congenital causes of aortic stenosis are more common in younger patients and usually present before the age of 50 years. Rheumatic and degenerative (senile) aortic stenoses are the two most common types of acquired aortic stenosis. In rheumatic aortic stenosis, the cusps and commissures become fused from an inflammatory response initiated by group A *Streptococcus* infection that results in retraction and stiffening of the cusps. Therefore, rheumatic aortic stenosis is often accompanied by aortic regurgitation. It is also unusual to have rheumatic aortic stenosis without involvement of the mitral valve. Degenerative, or senile, calcific aortic stenosis, the most common type in adults, is a result of normal mechanical wear and tear. Calcium is deposited at the base of the cusps and prevents the valve cusps from opening normally during systole.

Table 4-1
Causes of Aortic Stenoses

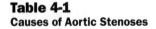

Congenital		Unicuspid valve
		Bicuspid valve
		Fused commissures
Acquired		Rheumatic heart disease
		Degenerative (senile) calcific aortic valve disease

Pathophysiology. The normal aortic valve area is approximately 2.5–3.5 cm². As the orifice of the aortic valve progressively narrows, a pressure gradient develops between the left ventricle and the aorta (Figs. 4-9 and 4-10). One might expect to see both a rise in the left ventricular pressure and a fall in the aortic pressure as the valve progressively narrows, but the compensatory mechanisms that control the pressures in the systemic arterial circulation tend to maintain mean aortic pressure at or near a normal level. However, the pulse pressure in patients with aortic stenosis is somewhat reduced as a result of the prolonged ejection phase of ventricular contraction. For this reason, the main abnormalities seen in aortic stenosis are a rise in left ventricular pressure during systole and a decreased cardiac output (CO).

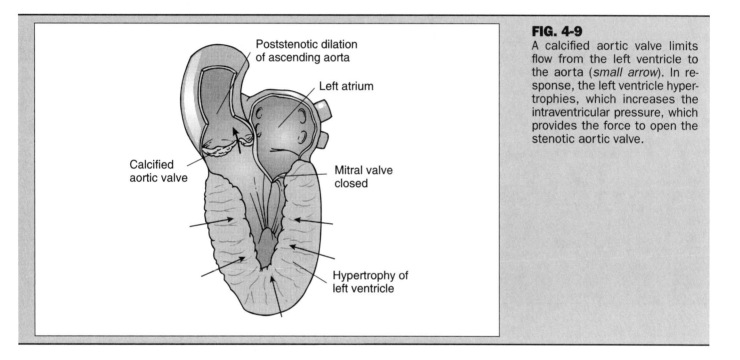

FIG. 4-9
A calcified aortic valve limits flow from the left ventricle to the aorta (*small arrow*). In response, the left ventricle hypertrophies, which increases the intraventricular pressure, which provides the force to open the stenotic aortic valve.

The left ventricle responds to this pressure gradient and pressure overload by becoming hypertrophic to maintain forward CO. This compensatory mechanism allows the left ventricle to sustain a large pressure gradient across the aortic valve for many years with only minimal reduction in CO and without left ventricular dilatation or the development of symptoms. The compensatory mechanism seen in aortic stenosis can be better understood by examining Laplace's law for a sphere, where wall stress (σ) is proportional to the product of pressure (p) and cavitary radius (r) and inversely proportional to wall thickness (h):

$$\sigma = \frac{p \times r}{2h}$$

Wall stress increases as the pressure gradient across the aortic valve increases. The left ventricle compensates for this increased wall stress by increasing wall thickness while the radius remains unchanged, therefore keeping increases in wall stress to a minimum. However, this compensatory mechanism is not without its cost. Left ventricular compliance decreases as wall thickness increases, resulting in a significant increase in left ventricular end-diastolic pressure, prolonged ejection phase, and shortened diastole. This is illustrated in Fig. 4-11, a pressure–volume curve for a patient with severe aortic stenosis. As illustrated, the decrease in left ventricular compliance results in the diastolic portion of the pressure–volume curve becoming steeper, thus resulting in a higher end-diastolic pressure for a given end-diastolic volume. These changes eventually lead to a decrease in coronary perfusion gradient and perfusion time as well as increased oxygen demand, eventually producing angina. Elevated end-diastolic pressure leads to left atrial

FIG. 4-10

RELATIONSHIPS AMONG LEFT VENTRICULAR PRESSURE, AORTIC PRESSURE, ELECTROCARDIOGRAM, AND HEART SOUNDS IN AORTIC STENOSIS. The obstruction to blood flow across the stenotic aortic valve causes a systolic pressure gradient and marked elevation in systolic ventricular pressure. The mean arterial pressure in aortic stenosis is usually normal, but the upstroke is delayed. The flow of blood across the stenotic valve results in a harsh systolic murmur (SM), and a fourth heart sound (S_4) is usually present, since the left atrium contracts against a stiff left ventricle. If the aortic valve is stenotic but still relatively compliant (congenital abnormality of the aortic valve), a high-frequency ejection click (EC) can sometimes be appreciated in early systole, just after the first heart sound (S_1).

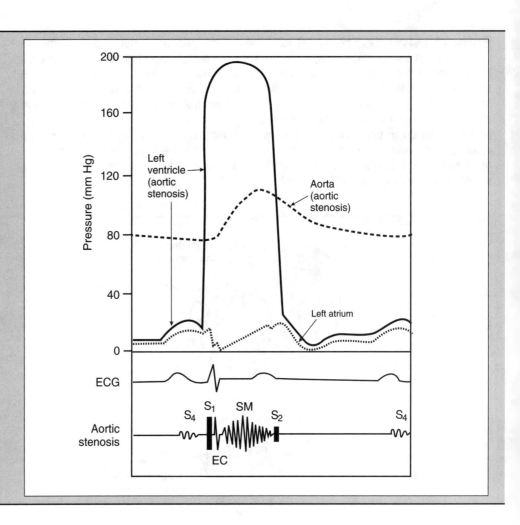

hypertension and eventually pulmonary venous hypertension, producing symptoms of dyspnea. This can be better understood by examining the pressure–volume curve for the normal heart and the heart with aortic stenosis. In the patient with aortic stenosis, the compliance of the ventricle decreases; therefore, for the same change in volume, the pressure curve rises more steeply as the ventricle fills. This also results in a slight reduction in the ventricular volume at end diastole, resulting in a lower stroke volume (SV). In addition, the ventricle has to work harder in order to achieve this level of forward output. However, as the aortic stenosis worsens, systolic ventricular function also begins to fail and the systolic portion of the pressure–volume curve becomes less steep, resulting in a higher end-systolic volume and therefore a smaller SV [Fig. 4-12].

Clinical Presentation Patients with aortic stenosis remain asymptomatic during the long latent phase of the disease. Symptoms develop as the valve orifice gradually narrows and the obstruction results in an ever increasing pressure load to the left ventricle. The most common presenting symptom is *angina*, followed by *syncope*, then *congestive heart failure (CHF)*. The presence of symptoms usually indicates clinically severe stenosis (aortic valve area < 0.8 cm2), which portends a poor outcome if left untreated. Typically, angina is caused by obstruction of blood flow in the coronary arteries by atherosclerotic plaques (see Chap. 3). However, only half of the patients with aortic stenosis who present with angina have clinically significant coronary artery disease. Angina in the other half of patients is due to increased oxygen demand by increased myocardial wall thickness and tension resulting from increases in intraventricular pressure (Fig. 4-13). This rise in intraventricular pressure decreases the coronary perfusion gradient, resulting in decreased coronary blood flow.

Syncope (transient loss of consciousness) in patients with aortic stenosis is usually brought on by exertion. This is a result of systemic vasodilatation in response to exercise in the presence of a fixed CO; therefore, the patient is unable to maintain an adequate cerebral perfusion pressure, resulting in syncope. Syncope at rest is much less common and is probably related to transient arrhythmias, including atrial fibrillation and ventricular tachycardia and fibrillation. Sudden death in previously asymptomatic patients is very rare. The presence of CHF suggests very advanced disease with ventricular dysfunction and is related to a very poor prognosis when compared to those patients with angina or syncope (Fig. 4-14).

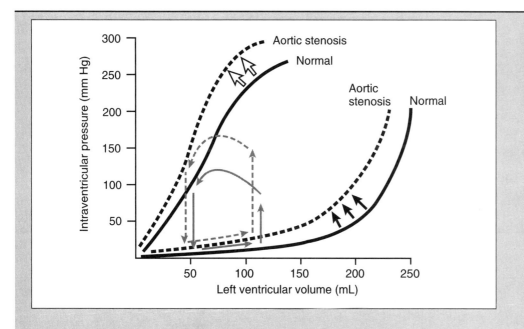

FIG. 4-11
PRESSURE–VOLUME CURVE UNDER NORMAL CONDITIONS (*SOLID LINE*) AND IN COMPENSATED AORTIC STENOSIS (*DASHED LINE*). In aortic stenosis, the left ventricle must contract against the narrowed aortic valve (increased afterload). Ejection begins only when intraventricular pressure becomes high enough to open the stenotic aortic valve (150 mm Hg). To maintain adequate stroke volume, the left ventricle hypertrophies, which shifts the isovolumic systolic pressure curve to the left (*open arrows*). Left ventricular hypertrophy causes the diastolic filling curve to shift upward (*filled arrows*), which leads to elevated end-diastolic pressures. The left ventricle maintains an adequate cardiac output by increasing its wall thickness and systolic function. This shifts the diastolic filling curve up and the systolic curve to the left, resulting in higher end-diastolic and -systolic pressures.

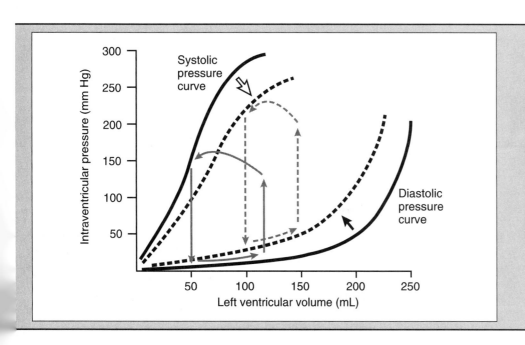

FIG. 4-12
PRESSURE–VOLUME CURVE IN DECOMPENSATED AORTIC STENOSIS (*DASHED LINES*). The systolic function of the left ventricle wanes, which shifts the systolic pressure curve to the right. The left ventricle is not able to generate enough force, which leads to reduced stroke volume (140 mL − 100 mL = 40 mL) and elevated end-diastolic pressures (approximately 40 mm Hg). Both of these changes result in clinical symptoms of heart failure.

FIG. 4-13

DIAGRAMMATIC REPRESENTATION OF THE PATHOPHYSIOLOGY OF AORTIC STENOSIS. The increased obstruction to left ventricular (LV) outflow results in an increased left ventricular systolic pressure, increased left ventricular diastolic pressure, and decreased aortic pressure. This results in an increase in left ventricular mass, increased oxygen consumption, and eventually, myocardial ischemia and left ventricular failure.

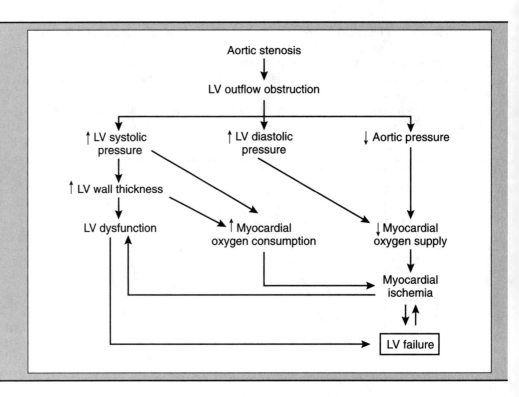

FIG. 4-14

NATURAL HISTORY OF AORTIC STENOSIS WITHOUT SURGICAL TREATMENT. Once symptoms develop, the prognosis is poor if the patient is untreated. (*Source:* Ross J Jr, Braunwald E: Aortic stenosis. *Circulation* 38 (Suppl V): 61, 1968.)

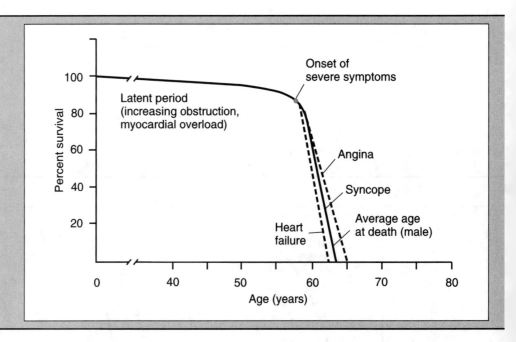

Physical Examination

Arterial Pulses. In severe aortic stenosis, the arterial pulse is slow to peak and is weak and sustained and is termed *pulsus tardus et parvus* (late and weak). Pulsus tardus may be detected by simultaneously palpating the apex and the carotid artery, which reveals a distinct lag in transmission of the arterial pulse from the left ventricle to the carotid arteries. Pulsus parvus manifests as decreased pulse and systolic pressures. However, the pulse pressure may be normal in patients with concomitant aortic regurgitation or in older patients with an inelastic arterial bed.

Venous Pressure. Inspection of the jugular venous pressure may reveal a prominent *a* wave resulting from a decrease in right ventricular compliance as a result of septal hypertrophy. In advanced aortic stenosis, pulmonary hypertension develops and is followed by right ventricular failure and tricuspid regurgitation, which results in a prominent *v* wave.

Auscultation. The first heart sound (S_1) is normal or soft in aortic stenosis. The second heart sound (S_2) undergoes several characteristic changes in the presence of aortic stenosis.

S_2 is made up of two components: an aortic component produced by aortic valve closure (A_2) and a pulmonic component produced by pulmonic valve closure (P_2) [Fig. 4-15]. During expiration, the P_2 is normally only 10–30 msec after the A_2, and the clinician normally can apprehend only a single S_2. However, since the late 1860s, it has been appreciated that with inspiration, S_2 normally splits (two distinct sounds can be heard). With inspiration, the pulmonary vascular bed becomes more compliant, and reduced pulmonary artery pressure causes a delayed P_2. In aortic stenosis, the aortic component of A_2 becomes progressively delayed as the degree of aortic stenosis worsens and the left ventricular ejection period becomes progressively longer. As A_2 becomes progressively delayed, paradoxic splitting of S_2 (two distinct sounds heard at expiration rather than inspiration) will occur. Paradoxic splitting can be heard in any condition that causes relative delay in aortic valve closure (e.g., left bundle branch block, LBBB). In addition to the abnormal pattern of S_2, the character of S_2 components changes in aortic stenosis. The A_2 becomes softer, since the excursion or valve mobility becomes progressively limited and the valve can no longer snap shut with enough force to generate an A_2 of normal intensity. P_2 increases in intensity as left heart failure leads to progressive pulmonary hypertension.

Auscultatory Findings in Aortic Stenosis
Paradoxically split S_2
Fourth heart sound (S_4)
Ejection click (congenital aortic stenosis only)
Systolic murmur ("diamond-shaped," harsh, radiates to the neck)

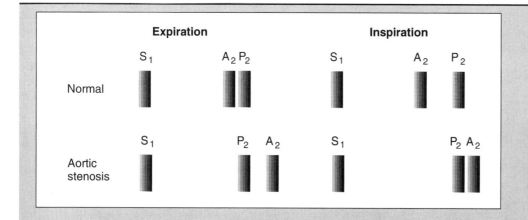

FIG. 4-15
DIAGRAMMATIC REPRESENTATION OF PHYSIOLOGIC VERSUS PARADOXIC SPLITTING OF THE SECOND HEART SOUND (S_2). Under normal conditions during expiration, the portion of S_2 produced by pulmonic valve closure (P_2) and the portion of S_2 produced by aortic valve closure (A_2) are superimposed. With inspiration, compliance in the pulmonary arterial bed decreases, normally causing a delay in P_2. In aortic stenosis, left ventricular hypertrophy and an increase in the ejection period causes A_2 to become delayed. P_2 still is delayed during inspiration, but because A_2 is delayed at baseline, S_2 "splits" during expiration.

In addition to changes in the pattern and character of S_2, aortic stenosis is associated with a prominent S_4 resulting from vigorous left atrial contraction against a stiff, high-pressure left ventricle (see Fig. 4-10). An aortic ejection sound (commonly called an "ejection click") may also be present early in the natural history of aortic stenosis. The ejection click is caused by the sudden opening of a stiff aortic valve early in ventricular systole; it is dependent on valve mobility and eventually disappears as the valves become calcified and fixed. Therefore, an ejection click related to aortic stenosis is most often present in children with congenital aortic stenosis. This sound is high pitched and occurs approximately 60 msec after S_1; it is heard best at the left sternal border with the diaphragm of the stethoscope.

The murmur of aortic stenosis is classically described as a "harsh" systolic murmur; it is best heard at the base of the heart and is transmitted to the carotid arteries. Unlike the murmur of mitral regurgitation, the murmur of aortic stenosis is not holosystolic. In the normal cardiac cycle there is an isovolumic contraction and relaxation period at the beginning and at the end of systole, respectively. During these periods there is no flow of blood across the aortic valve and therefore no murmur can be generated. This is the physiologic reason why the murmur of aortic stenosis starts a few milliseconds after S_1 and ends prior to S_2. The murmur characteristically has a "diamond-shaped" pattern, where the murmur's peak intensity is heard during midsystole. The murmur peaks later in systole as the degree of stenosis worsens, since a larger pressure gradient and therefore a longer ejection period are required to open the aortic valve. When the left ventricle begins to fail, the CO decreases, and the murmur becomes softer; therefore, the intensity of the murmur does *not* necessarily correlate with the severity of stenosis. Aortic stenosis murmurs increase in intensity with increases in SV; therefore, the murmur is louder with leg raising, which increases the volume of the ventricle at end diastole by increasing venous return. On the other hand, standing suddenly decreases the intensity of the murmur by reducing venous return, which in turn decreases SV by decreasing the volume at end diastole.

AORTIC REGURGITATION

Etiology. The etiology of aortic regurgitation in developed countries has changed significantly with the decline of rheumatic heart disease and syphilis. Aortic regurgitation can be caused by either primary disease of the leaflets or aortic root dilation (Fig. 4-16).

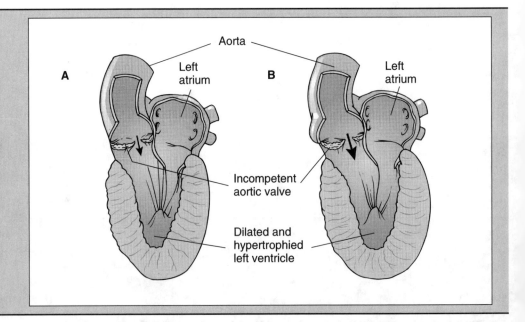

FIG. 4-16
CAUSES OF AORTIC REGURGITATION. (A) Scarring of the aortic valve has caused the leaflets to coapt incorrectly, which leads to regurgitation of blood (*arrow*) into the left ventricle during diastole. The volume load placed on the heart causes the left ventricle to dilate. (B) Dilation of the aortic root causes the leaflets of a normal aortic valve to separate, which results in poor leaflet coaptation and regurgitation of blood into the left ventricle.

Aorta

Left atrium

A

B

Left atrium

Incompetent aortic valve

Dilated and hypertrophied left ventricle

The presentation of **aortic regurgitation** depends on whether it develops acutely or chronically.

Pathophysiology. Aortic regurgitation is a problem related to left ventricular volume overload. Normally, no volume flows back into the left ventricle during diastole because the aortic valve is closed. In aortic regurgitation, however, some portion of the forward CO leaks back into the left ventricle during diastole, resulting in a decrease in the diastolic arterial pressure and an increase in diastolic pressure in the left ventricle (Fig. 4-17). The pathophysiology of aortic regurgitation depends on whether the leakage occurs suddenly (acute aortic regurgitation) or relatively slowly (chronic aortic regurgitation) over time.

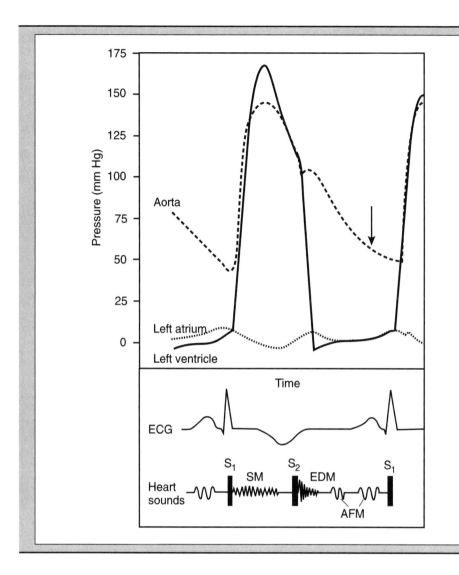

FIG. 4-17
RELATIONSHIPS AMONG LEFT VENTRICULAR PRESSURE, AORTIC PRESSURE, ELECTROCARDIOGRAM (ECG) AND HEART SOUNDS IN AORTIC REGURGITATION. Regurgitation of blood through the aortic valve during diastole causes the aortic pressure to fall dramatically (*arrow*). The regurgitant flow yields two murmurs. First, a high-frequency, early diastolic murmur (EDM) resulting from the turbulent regurgitant flow can be heard. Second, the regurgitant flow causes partial mitral valve closure, which can cause turbulent flow through the mitral valve. This functional "mitral stenosis" causes a mid- or late diastolic rumble (Austin Flint murmur, AFM), which was first described by Austin Flint in the early 1860s. Aortic and left ventricular pressures are increased during systole because the regurgitant volume during diastole increases the stroke volume (SV), which now must be ejected by the left ventricle. This increase in SV often causes a soft systolic ejection murmur (SM).

In patients with severe *acute aortic regurgitation*, the ventricle has not had time to adapt to the increased volume load. Therefore, the left ventricular end-diastolic pressure increases significantly as the additional volume to the left ventricle from the regurgitant fraction pushes the patient up the diastolic pressure curve. The net result is elevated left ventricular and left atrial pressure and pulmonary congestion. Fig. 4-18 represents the pressure–volume relationship in a typical patient with acute aortic regurgitation. Since the left ventricle has not had enough time to adjust to the sudden large increase in diastolic volume, increased ventricular filling rises on the diastolic pressure curve from point A to B. The significant increase in left ventricular end-diastolic pressure from 8 mm Hg to 50 mm Hg causes increased left atrial pressure (since the mitral valve is open), which leads to acute pulmonary edema. Elevated left ventricular end-diastolic pressure also results in an increase in left ventricular wall stress and myocardial oxygen demand, which may result in angina. Finally, while the stroke volume is increased to 125 mL (175 mL − 50 mL; see Fig. 4-18), since a large portion leaks back into the left ventricle (80 mL), the effective forward stroke volume is markedly reduced (45 mL).

In *chronic aortic regurgitation*, the ventricle has had time to adapt to the increased volume overload and is able to function as an efficient, high-compliance pump that handles high end-diastolic and SVs without significant increases in end-diastolic pressure. Fig. 4-19 represents the pressure–volume curve in chronic aortic regurgitation. Left ventricular dilation shifts the diastolic filling curve to the right, so that the left ventricle can tolerate large end-diastolic volumes without an accompanying increase in intraventricular pressure. The increased end-diastolic volume results in an increase in total

FIG. 4-18
(A) PRESSURE–VOLUME CURVE IN ACUTE, SEVERE AORTIC REGURGITATION. The heart has not had time to compensate, and the regurgitation of blood into the left ventricle moves the patient's end-diastolic volume from A to B, which leads to an elevated end-diastolic pressure.
(B) A SCHEMATIC OF THE ABNORMALITIES SHOWN FOR NORMAL PHYSIOLOGY AND AORTIC REGURGITATION. In aortic regurgitation, the end-diastolic volume and pressure are increased. While 125 mL is ejected from the left ventricle with each contraction, 80 mL leaks backwards, yielding an effective stroke volume of only 45 mL.

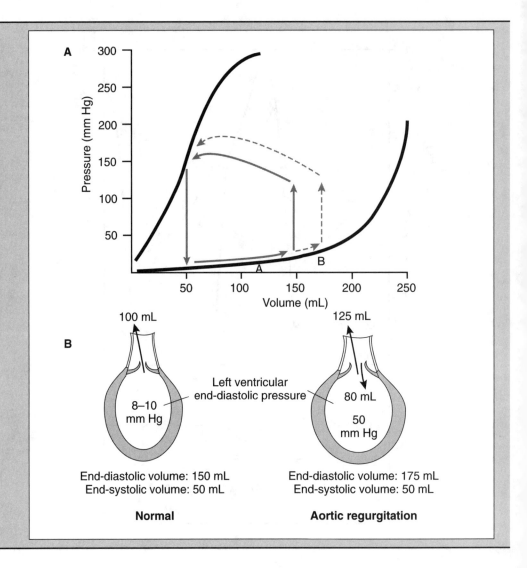

SV and preservation of forward CO (100 mL) despite a large regurgitant fraction. As the patient exercises, the peripheral vascular resistance falls, decreasing afterload, and the diastolic period shortens with increased heart rate (HR). Both of these mechanisms help to reduce the amount of regurgitation, resulting in few or no symptoms. This is often referred to as the "honeymoon" period of aortic regurgitation. This period can last for many years until the left ventricular systolic function begins to decline.

In chronic decompensated aortic regurgitation, the adaptive mechanisms of the left ventricle ultimately fail, and the systolic pressure curve shifts to the left. The decline in left ventricular systolic function results in an increase in end-systolic volume and an increase in end-diastolic volume as the ventricle further dilates. However, the increase in end-systolic volume is much higher relative to the increase in end-diastolic volume. This is depicted in Fig. 4-20, which represents the pressure–volume curve for a patient with chronic decompensated aortic regurgitation. The heart tries to compensate by increasing the end-diastolic volume, shifting the diastolic filling curve to the right, but this increase is not enough to preserve forward CO. Eventually there is a decline in ejection fraction, SV, forward SV, and elevation in left ventricular end-diastolic pressure and wall stress. At this point, patients begin developing symptoms of angina, pulmonary congestion, and fatigue.

Clinical Presentation. Patients with chronic aortic regurgitation often remain asymptomatic for many years despite severe left ventricular volume overload. Eventually, symptoms of angina or dyspnea occur as the ventricle dilates and myocardial dysfunction ensues. Patients often complain of increased fatigability, dyspnea on exertion, paroxys-

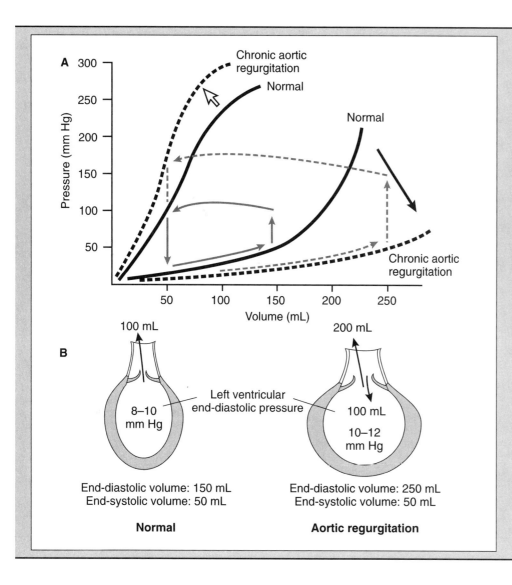

mal nocturnal dyspnea, and night sweats. Syncope and angina occur rarely. Patients more commonly complain of palpitations, pounding in the chest, head pounding, and an uncomfortable awareness of their heart beating before symptoms of ventricular dysfunction develop. By the time those symptoms of ventricular dysfunction occur, many patients are unable to benefit from surgical repair because of irreversible ventricular dysfunction. Therefore, it is very important to diagnose this condition early in its course.

In contrast, patients with severe acute aortic regurgitation are not able to tolerate the sudden rise in increased volume load over a prolonged period and present with signs and symptoms of cardiovascular collapse. These patients appear acutely ill and have evidence of cardiogenic shock and pulmonary edema.

Physical Examination

Arterial Pulses. The diagnosis of chronic aortic regurgitation is associated with many physical examination findings, each with specific eponyms. Most of the findings are related to increased SV and rapid diastolic runoff (regurgitation of blood into the left ventricle). This results in a widened pulse pressure (pulse pressure greater than diastolic pressure) characterized by a rapid rise and sudden collapse (water-hammer pulse). For this reason, severe chronic aortic regurgitation is associated with reduced diastolic blood pressure (usually less than 70 mm Hg) and increased systolic blood pressure (often greater than 160 mm Hg). Several peripheral signs resulting from the widened pulse pressure have been described by physicians in the past. Traube's sign (pistol-shot sounds) is a booming systolic and diastolic sound heard over the femoral arteries.

FIG. 4-20
(A) PRESSURE–VOLUME CURVE AND HEMODYNAMIC CHANGES IN CHRONIC DECOMPENSATED AORTIC REGURGITATION. As the ventricle begins to fail, the systolic pressure curve shifts to the right, resulting in an increased end-systolic volume and a decreased effective stroke volume (SV). The ventricle tries to compensate for the decrease in SV by increasing the end-diastolic volume, but this results in a higher end-diastolic pressure because the ventricle is not able to dilate any further.
(B) SCHEMATIC OF THE ABOVE EVENTS. As the patient's ventricle decompensates, end-systolic volume increases and effective SV decreases (150 mL to 100 mL).

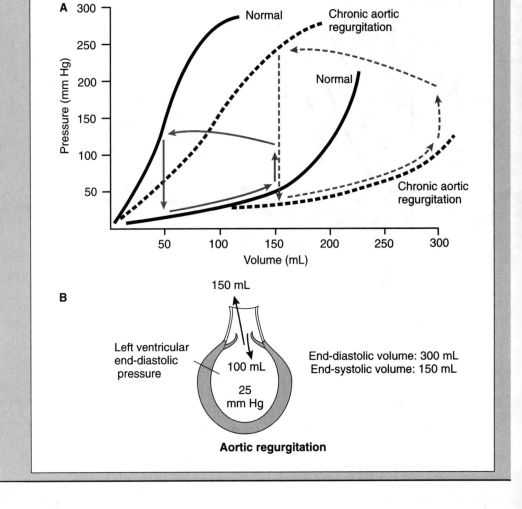

Auscultatory Findings in Aortic Regurgitation
Early diastolic murmur (blowing and high pitched)
Mid- to late diastolic murmur (Austin Flint murmur, low-frequency "rumble")
Midsystolic murmur

Duroziez's sign is a to-and-fro murmur heard over the femoral artery when it is compressed with the head of the stethoscope. Both of these signs are due to the large SV in both the forward and reverse directions because of the incompetent aortic valve. Dancing or bobbing of the uvula (Müller's sign) and head-bobbing (de Musset's sign), which coincide with systolic pulsations, can be observed.

Venous Pulse. The jugular venous pulse is not affected until late in the natural history of aortic regurgitation, when left ventricular dysfunction leads to heart failure and elevated jugular venous pressure.

Auscultation. The cardinal finding of aortic regurgitation is a high-frequency decrescendo early diastolic murmur, heard best along the mid left sternal border, apex, or over the aortic area (see Fig. 4-17). The murmur starts with S_2 and diminishes by mid- to late diastole. It is described as a "blowing" murmur and is best appreciated with the patient sitting up and leaning forward with the breath held at end expiration. The intensity of the murmur increases with any maneuver that increases afterload, such as vasopressor infusion, squatting, or isometric exercise. Conversely, vasodilation may lessen the intensity of the murmur; this is often seen during pregnancy and amyl nitrate infusion. The severity of the lesion is more closely correlated with the duration of the murmur rather than its intensity; in severe aortic regurgitation, the murmur may be heard throughout diastole (holodiastolic).

A low-frequency, mid- to late diastolic murmur is also commonly heard in patients with severe aortic regurgitation. Known as the Austin Flint murmur, it probably is due to turbulence below the mitral valve that is generated when the aortic regurgitant jet pushes the anterior mitral leaflet into the mitral inflow stream (Fig. 4-21). Amyl nitrate is useful in distinguishing the Austin Flint murmur from the murmur of mitral stenosis; amyl nitrate causes the Austin Flint murmur to decline in intensity, while it increases the intensity of the mitral stenosis murmur.

Amyl nitrate is an arterial vasodilator and therefore reduces the severity of aortic regurgitation.

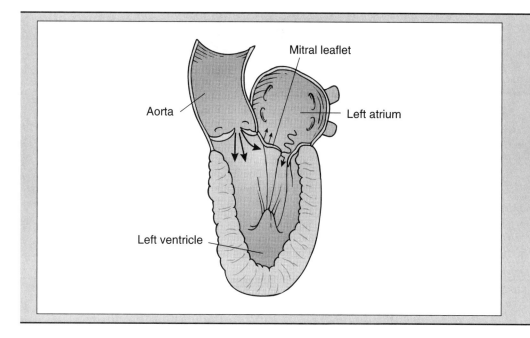

FIG. 4-21
DIAGRAMMATIC REPRESENTATION OF THE AUSTIN FLINT MURMUR IN AORTIC REGURGITATION. The regurgitant aortic jet (*large arrows*) pushes the anterior mitral leaflet into the mitral inflow stream (*small arrows*), generating an obstruction to left ventricular filling (*wavy arrow*).

Finally, a midsystolic murmur resulting from increased SV passing through the aortic valve can sometimes be appreciated in patients with aortic regurgitation.

▋DISEASES OF THE MITRAL VALVE

The mitral valve separates the left atrium and ventricle and is much more complex than the aortic valve. Unlike the other valves of the heart, the mitral valve has two leaflets: a longer tongue-like anterior leaflet and a cup-like posterior leaflet (see Fig. 4-4). The proper function of the mitral valve is dependent not only on the valve itself but also on the rest of the mitral apparatus, which consists of the posterior left atrial wall, the mitral annulus and leaflets, the chordae tendineae, papillary muscles, and left ventricular free wall. Abnormalities in any of these components can lead to a dysfunctional mitral valve. Mitral valve disease can be classified by whether there is obstruction to left ventricular filling (mitral stenosis) or ineffective closure resulting in leaking (mitral regurgitation).

Mitral valve disease can be classified as mitral stenosis or mitral regurgitation.

MITRAL STENOSIS

Etiology. Mitral stenosis is usually a sequela of rheumatic heart disease. Only 60% of patients with symptomatic mitral stenosis have a known history of acute rheumatic fever (approximately 15–25 years before presentation). However, virtually all adults with mitral stenosis have evidence of rheumatic deformities on pathologic examination of the valve. Therefore, a history of rheumatic fever cannot reliably be used as a guide to the likely presence or absence of this disease. The incidence of mitral stenosis has declined significantly in the developed countries as a result of the effective use of antibiotic therapy. However, mitral stenosis is still very common in the developing nations.

Pathophysiology. In the normal heart, the flow of blood from the left atrium to the left ventricle is unrestricted, and no pressure gradient exists. The normal mitral valve area is 4–6 cm² and as the mitral orifice narrows and becomes stenotic (< 2 cm²), the flow becomes restricted and a pressure gradient between the left atrium and left ventricle is generated (Figs. 4-22 and 4-23). This gradient causes the left atrial pressure to rise so that blood flow across the mitral valve can be maintained. The increase in left atrial pressure results in the development of increased pulmonary venous and capillary pressures, resulting in pulmonary congestion and symptoms of dyspnea. Hemoptysis may

FIG. 4-22
In mitral stenosis, thickening of the mitral valve restricts filling of the left ventricle (*wavy arrow*). Left atrial pressure increases, which causes left atrial dilation.

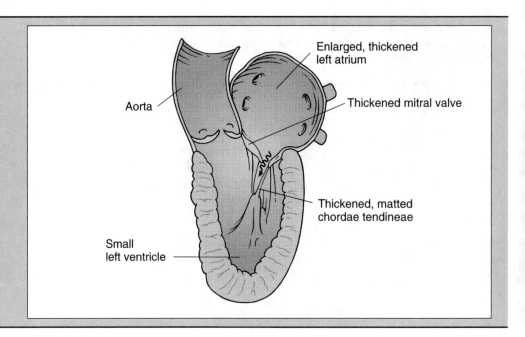

FIG. 4-23
RELATIONSHIPS AMONG LEFT VENTRICULAR PRESSURE, AORTIC PRESSURE, ELECTROCARDIOGRAM, AND HEART SOUNDS IN MITRAL STENOSIS. The stenotic mitral valve results in an elevated left atrial pressure and an abnormal pressure gradient across the mitral valve. The resulting turbulent flow across the valve results in a low-pitched diastolic (DM) murmur. The thicker and stiffer mitral valve now causes an audible opening snap (OS) and a louder first heart sound (S_1).

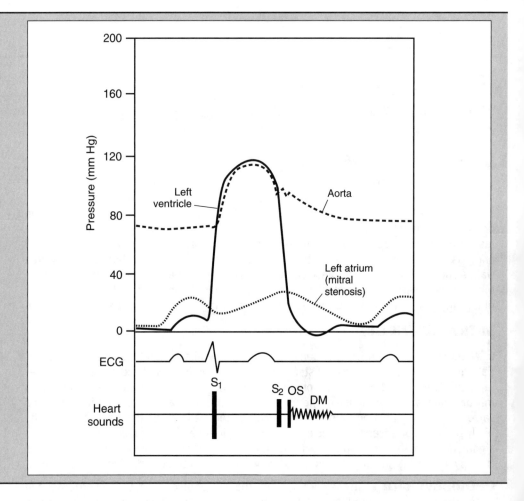

develop in severe cases of pulmonary hypertension as a result of migration of the red blood cells into the pulmonary interstitium and alveolar spaces. Pulmonary hypertension can develop in patients with mitral stenosis as a response to the elevated left atrial pressure, which is transmitted to the pulmonary circulation. As the pulmonary pressures gradually rise, reactive changes (medial hypertrophy and intimal fibrosis) on the pulmonary arteriolar bed frequently develop and pose a progressive obstruction to blood flow in the lungs, eventually resulting in an enormous pressure load in the right ventricle, causing it to dilate and fail. Therefore, patients with mitral stenosis and pulmonary hypertension are often said to have a "double stenosis," one at the mitral valve and the other at the level of the pulmonary arterioles.

As the blood flow across the mitral valve decreases, so does forward CO. This is because mitral stenosis affects the preload conditions of the left ventricle by decreasing end-diastolic volume and, therefore, SV. The pressure–volume changes observed in mitral stenosis are summarized in Fig. 4-24. Since the left ventricle is not diseased, the slope and position of the diastolic pressure curve does not change. However, restricted filling of the left ventricle leads to a smaller end-diastolic volume, which results in a smaller SV. Therefore, left ventricular size is usually normal or smaller than normal in patients with mitral stenosis, and the left ventricle is often referred to as the "protected" chamber, since it is not exposed to abnormally high pressures or volumes.

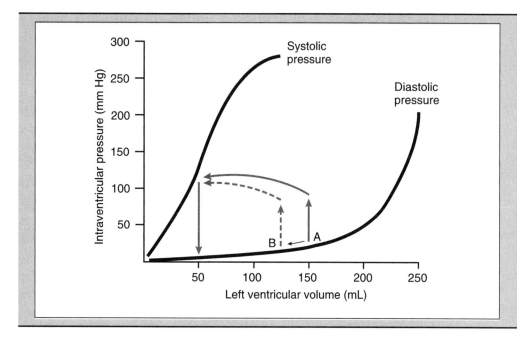

FIG. 4-24
PRESSURE–VOLUME CURVE IN MITRAL STENOSIS. The left ventricular end-diastolic volume is shifted from point A to B, since ventricular filling is restricted by the stenotic mitral valve. Reduced ventricular filling results in a smaller stroke volume.

Clinical Presentation. The clinical presentation of mitral stenosis is largely dependent on the degree of stenosis and the severity of the reduced valve area. Patients usually present with symptoms of typical left-sided heart failure. For example, as mitral stenosis worsens, patients develop shortness of breath resulting from pulmonary venous congestion from increasing left atrial and pulmonary venous pressures. In the early stages, dyspnea is noticeable only on exertion. Later, increasing fatigue and signs of pulmonary congestion occur with less activity and at rest, and patients often complain of orthopnea and paroxysmal nocturnal dyspnea. Pulmonary hypertension, hemoptysis, and right-sided heart failure symptoms (hepatomegaly, ascites, peripheral edema) develop as the stenosis continues to worsen and left atrial pressures become more elevated.

Symptoms of mitral stenosis may be exacerbated by any condition associated with increased HR. Increased HR decreases the diastolic period and the amount of time available in diastole for the blood to flow across the stenotic valve, which worsens pulmonary venous congestion. This is the reason why patients with mitral stenosis may be asymptomatic at rest but develop dyspnea on exertion as the CO and HR increase. Any conditions that increase the HR can exacerbate the symptoms of mitral stenosis; these include fever, anemia, hyperthyroidism, pregnancy, and tachycardias. Atrial fibrillation is particularly common in patients with mitral stenosis, probably a result of left atrial dilatation in response to the elevated left atrial pressure.

Since patients with mitral stenosis develop an enlarged left atrium and have reduced blood flow across the mitral valve, they are prone to developing stasis of blood flow and thrombi in the left atrium. This increases the risk of developing systemic thromboembolism. The risk for thromboembolism increases with decreased CO, increasing age, the size of the left atrial appendage, and the presence of atrial fibrillation. Prior to the development of modern surgical and anticoagulant therapy, approximately 25% of all deaths related to mitral stenosis were the result of an embolic event. The low-flow state and the abnormalities found on the valve surface also make the mitral valve an ideal host for bacteria in the bloodstream, increasing the risk of infective endocarditis in these patients. Patients may also complain of hoarseness, which results from the compression of the recurrent laryngeal nerve by a greatly dilated left atrium (Ortner's syndrome).

Physical Examination. The classic appearance of a patient with mitral stenosis is exhibition of a ruddy, pinkish-purplish patch over the malar area often referred to as the mitral facies (livedo reticularis of the malar area). This is attributed to decreased CO and systemic vasoconstriction.

Pulses. The arterial pulses are usually normal but may be small in volume in those patients where the SV is reduced. Palpation of the precordium often reveals a right ventricular tap, the result of increased right ventricular pressures. The jugular venous pulse is usually normal until pulmonary hypertension develops.

Auscultation. The classic murmur of mitral stenosis is the *diastolic rumble* that immediately follows an opening snap (see Fig. 4-23). The murmur is due to turbulent flow across the narrowed mitral valve orifice. It is a low-frequency diastolic murmur that is heard best at the apex of the heart with the bell of the stethoscope while the patient is lying in the left lateral recumbent position. The murmur is often difficult to hear and sometimes is localized to a very specific place on the precordium near the apex. However, as the murmur increases in intensity it can often be heard over the axilla and the lower left sternal area. Because the intensity of the murmur does not correlate with the severity of the stenosis, the duration of the murmur may better represent the severity of the stenosis.

In mitral stenosis, the S_1 is characteristically loud because the mitral valve is held in the open position by the increased transmitral gradient until the force of ventricular systole is large enough to close the valve. The P_2 becomes louder as the pulmonary pressure increases and results in an accentuation of the pulmonic valve closure. As pulmonary pressure further increases, a Graham Steell's murmur of pulmonic valve regurgitation may be heard (not shown in Fig. 4-23). After the S_2, a high-pitched *opening snap* can be heard. The opening snap is thought to be secondary to a sudden tensing of the valve leaflets after the valve has fully opened. The interval between the opening snap and S_2 is inversely related to the severity of the stenotic lesion; that is, as the stenosis worsens, left atrial pressure increases and the gradient between left atrial and left ventricular pressures increases, forcing the mitral valve open sooner (a shorter S_2–opening snap interval). The opening snap can be confused sometimes with a P_2 but usually occurs later in diastole.

Auscultatory Findings in Mitral Stenosis
Diastolic murmur (low pitched)
Opening snap after S_2
Loud S_1

Case Study: Continued

This patient's initial symptoms can be attributed to pulmonary edema secondary to mitral stenosis. She probably had had rheumatic fever in the past and was asymptomatic until this episode. The mitral stenosis progressively worsened over time and eventually led to the symptoms of fatigue and shortness of breath with exertion. The sudden worsening of her symptoms days prior to presentation was due to the sudden onset of atrial fibrillation and a rapid HR, which shortened the diastolic filling period. As shown in Fig. 4-1, the patient did not have discrete P waves, only an undulatory baseline resulting from fibrillatory activity of the atria (wandering wavelets of activation in the atria). Since the AV node was engaged irregularly, the QRS complexes are also irregular. Other than the atrial fibrillation, the ECG is normal.

The patient refused treatment and further evaluation after her first hospitalization 1 year ago. She had felt well during the year until 1 week ago when she developed fever, chills, malaise, and worsening shortness of breath. Her physical examination was now significant for a fever of 102.5°F, a rapid HR, and a new holosystolic murmur heard best at the apex and radiating to the axilla. Laboratory tests revealed an elevated white blood cell (WBC) count and erythrocyte sedimentation rate (ESR). What are the possible reasons for this woman's acute decompensation?

MITRAL REGURGITATION

Normal closure of the mitral valve requires the proper function of all of the components of the mitral apparatus. Dysfunction in one or many components leads to malcoaptation of the two mitral leaflets and results in mitral regurgitation.

Etiology. For the mitral valve to close properly, separate components of the mitral valve apparatus must work in coordination. Any abnormality in the mitral valve, papillary muscle, chordae tendineae, or the mitral annulus may lead to incomplete valve closure and mitral regurgitation. The most common causes of mitral regurgitation include ischemia, infective endocarditis, myxomatous degeneration of the mitral valve (including the mitral prolapse syndrome), collagen vascular disease, spontaneous rupture of the chordae tendineae, and rheumatic fever (Table 4-2).

Table 4-2
Causes of Acute and Chronic Mitral Regurgitation

ACUTE	CHRONIC
Mitral annulus disorders	Inflammatory
Infective endocarditis (abscess formation)	Rheumatic heart disease
Trauma (valvular heart surgery)	Systemic lupus erythematosus
Paravalvular leak resulting from interruption (surgical technical problems or infective endocarditis)	Scleroderma
	Degenerative
Mitral leaflet disorders	Myxomatous degeneration of mitral valve leaflets (Barlow's click-murmur syndrome, prolapsing leaflet, mitral valve prolapse)
Infective endocarditis (perforation or interfering with valve closure by vegetation)	Marfan's syndrome
Trauma (tear during percutaneous mitral balloon valvotomy or penetrating chest injury)	Ehlers-Danlos syndrome
Tumors (atrial myxoma)	Pseudoxanthoma elasticum
Myxomatous degeneration	Calcification of mitral valve annulus
Systemic lupus erythematosus (Libman-Sacks lesion)	Infective
	Infective endocarditis affecting normal, abnormal, or prosthetic mitral valves
Rupture of chordae tendineae	
Idiopathic (e.g., spontaneous)	Structural
Myxomatous degeneration (mitral valve prolapse, Marfan's syndrome, Ehlers-Danlos syndrome)	Ruptured chordae tendineae (spontaneous or secondary to myocardial infarction, trauma, mitral valve prolapse, endocarditis)
Infective endocarditis	Rupture or dysfunction of papillary muscle (ischemia or myocardial infarction)
Acute rheumatic fever	Dilatation of mitral valve annulus and left ventricular cavity (congestive cardiomyopathies, aneurysmal dilatation of the left ventricle)
Trauma (percutaneous balloon valvotomy, blunt chest trauma)	Hypertrophic cardiomyopathy
	Paravalvular prosthetic leak
Papillary muscle disorders	
Coronary artery disease (causing dysfunction and, rarely, rupture)	Congenital
Acute global left ventricular dysfunction	Mitral valve clefts or fenestrations
Infiltrative diseases (amyloidosis, sarcoidosis)	Parachute mitral valve abnormality in association with:
Trauma	Endocardial cushion defects
	Endocardial fibroelastosis
Primary prosthetic mitral valve disorders	Transposition of the great arteries
Porcine cusp perforation (endocarditis)	Anomalous origin of the left coronary artery
Porcine cusp degeneration	
Mechanical failure (strut fracture)	
Immobilized disk or ball of the mechanical prosthesis	

Pathophysiology. In mitral regurgitation, forward left ventricular SV is reduced since a significant portion of the left ventricular SV is ejected into the low-pressure left atrium (Fig. 4-25). The regurgitant blood in the left atrium increases left atrial pressure, particularly during systole (Fig. 4-26). A volume-related stress is placed on the left ventricle as the regurgitated volume is returned to the left ventricle during diastole. The left ventricle eventually dilates to increase its SV and maintain forward SV. The hemodynamic effects of mitral regurgitation are determined by size of the regurgitant orifice, the pressure gradient between the left ventricle and atrium, the left atrial compliance, and the duration of systole. For example, the gradient between left ventricle and atrium increases with any state that increases systemic blood pressure or restricts flow of blood out of the ventricle (e.g., aortic stenosis) and worsens mitral regurgitation (Fig. 4-27). The increased left ventricular afterload associated with both of these conditions favors regurgitation of blood into the low-pressure left atrium.

Left atrial compliance is an important determinant for how well patients tolerate mitral regurgitation. In *acute* severe mitral regurgitation, the left atrium is normal in size and relatively noncompliant. The increased blood in the left atrium leads to a significant

FIG. 4-25
MITRAL REGURGITATION. During systole, blood is ejected into the aorta via the open aortic valve and regurgitates back into the left atrium (*arrows*).

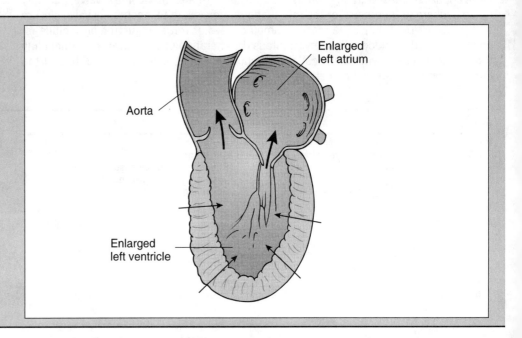

FIG. 4-26
RELATIONSHIPS AMONG LEFT VENTRICULAR PRESSURE, AORTIC PRESSURE, ELECTROCARDIOGRAM, AND HEART SOUNDS IN MITRAL REGURGITATION. Regurgitation of blood into the left atrium during ventricular systole causes the left atrial pressure to rise rapidly (prominent *v* wave) and produces a murmur that lasts throughout systole (SM). The increased left atrial pressure and volume at the onset of diastole increases the rapid filling rate, which accentuates the third heart sound (S_3). S_1 = first heart sound; S_2 = second heart sound.

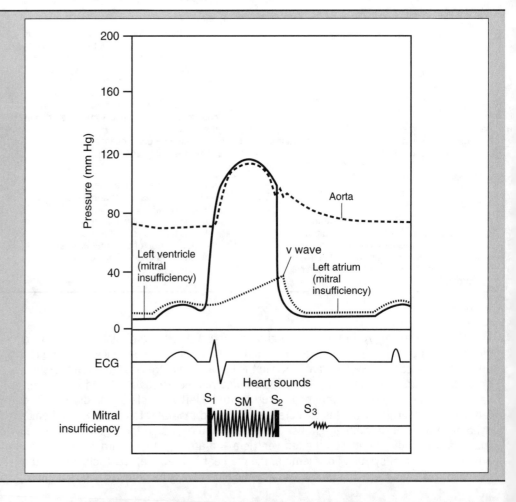

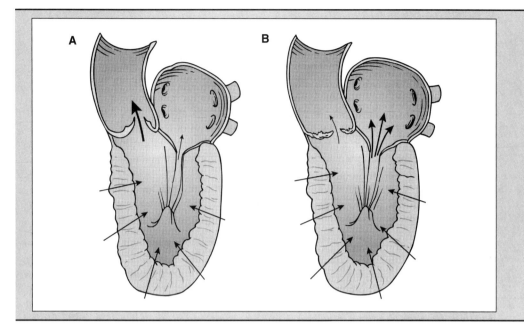

FIG. 4-27
The amount of mitral regurgitation present is dependent on the gradient between the left atrium and left ventricle. (A) In the left schematic, there is no obstruction to aortic valve flow during systole, and there is very little accompanying mitral regurgitation. (B) In the right schematic, flow through the aortic valve is restricted (moderate aortic stenosis is present), which causes more blood to be regurgitated into the left atrium.

increase in left atrial pressure. In addition, the left ventricle has not had time to compensate for the increased volume load. The pressure–volume relationship in acute mitral regurgitation is shown in Fig. 4-28. The increased volume load changes the end-

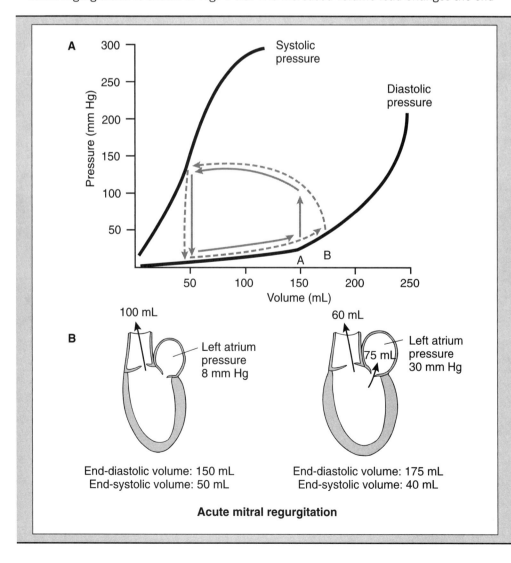

Acute mitral regurgitation

FIG. 4-28
(A) PRESSURE–VOLUME CURVE IN ACUTE MITRAL REGURGITATION. In acute mitral regurgitation, the regurgitant volume of blood, which was ejected into the left atrium in systole, returns to the left ventricle, increasing both the left ventricular end-diastolic volume and pressure.
(B) SCHEMATIC OF ACUTE MITRAL REGURGITATION. In acute mitral regurgitation, 75 mL of blood leaks back into the noncompliant left atrium, which leads to marked elevation in left atrial pressure (LAP) to 30 mm Hg. Effective forward flow is reduced to 60 mL, which leads to reduced arterial pressure.

diastolic volume from A to B. While this increases the SV to approximately 135 mL, 75 mL regurgitates into the left atrium and leads to an effective "forward" SV of 60 mL. Patients with acute mitral regurgitation present with pulmonary edema (elevated left atrial pressure) and low arterial pressures (low effective CO).

In contrast, a patient with *chronic* mitral regurgitation has time to undergo compensatory changes that allow the left atrium and the left ventricle to dilate and become more compliant. Fig. 4-29 illustrates the changes in the pressure–volume curve for the left ventricle in chronic mitral regurgitation. A rightward shift of the diastolic pressure curve allows the increased volumes to be handled with little increase in left atrial pressure. However, this compensatory mechanism is not without cost. The left ventricle must dilate significantly to increase SV substantially to compensate for the large regurgitant volume and maintain forward CO. If mitral regurgitation goes untreated for a long period of time, the chronic volume overload eventually leads to left ventricular systolic dysfunction (rightward shift of the isovolumic systolic pressure curve) and heart failure.

Clinical Presentation. The symptoms with which a patient with mitral regurgitation presents depend on the severity of the regurgitation as well as the rapidity of its onset. A patient with severe acute mitral regurgitation presents with pulmonary edema and respiratory extremus. On the other hand, a patient with progressive chronic mitral regurgitation may remain asymptomatic for a long time. Fatigue and weakness resulting from low forward CO are usually the initial symptoms, since the left atrium and pulmonary vasculature have sufficient time to develop compensatory mechanisms in response

Acute Mitral Regurgitation (e.g., Ruptured Chordae)
Normal left atrial and left ventricular size
Acute pulmonary edema resulting from elevated left atrial pressure
Reduced "forward" SV

Chronic Mitral Regurgitation
Enlarged left ventricle
Markedly enlarged left atrium
Slightly elevated left atrial pressure

FIG. 4-29
(A) PRESSURE–VOLUME CURVE IN CHRONIC MITRAL REGURGITATION. The ventricle has had adequate time to adjust to the added regurgitant volume by shifting the diastolic filling curve to the right. Therefore, the ventricle is now able to handle a larger end-diastolic volume without a significant increase in end-diastolic pressure. (B) Cardiac output is preserved as a result of the left ventricular enlargement despite the large amount of regurgitant blood (110 mL). Left atrial enlargement keeps left atrial pressure (LAP) relatively low. These compensatory mechanisms ultimately fail.

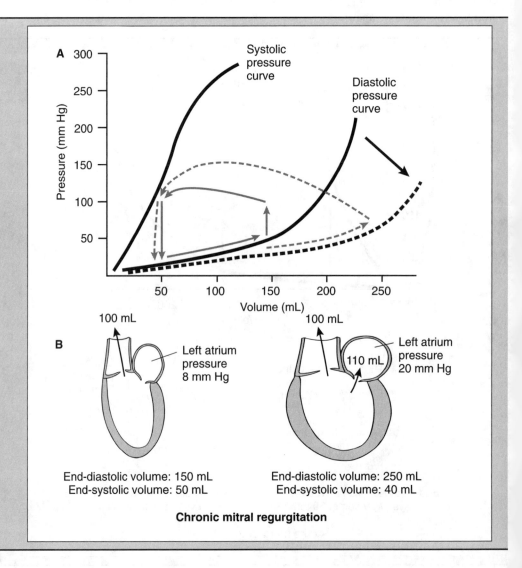

to the increased volume and pressure. The most important compensatory mechanism is increased compliance of the left atrium and pulmonary venous system, mediated mainly by a marked increase in left atrial size.

As mitral regurgitation worsens over time, the left ventricle begins to fail. The patient can no longer compensate for the increased left atrial volume and pressure and eventually develops symptoms of pulmonary congestion. Patients may also develop atrial fibrillation as a result of left atrial enlargement.

Physical Examination

Arterial Pulse. The examination of the arterial pulse may be very helpful in distinguishing the murmur of mitral regurgitation from aortic stenosis, both of which are associated with prominent systolic murmurs. The carotid upstroke is brisk in severe mitral regurgitation and delayed in aortic stenosis.

Auscultation. The holosystolic murmur is the most prominent physical finding in mitral regurgitation. The murmur is holosystolic because the ventricle no longer has a period of isovolumic contraction or relaxation (see Fig. 4-27). Since the mitral valve is leaky and the left atrium is a low-pressure chamber, the ventricle ejects blood into the left atrium as soon as the ventricle begins to contract. This increases the pressure in the left atrium, and diastole begins without a period of isovolumic relaxation. Therefore, the murmur starts with S_1 and ends with S_2, is usually high-pitched, and classically radiates to the axilla. The presence of a S_3 is suggestive of severe disease. While a S_3 is usually associated with CHF (see Chap. 1), the presence of a S_3 in mitral regurgitation does not necessarily indicate CHF since it can be caused by rapid filling of the left ventricle by the large volume of blood stored in the left atrium in diastole. If the mitral regurgitation is predominantly from abnormalities in the posterior leaflet, the mitral regurgitation jet is directed toward the aortic root, and the murmur is best heard at the upper sternum. On the other hand, if the anterior leaflet is involved, the mitral regurgitation jet is directed posteriorly, and the murmur may radiate to the spine or even to the top of the head. Mitral regurgitation secondary to mitral valve prolapse often has a late systolic murmur following a systolic click. Pulmonary hypertension eventually develops as mitral regurgitation worsens, and a loud P_2 becomes evident later in the course. Patients with severe mitral regurgitation and left ventricular dilatation may present with "silent" mitral regurgitation because the CO is not great enough to generate turbulent flow across the mitral valve.

Auscultatory Findings in Mitral Regurgitation
Holosystolic murmur
Third heart sound (S_3) may be present

The chest x-ray revealed pulmonary edema, and an echocardiogram revealed findings consistent with rheumatic heart disease, mitral stenosis, and mitral regurgitation. There was also a mass noted on the mitral valve consistent with vegetation. Blood cultures grew Streptococcus viridans.

Case Study:
Continued

MITRAL VALVE PROLAPSE

Mitral valve prolapse is a relatively common and often asymptomatic "billowing" of the mitral valve into the left atrium as a result of diverse pathogenic mechanisms (Fig. 4-30). It is the most prevalent valvular abnormality and is estimated to affect 3%–5% of the general population; it is believed to be more common in women. Mitral valve prolapse is synonymous with systolic-click–murmur syndrome, billowing mitral valve syndrome, Barlow's syndrome, myxomatous mitral valve, and floppy valve syndrome. Most cases of mitral valve prolapse occur as a primary condition. In about 5% of cases, a primary cause is known and is usually related to connective tissue disorders such as Marfan's syndrome. Postmortem evaluation of patients with mitral valve prolapse reveals a myxomatous proliferation of the spongiosa (middle layer of the leaflet) component of the valve, which seems to be related to abnormalities in collagen metabolism.

Clinical Presentation Patients with mitral valve prolapse are usually asymptomatic. Many patients with mitral valve prolapse, however, present with nonspecific symptoms such as fatigability, palpitations, syncope, presyncope, chest discomfort,

Auscultatory Findings in Mitral Valve Prolapse
Midsystolic click
Systolic murmur may be present

FIG. 4-30
MITRAL VALVE PROLAPSE. The leaflets of the mitral valve are redundant and "billow" back into the left atrium.

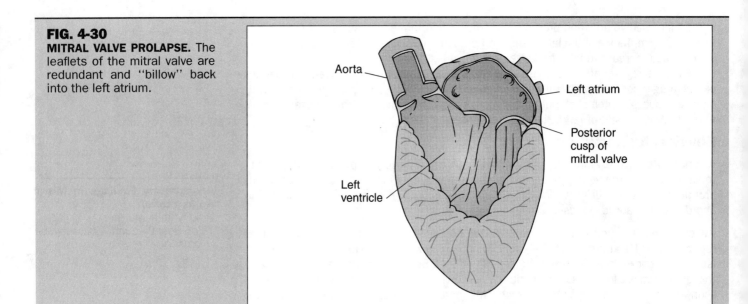

anxiety, and autonomic dysfunction. It is not known whether these symptoms are related to the presence of mitral valve prolapse or are coincidental. If the prolapse of the leaflet is severe enough, mitral regurgitation occurs. Patients usually remain asymptomatic until the regurgitation becomes hemodynamically significant. Patients with mitral valve prolapse are also more susceptible to chordal rupture and occasionally present with the sudden development of severe mitral regurgitation. Like patients with other valvular lesions, patients with mitral valve prolapse should be instructed regarding the risk of endocarditis and prophylaxis with antibiotics prior to invasive procedures.

Physical Examination. There is a higher than normal prevalence of straight back syndrome, scoliosis, pectus excavatum, and shallow chest associated with mitral valve prolapse. The hallmark physical finding of mitral valve prolapse is a midsystolic click heard on auscultation. This is a high-frequency sound and therefore is best appreciated with the diaphragm of the stethoscope with the patient in the left lateral decubitus position. The click is believed to be produced by a sudden tensing of the prolapsing leaflet and is sometimes followed by a mid- to late systolic murmur (if mitral regurgitation is present).

Any provocative maneuver that reduces the left ventricular volume causes the leaflets to prolapse earlier, and the click and the murmur occur earlier and move closer to S_1. Therefore, the click and murmur occur sooner during a Valsalva maneuver, on sudden standing, and with the inhalation of amyl nitrate and occur later with squatting, leg raising, and isometric exercise. These maneuvers aid in distinguishing the findings of mitral valve prolapse from other valvular lesions.

■ DISEASES OF THE TRICUSPID VALVE

TRICUSPID STENOSIS

The tricuspid valve is the trileaflet valve that separates the right atrium and ventricle. Tricuspid stenosis is almost always related to rheumatic heart disease and is rarely an isolated finding. If there is rheumatic involvement of the tricuspid valve, the aortic and mitral valves are usually also involved. Other, rarer causes of tricuspid stenosis include congenital tricuspid atresia and carcinoid syndrome. Patients with significant tricuspid stenosis usually present with signs and symptoms of right heart failure, fatigue, abdominal pain, decreased appetite, and lower extremity swelling. A diastolic gradient develops across the tricuspid valve as the stenosis worsens and is responsible for the development of a low, cardiac output state. This leads to the congestion of the venous system and elevated right heart filling pressures, which are responsible for these symptoms. The murmur and opening snap of tricuspid stenosis are similar to those found in patients with mitral stenosis and often are misdiagnosed as the latter. Differences in venous pulsation and dynamic auscultation can help in differentiating the two murmurs. The diastolic murmur and opening snap of tricuspid stenosis are best heard at the lower left sternal border. They increase in intensity with maneuvers that increase venous return and with inspiration (Carvallo's sign) as do most right-sided heart sounds, and there is a distinct difference in the venous pulsations. The *a* wave of the jugular venous pulse is tall, sharp, and prominent as a result of the right atrium contracting against a stenotic tricuspid valve. Since mitral stenosis usually accompanies tricuspid stenosis and the auscultatory findings of mitral stenosis can predominate, close examination of the neck veins may be the only clue that concomitant tricuspid stenosis exists.

TRICUSPID REGURGITATION

Tricuspid regurgitation is usually secondary and is due to the dilatation of the right ventricle and the tricuspid annulus rather than to intrinsic involvement of the valves. Any causes of right ventricular enlargement and failure resulting from pressure or volume overload can be the culprit. Tricuspid regurgitation is also the most common valvular lesion in intravenous drug abusers who present with endocarditis, since the left-sided valves are protected by the lungs, which act as a filter. Primary causes of tricuspid regurgitation are rare and usually are congenital in nature, the most common being Ebstein's anomaly. In Ebsteins's anomaly, the tricuspid annulus and valve are downwardly displaced into the right ventricle because of anomalous attachment of the tricuspid leaflets. Therefore, the proximal portion of the right ventricle is made up of atrial tissue, leaving a small ventricular chamber. Rheumatic involvement of the tricuspid valve may cause regurgitation, but isolated tricuspid regurgitation without stenosis is rare. Patients with significant tricuspid regurgitation have evidence of right heart failure as outlined above. The holosystolic murmur of tricuspid regurgitation is very similar to the murmur of mitral regurgitation, but as stated above, it increases in intensity with maneuvers that increase right-sided filling. The murmur of tricuspid regurgitation is best heard at the fourth intercostal space in the parasternal area rather than the apex, and examination of the neck veins is also helpful in differentiating it from mitral regurgitation. Inspection of the jugular venous pulsation reveals a prominent *v* wave as a result of a significant portion of the right ventricular SV being directed into the right atrium, which is then transmitted directly to venous system. The normal *x* descent also disappears, since the right atrium is already volume loaded from the regurgitant volume, and therefore passive filling of the right atrium is negligible. As in tricuspid stenosis, careful examination of the neck veins and dynamic auscultation may be very helpful in differentiating tricuspid regurgitation from mitral regurgitation.

■ DISEASES OF THE PULMONIC VALVE

PULMONIC STENOSIS

Pulmonic stenosis is almost always due to congenital deformity of the valve (see Chap. 6). Rheumatic involvement of the pulmonic valve is very rare and, if present, almost always involves other valves as well. Carcinoid syndrome can affect the pulmonic valve and the right ventricular outflow tract, causing constriction of the valve ring and fusion of the leaflets. As with aortic stenosis, a pressure gradient develops across the right ventricular outflow tract, which eventually leads to right ventricular failure.

PULMONIC REGURGITATION

The most common cause of pulmonic regurgitation is dilatation of the valve ring secondary to pulmonary hypertension or to dilatation of the pulmonary artery resulting from connective tissue diseases such as Marfan's syndrome. The next most common cause of pulmonic regurgitation is infective endocarditis. Other causes include congenital malformations (especially tetralogy of Fallot), carcinoid syndrome, trauma, and syphilis. Pulmonic regurgitation causes a volume overload on the right ventricle and eventually results in right ventricular failure. Palpation of the precordium may reveal a right ventricular heave, and auscultation may reveal a high-pitched blowing decrescendo murmur best heard at the upper left sternal border (Graham Steell's murmur). A wide splitting of S_2

may also be present as a result of the increased right ventricular diastolic volume. Like all right-sided murmurs, the murmur of pulmonic regurgitation increases in intensity with inspiration.

▮ SUMMARY

Normal cardiac function requires efficient action of the four cardiac valves. The valves provide unidirectional flow between the atria and ventricles (tricuspid valve and mitral valve) and between the ventricles and great vessels (pulmonic valve and aortic valve). All four valves can be associated with abnormal function due to obstruction to flow (stenosis) or regurgitation of flow. The pathophysiologic cardiac consequences depend on the valve and the functional abnormality. For example, while aortic stenosis places an abnormal pressure load on the left ventricle, aortic regurgitation and mitral regurgitation subject the left ventricle to abnormal volume loads, and mitral stenosis places no abnormal loads on the left ventricle. The signs and symptoms of valvular abnormalities also depend on how quickly the abnormality develops. If mitral regurgitation develops suddenly (e.g., a torn chordae tendineae), the patient often presents with rapidly progressive profound heart failure; conversely, chronic mitral regurgitation resulting from rheumatic heart disease may be asymptomatic for many years because of compensatory left ventricular and left atrial dilatation.

The pathophysiology of these different abnormalities can be best understood by evaluating pressure–volume loops and pressure–time analysis. Pressure–volume loops and pressure–time analysis also help the student understand the pathophysiologic basis for the characteristic physical examination findings associated with each valvular abnormality. In aortic stenosis, a narrowed aortic valve orifice is associated with turbulent flow during systole, which produces a systolic heart murmur. However, since the aortic valve is normally closed during diastole, a diastolic murmur is not heard unless there is associated aortic regurgitation.

Valvular heart diseases are commonly encountered in all branches of clinical medicine. Valvular heart diseases place abnormal hemodynamic burdens on the heart and may ultimately lead to heart failure if not treated appropriately. Accurate diagnosis and treatment of valvular heart diseases require a thorough understanding of the underlying pathophysiology.

KEY POINTS

- Ventricular and valvular function can be assessed by using the closely related methods of pressure–time analysis and pressure–volume analysis.
- All valvular abnormalities can be grouped pathophysiologically into either stenotic or regurgitant problems.
- Abnormalities can be present for any of the four valves: aortic, mitral, tricuspid, and pulmonic.
- *Aortic stenosis* causes a pressure overload on the left ventricle, which leads to left ventricular hypertrophy and is associated with a systolic murmur. *Aortic regurgitation* places a volume load on the left ventricle, which leads primarily to left ventricular enlargement and is associated with a diastolic murmur.
- *Mitral stenosis* does not put any abnormal loads on the left ventricle (but a pressure load on the left atrium) and is associated with a diastolic murmur. *Mitral regurgitation* places a volume load on the left ventricle, which leads to left ventricular dilatation in longstanding cases and is associated with a systolic murmur.

Case Study:
Resolution

The patient was admitted to the hospital and started on intravenous antibiotics for presumed infective endocarditis. She was later referred to surgery for a mitral valve replacement when she continued to have CHF secondary to severe mitral regurgitation despite medical therapy. At surgery, her valve was seen to be severely scarred and calcified. The mitral valve was excised and an artificial St. Jude Medical® mechanical heart valve (Fig. 4-31) was emplaced. She was discharged from the hospital after a full course of antibiotic therapy and continued to do well afterwards.

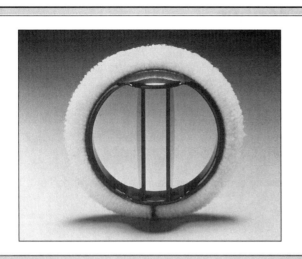

FIG. 4-31
The St. Jude Medical® mechanical heart valve can replace either the mitral valve or the aortic valve. The valve is shown in face with the two leaflets open. Two leaflets open and allow excellent flow through the orifice. (*Source:* Courtesy of Vince Gilbert, St. Jude Medical, St. Paul, Minnesota.)

▮ REVIEW QUESTIONS

Directions: For each of the following questions, choose the **one best** answer.

1. In which phases of the cardiac cycle is the mitral valve open?

    (A) Ejection period, early filling, diastasis
    (B) Isovolumic relaxation, early filling, diastasis, atrial systole
    (C) Early filling, diastasis, atrial systole
    (D) Ejection period
    (E) Isovolumic relaxation, early filling, diastasis

2. Which of the following conditions causes pressure overload of the left ventricle?

    (A) Aortic stenosis
    (B) Aortic regurgitation
    (C) Mitral stenosis
    (D) Mitral regurgitation

3. David Singer, 47 years old, passed out (syncope) while surfing 4 days ago. On examination, he is noted to have a midsystolic murmur. His left ventricular impulse is sustained. Mr. Singer's symptoms indicate which one of the following conditions?

    (A) Aortic stenosis
    (B) Aortic regurgitation
    (C) Mitral stenosis
    (D) Mitral regurgitation

■ ANSWERS AND EXPLANATIONS

1. The answer is C. An open mitral valve allows filling of the left ventricle. The left ventricle begins filling when the mitral valve opens at the end of the isovolumic filling period. The mitral valve is open during the early filling period, diastasis, and atrial systole. The mitral valve closes when ventricular contraction increases ventricular pressure to a level greater than atrial pressure. Mitral valve closure signals the beginning of systole, which is composed of the isovolumic contraction period and the ejection period.

2. The answer is A. Aortic stenosis causes pressure overload on the left ventricle because the left ventricle must expel blood across a narrowed orifice. Mitral regurgitation and aortic regurgitation cause the ventricle to face an increased volume load. In mitral stenosis, the left ventricle is not exposed to any abnormal loads.

3. The answer is A. Mr. Singer has aortic stenosis. One of the symptoms of aortic stenosis is syncope associated with physical exertion. Exertional syncope can be due to arrhythmias (usually a tachycardia) or valvular abnormalities. The physical examination findings are consistent with aortic stenosis. Aortic regurgitation and mitral stenosis are associated with diastolic murmurs. Mitral regurgitation normally causes a holosystolic murmur.

■ REFERENCES

Baim DS, Grossman W: *Cardiac Catheterization, Angiography and Intervention.* Baltimore, MD: Williams & Wilkins, 1996, pp 151–167.

Carabello BA, Crawford FA: Valvular heart disease. *N Engl J Med.* 337:32–41, 1997.

Guyton AC: *Textbook of Medical Physiology.* Philadelphia, PA: W. B. Saunders, 1986.

Honig CR: *Modern Cardiovascular Physiology.* Boston, MA: Little, Brown, 1988.

Kusumoto FM: Cardiovascular disorders: heart disease. In *Pathophysiology of Heart Disease.* Edited by McPhee SJ, Lingappa VR, Ganong WF, et al. Stamford, CT: Appleton & Lange, 1997, pp 237–246.

Walmsey R, Watson H: *Clinical Anatomy of the Heart.* New York, NY: Churchill Livingstone, 1978.

Chapter 5

PERICARDIAL DISEASES

Fred M. Kusumoto, M.D.

■ CHAPTER OUTLINE

Case Study:
Introduction

Steve Mickelsen was a 29-year-old healthy man who developed a cough and fever several days previously. Over the last 24 hours he had developed severe chest pain. He described the chest pain as sharp, worse with a deep breath, and worse when he lay down. Mr. Mickelsen's physical examination was significant for a loud scratchy sound heard throughout the precordium on auscultation. His physical examination was otherwise normal and his electrocardiogram (ECG) is shown in Fig. 5-1. What was wrong with Mr. Mickelsen?

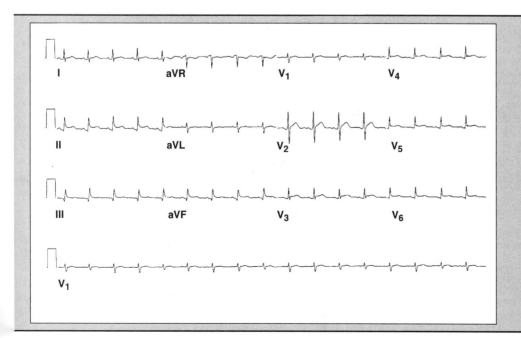

FIG. 5-1
MR. MICKELSEN'S 12-LEAD ELECTROCARDIOGRAM.

I   aVR   V₁   V₄

II   aVL   V₂   V₅

III   aVF   V₃   V₆

V₁

▊ INTRODUCTION

Since the time of Hippocrates, it has been known that the heart is surrounded by a "smooth mantle filled with fluid resembling urine." In fact, during antiquity, philosopher scientists felt that a heart covered by "hair" (possibly fibrinous deposits in the pericardial space) was associated with bravery and extreme cunning. While congenital absence of the pericardium is associated with minimal hemodynamic sequelae, diseases of the pericardium can produce catastrophic consequences. This chapter first reviews the basic anatomy and physiology of the pericardium and then discusses the two commonly encountered pathophysiologic processes associated with the pericardium: inflammation of the pericardium (*pericarditis*) and abnormal accumulation of fluid in the pericardial space (*pericardial effusion*).

▊ NORMAL PERICARDIAL ANATOMY AND PHYSIOLOGY

ANATOMY AND HISTOLOGY

___

Pericardial Anatomy

- Parietal pericardium
  Mesothelial layer
  Fibrous layer
- Visceral pericardium

Embryologically, at approximately 23 days, the right and left endocardial tubes fuse and invaginate into the pericardial cavity like a fist pushing into a balloon (Fig. 5-2). In the adult heart this sac becomes closely applied to the heart and extends to partially cover the proximal great arteries (Fig. 5-3). The outer surface of the pericardium (Fig. 5-4) is composed of two layers, a strong, thick fibrocollagenous outer layer lined by a single layer of mesothelial cells. These two layers form the parietal pericardium, which is attached to the sternum and diaphragm by dense ligaments. The parietal pericardium fuses into the adventitial connective tissue of the great arteries and veins. These attachments allow the parietal pericardium to limit the movement of the heart in the chest cavity with changes in position or posture. The inner surface of the pericardium, called the visceral pericardium, is composed of a single layer of mesothelial cells that is closely apposed to the epicardial surface of the heart.

FIG. 5-2
EMBRYO AT THE 10-SOMITE STAGE (APPROXIMATELY 23–25 DAYS), SHOWING THE HEART PUSHING INTO THE PERICARDIAL CAVITY. (*Source:* Adapted with permission from Netter FH: *The Ciba Collection of Medical Illustrations: Heart,* vol 5. East Hanover, NJ: Novartis Pharmaceuticals, 1992, p 118.)

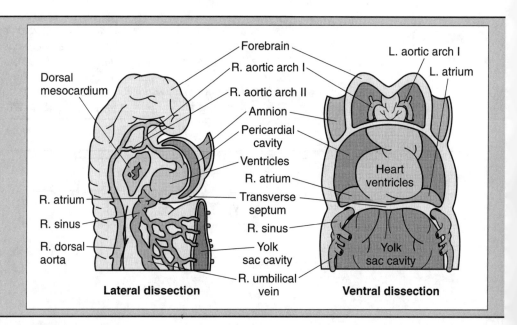

The pericardial space formed by the visceral and parietal pericardium is filled with approximately 15–50 mL of clear fluid that appears to be an ultrafiltrate of plasma. There is constant turnover of pericardial fluid; labeled erythrocytes placed in the pericardium can be observed in the bloodstream within several hours, although it takes several days for all of the cells to be removed. Pericardial fluid contains phospholipids, which may act as a lubricant between the pericardial layers. Several studies have shown that the parietal pericardium produces various prostaglandins that can exert significant physiologic effects, which may be important for circulatory regulation.

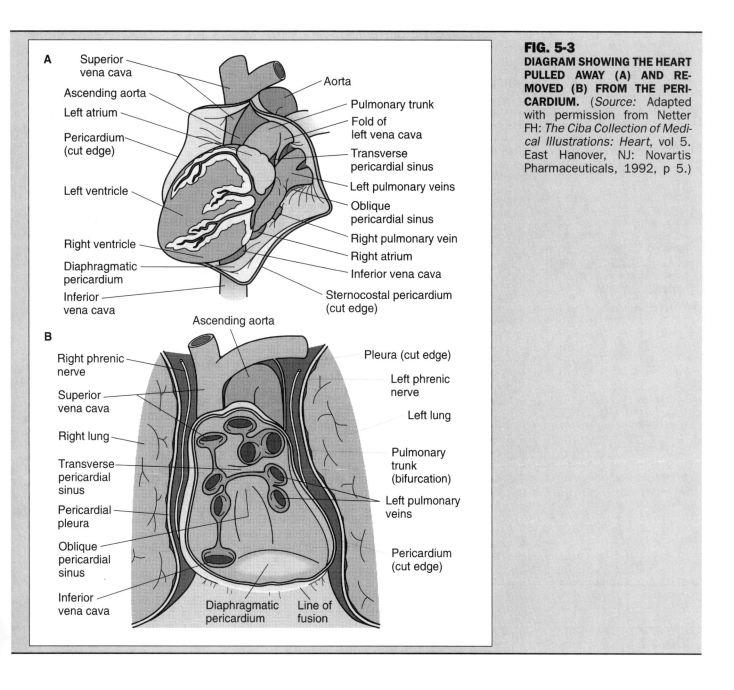

FIG. 5-3
DIAGRAM SHOWING THE HEART PULLED AWAY (A) AND RE-MOVED (B) FROM THE PERICARDIUM. (*Source:* Adapted with permission from Netter FH: *The Ciba Collection of Medical Illustrations: Heart*, vol 5. East Hanover, NJ: Novartis Pharmaceuticals, 1992, p 5.)

The fibrous layer of the parietal pericardium is principally made up of collagen with a small amount of elastin. Fig. 5-4 shows an electron micrograph of the fibrous layer of the parietal pericardium. Layers of wavy bands of collagen bundles that are arranged in a crisscross pattern can be observed (Fig. 5-5). The fibrous layer is thickest at the thinnest portions of the heart, such as the right atrium, and at points of attachment at the great vessels, sternum, and diaphragm.

The mesothelial surfaces of the inner parietal pericardium and the visceral pericardium are very complex (see Fig. 5-4). The cell surfaces facing the pericardial surface are covered by numerous microvilli and long cilia, which appear to provide specialized low-friction surfaces and to increase the cell surface area available for fluid transport.

PHYSIOLOGY

The pericardium forms a sac around the heart that limits its expansion. The parietal pericardium is responsible for the characteristic properties of the pericardium. Initially, as volume in the pericardial space (the sum of the volume of the heart and the pericardial fluid) is increased, pressure remains at a low, constant level as the wavy collagen bundles

Pericardial Physiology

At low volumes: compliant
At high volumes: noncompliant

FIG. 5-4
ELECTRON MICROGRAPH OF THE CROSS SECTION OF THE PARIETAL PERICARDIUM. The thin mesothelial layer is indicated by the *arrowheads*. The thick fibrous pericardium is composed of wavy bands of collagen oriented at different angles. The *inset* shows a scanning electron micrograph of the complex inner surface of the parietal pericardium covered by numerous cilia and microvilli. (*Source:* Adapted with permission from Ishihara T, Ferrans VJ, Jones M, et al: Histologic and ultrastructural features of normal human parietal pericardium. *Am J Cardiol* 46:745, 1980.)

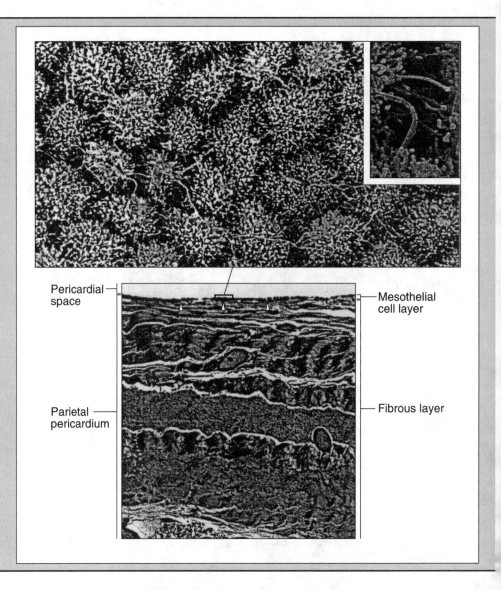

FIG. 5-5
SCHEMATIC DIAGRAM SHOWING THE CRISSCROSS ORIENTATION OF COLLAGEN FIBERS IN THE PARIETAL PERICARDIUM. (*Source:* Adapted with permission from Elias H, Boyd LJ: Notes on the anatomy, embryology, and histology of the pericardium. *J New York Med Coll* 2:50, 1960.)

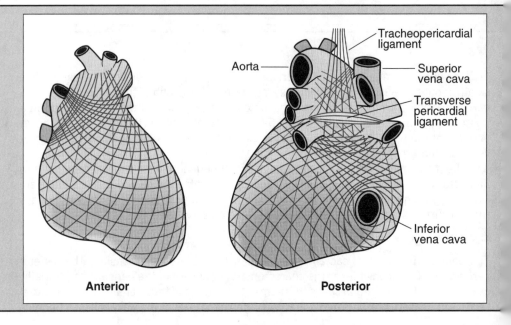

"straighten." However, with continued volume increases, the collagen matrix of the pericardium prevents further volume expansion, pericardial compliance decreases, and the intrapericardial pressure increases dramatically (Fig. 5-6). The pericardium thus has relatively little effect at small cardiac volumes, but if cardiac volume increases acutely (either from rapid heart enlargement or increased pericardial fluid), the pericardium exhibits a tremendous restraining effect. Under normal conditions the parietal pericardium can be envisioned as a loosely fitting sac around the heart.

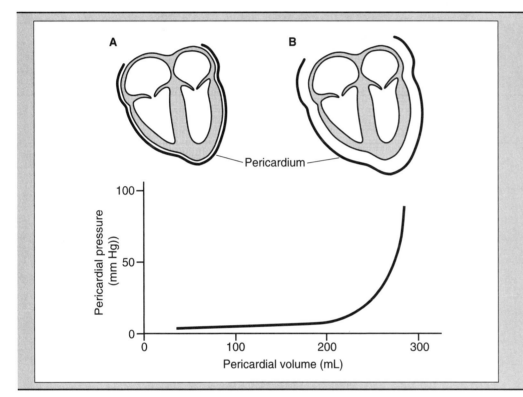

FIG. 5-6
PRESSURE–VOLUME RELATION-SHIP OF THE CANINE PERICARDIUM. As intrapericardial volume is increased (by the addition of fluid into the pericardial space as shown in the right schematic [B]), the pericardium is initially very compliant; however, when the total volume encompassed by the pericardium becomes greater than 200 mL, the pericardium becomes very noncompliant, and intrapericardial pressure increases dramatically.

The measurement of pressure within the pericardial space has been the subject of some controversy. With the use of conventional end-hole catheters, the intrapericardial pressure has been estimated to be zero and virtually identical to intrathoracic pressure. Using specially designed balloon catheters, other investigators have suggested that the pericardium actually exerts a significant constraining effect and that at end diastole the pericardial pressure is equal to right atrial and right ventricular diastolic pressures. While there is some controversy about the precise point at which the pericardium affects cardiac filling, all investigators agree that the pericardium prevents acute distention of the heart.

In summary, it appears that the pericardium (1) provides a relatively inelastic envelope that protects against sudden cardiac dilatation, (2) limits cardiac displacement within the chest, and (3) may provide a relatively low-friction surface for efficient cardiac contraction.

■ PERICARDITIS

ACUTE PERICARDITIS

The most common disorder of the pericardium is acute inflammation of the pericardium (*acute pericarditis*). As shown in Fig. 5-7, inflammation of the pericardium is often associated with fibrinous exudates that coat the lining of the pericardial space (the hairy heart?). There are a number of common causes of acute pericardial inflammation, which are summarized in Table 5-1.

Clinical Characteristics of Acute Pericarditis

1. Positional chest pain
2. Friction rub
3. ST-segment elevation

FIG. 5-7

ANATOMIC SPECIMEN SHOWING THE FIBRINOUS EXUDATE COVERING THE VISCERAL PERICARDIUM AND THE INNER SIDE OF THE PARIETAL PERICARDIUM FROM ACUTE PERICARDITIS. (*Source:* Reprinted with permission from Hurst JW: *Atlas of the Heart.* New York, NY: McGraw-Hill, 1988, Fig. 7.1.)

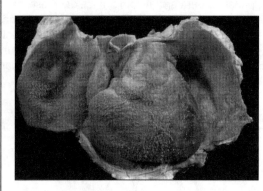
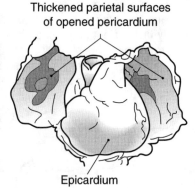

Thickened parietal surfaces of opened pericardium

Epicardium

Table 5-1

Causes of Acute Pericarditis

CAUSE	COMMENT
Idiopathic	Most commonly, the specific cause of pericarditis cannot be determined.
Viral	Coxsackie A and B viruses, adenovirus, cytomegalovirus, Epstein-Barr virus, hepatitis B virus, and human immunodeficiency virus can be associated with pericarditis.
Bacterial infection	Pneumococcal, staphylococcal, neisserial, and tubercular infections may be associated with pericarditis.
Fungal	Histoplasmosis, coccidioidomycosis, and *Candida* fungal infections can uncommonly be associated with pericarditis.
Other infection	Toxoplasmosis, amebiasis, and mycoplasmas can be associated with pericarditis.
Myocardial infarction	Acutely during myocardial infarction; autoimmune reaction after myocardial infarction (Dressler's syndrome).
Uremia	Uremia is present in up to 20% of pericarditis patients; etiology is unclear, perhaps autoimmune.
Neoplastic disease	Pericarditis is present in 5%–15% of patients with malignant neoplasia; often it is associated with pericardial effusion.
Radiation	Radiation causes direct injury to the pericardium; the incidence depends on radiation dose and volume of the heart included in the radiation field.
Autoimmune disorders	Rheumatic fever, lupus erythematosus, rheumatoid arthritis, and polyarteritis nodosa are all associated with an autoimmune-mediated pericarditis in 10%–50% of patients.
Drugs	Procainamide, hydralazine, and methysergide are all associated with an autoimmune-mediated pericarditis.
Trauma	Pericardial injury is present in 50% of autopsy cases of nonpenetrating trauma to the heart. It is usually associated with other significant cardiac injury.

Symptoms of acute pericarditis include chest pain that is often positional in nature. Most commonly the pain is worsened by lying supine, coughing, or with deep inspiration. In addition, patients frequently complain of shortness of breath, mainly because they are unable to take a deep breath without severe pain.

On physical examination, a loud *pericardial friction rub* is the pathognomonic finding characteristic of acute pericarditis (Fig. 5-8). The rub is a high-pitched, often "scratchy" sound that has been compared to the "squeak of a new leather saddle." Traditionally, there are three components to the rub, which occur during (1) contraction of the atria, (2) contraction of the ventricles, and (3) rapid relaxation of the ventricles. The systolic component resulting from ventricular contraction is the loudest and most easily heard. Frequently, the early diastolic component resulting from ventricular relaxation and the late diastolic component produced by atrial contraction merge, resulting in a "to-and-fro" rub. The genesis of the rub is generally thought to be friction between the inflamed mesothelial surfaces of the visceral and parietal pericardium, although pericardial rubs

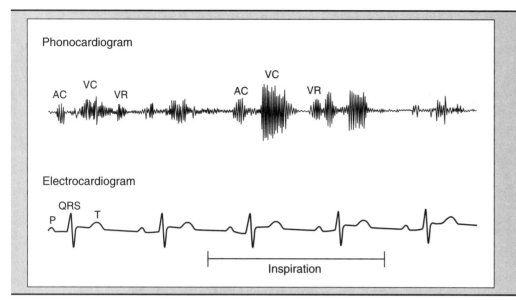

Phonocardiogram

Electrocardiogram

FIG. 5-8
THE THREE COMPONENTS OF THE PERICARDIAL RUB. A late diastolic component is due to atrial contraction (AC), a loud systolic component is due to ventricular contraction (VC), and a relatively soft early diastolic component is due to ventricular relaxation (VR). Notice that all components of the rub become louder with inspiration.

can sometimes be heard in the presence of a large amount of pericardial fluid. The pericardial rub is often evanescent and sometimes can only be heard in particular positions, such as with the patient leaning forward. In addition, the intensity of the rub changes with respiration, usually becoming louder with deep inspiration.

The ECG yields abnormal findings in approximately 90% of patients with acute pericarditis. Pericardial inflammation is often associated with diffuse ST-segment elevation in most of the leads. The exact mechanism for ST-segment elevation is unclear. Like the ST-segment elevation observed in myocardial infarction (see Chap. 3), it is thought that the ST-segment elevation in pericarditis is a combination of systolic and diastolic effects. Most investigators feel that pericardial inflammation causes widespread inflammation of the superficial epicardium, which leads to resting depolarization of the epicardial cardiac myocytes (makes the interior of the cell less negative and the surface of the cell more negative). As shown at the lower left of Fig. 5-9B, this leads to a current flow from the epicardium to the endocardium, which results in *absolute* TP-segment depression when measured from the surface ECG. After the ventricular myocardial cells are depolarized and all of the cells are at the plateau phase (phase 2), no current flows (see Fig. 5-9B). Since all commercially available ECGs zero the baseline to the TP segment, these changes result in *relative* ST-segment elevation. Actually, in addition to this diastolic effect, the epicardial tissue also repolarizes more quickly, which can directly cause ST-segment elevation. However, experimental data suggest that the diastolic effect produced by resting depolarization is much larger than the systolic effect of early repolarization (see discussion in Chap. 3).

Mr. Mickelsen's ECG was examined by the physician who noticed the diffuse ST-segment elevation. Mr. Mickelsen had acute viral pericarditis. To treat the inflammation he was given nonsteroidal anti-inflammatory drugs (NSAIDs). Unfortunately over the next several weeks, Mr. Mickelsen developed profound weakness and was now noted to have a very rapid heart rate (130 beats/min) and reduced blood pressure (84/44 mm Hg). With inspiration, his blood pressure dropped to 58/39 mm Hg. On physical examination, Mr. Mickelsen's heart sounds were muffled, and his jugular venous pressure was elevated. His chest radiograph is shown in Fig. 5-10.

Case Study:
Continued

CONSTRICTIVE PERICARDITIS

Rarely, acute pericarditis can progress to recurrent episodes of pericarditis or a festering chronic pericarditis. In general, the symptoms, physical examination findings, and ECG of patients with relapsing or chronic pericarditis are similar to those of acute pericarditis, but they may be more longstanding and can be subtler.

Constrictive pericarditis may develop if the pericardium is chronically inflamed (chronic pericarditis).

FIG. 5-9

(A) Normally, during diastole, cells of both the endocardium and epicardium have a resting membrane potential of −90 mV, and since no current flows, the electrocardiogram (ECG) is at baseline. Similarly, during systole, all of the cells are at the plateau phase with a membrane potential of 10–20 mV, and the ST segment is also usually isoelectric. (B) In pericarditis, at baseline the epicardial cells are partially depolarized, and a current flows from epicardium to endocardium, which causes TP-segment depression. During systole, all cells achieve similar membrane potentials, and no current flows. However, since the ECG machine defines the TP segment as zero, relative ST-segment elevation is observed.

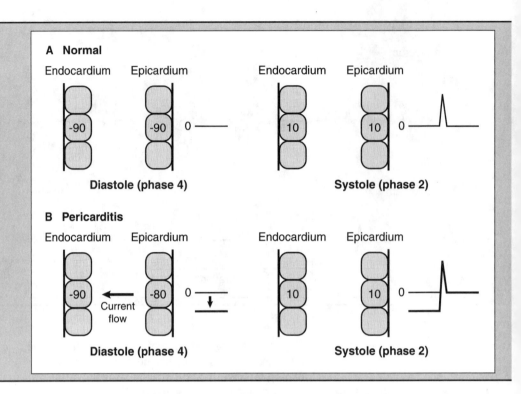

FIG. 5-10

MR. MICKELSEN'S CHEST RADIOGRAPH. Can you identify the abnormality?

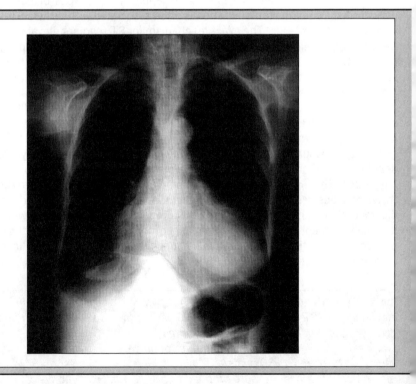

In some cases, chronic inflammation of the pericardium can lead to *constrictive pericarditis*. In this disease, chronic inflammation causes the pericardium to become thickened, with very little distensibility. Worldwide, the most common cause of constrictive pericarditis is tuberculosis. With chronic inflammation, frequently the visceral and parietal pericardial layers become fused and calcium is deposited (Fig. 5-11). The pericardium now acts as a fixed "case" over the heart that (1) causes abnormal filling of ventricles and (2) prevents changes in intrathoracic pressure from affecting the heart.

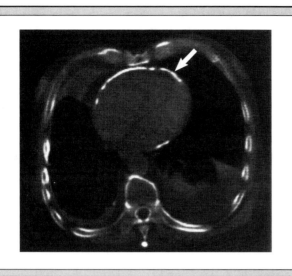

FIG. 5-11
COMPUTED TOMOGRAPHY OF THE CHEST IN A PATIENT WITH CONSTRICTIVE PERICARDITIS. The heavily calcified pericardium can be observed (*arrow*). (*Source:* Reprinted with permission from Shabetai R: Diseases of the pericardium. *Cardiol Clin* 8(4):655, 1990.)

In patients with constrictive pericarditis, filling of the left and right ventricles occurs normally in early diastole. However, once the ventricles fill to the limit of the pericardial space, ventricular filling comes to a rapid halt (Fig. 5-12), which leads to a characteristic "spike-and-plateau" morphology of the right and left ventricular pressure recording. The early diastolic "spike" corresponds to the normal (frequently supranormal) filling in early diastole while the "plateau" occurs during mid- and late diastole when there is little

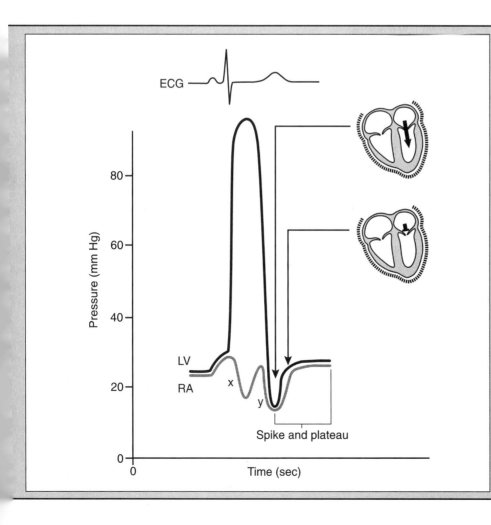

FIG. 5-12
DIAGRAM SHOWING THE HEMODYNAMIC CONSEQUENCES OF CONSTRICTIVE PERICARDITIS. Initially the left ventricle (LV) fills rapidly, but once the heart becomes constrained by the thick pericardium, left ventricular filling slows and left ventricular pressure markedly increases, which yields the characteristic "spike and plateau." ECG = electrocardiogram; RA = right atrium.

additional volume increase in the ventricles (as a result of pericardial restraint). The sudden cessation of ventricular filling can often produce a pericardial "knock." The pericardial knock usually occurs earlier and has a slightly higher pitch than the third heart sound described earlier for congestive heart failure (see Chapter 1).

Rapid filling of the ventricles during diastole leads to rapid filling of the atria via the vena cava and pulmonary veins. (Since the mitral and tricuspid valves are open, the atria serve as conduits.) Consequently, the atrial pressure tracings are characterized by a prominent *y* descent (analogous to the "spike" on the ventricular pressure recording). The systolic *x* descent is also prominent, which leads to a characteristic W configuration of the jugular venous pulse in patients with constrictive pericarditis (see Fig. 5-12).

Another important feature of the pathophysiology of constrictive pericarditis is the alteration in right-sided pressures in response to respiration. Normally, with inspiration, intrathoracic pressure decreases, and flow from the right-sided chambers into the pulmonary vascular bed increases, which causes a fall in right atrial pressure and the jugular venous pressure (Fig. 5-13A). As shown in Fig. 5-13B, the thickened pericardium prevents changes in intrathoracic pressure from affecting the intracardiac chambers so that patients with constrictive pericarditis do not have inspiratory fall of right atrial and jugular venous pressure. In fact, in 1873, Adolph Kussmaul described two patients with constrictive pericarditis who actually displayed increased jugular venous pressure with inspiration. While the reasons are not fully understood, it is thought that inspiratory increase in intra-abdominal pressure and subsequent increased venous return to the right-sided cardiac chambers are responsible for this finding (see Fig. 5-13B). Inspiratory increase of jugular venous pressure is now referred to as *Kussmaul's sign*.

Pathophysiology of Constrictive Pericarditis

1. Abnormal ventricular filling
2. Changes in intrathoracic pressure do not affect filling

Jugular venous pressure is used to estimate right atrial pressure.

FIG. 5-13
RESPIRATORY EFFECTS ON RIGHT ATRIAL PRESSURE. (A) Normally, with inspiration, negative intrathoracic pressures lead to increased flow of blood into the lung from the right chambers, which leads to reduced right atrial and jugular venous pressure. (B) In constrictive pericarditis, the thick pericardium prevents the transfer of intrathoracic pressure, which leads to no respiratory variability of right atrial pressure, or in some cases, inspiratory increase in right atrial pressure (Kussmaul's sign). In severe cases of constrictive pericarditis, the increased intra-abdominal pressure associated with inspiration causes increased return of blood to the right-sided chambers, which cannot be compensated for, and inspiratory increase in right atrial pressure is observed. LA = left atrium; RA = right atrium; LV = left ventricle.

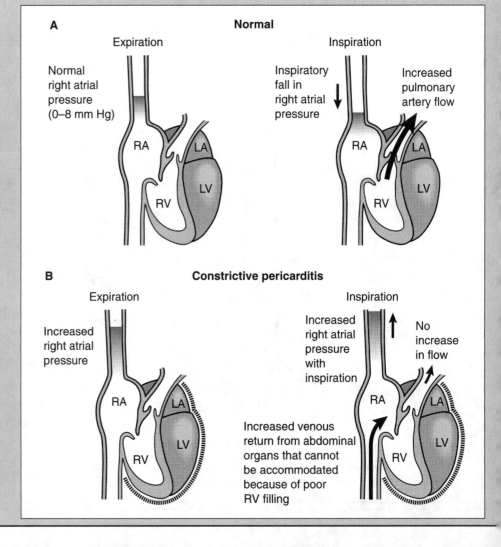

PERICARDIAL EFFUSION

Acute and chronic pericarditis are commonly associated with the accumulation of a small amount of fluid. However, in some cases, large amounts of fluid can accumulate in the pericardial space, which can significantly alter cardiac function. All forms of pericarditis can be associated with fluid accumulation, but most commonly, large pericardial effusions are associated with viral infections, neoplasia, trauma, and post-radiation.

The physiologic impact of increased pericardial fluid depends both on how much and how quickly fluid accumulates. If fluid accumulates slowly, the pericardial space can accommodate up to 2 L of fluid by increased stretch and size. In conditions that cause chronic dilatation of the heart (such as aortic and mitral regurgitation), pericardial mass increases slowly over time, paralleling the increase in cardiac mass. However, only 80–200 mL can be acutely added to the pericardial space before the pericardium begins to operate on the steep portion of its pressure–volume curve.

Pericardial fluid and the heart occupy a relatively fixed volume; if fluid is added to the pericardial space when the pericardium is operating on the steep portion of its pressure–volume curve, pericardial pressure, right ventricular diastolic pressure, and left ventricular diastolic pressure begin to rise. As more fluid accumulates, right ventricular diastolic pressure and pericardial pressures equilibrate, and then pericardial pressure and right ventricular diastolic pressure increase to equilibrate with left ventricular diastolic pressure. The increase and equilibration of chamber pressures with rapid accumulation of pericardial fluid are called *pericardial tamponade*, which leads to several profound, characteristic consequences.

First, increased right ventricular diastolic pressure leads to elevated right atrial pressures. As shown in Fig. 5-14, the right atrial pressure at end diastole is elevated (20 mm Hg, normal: 0–8 mm Hg). As the heart contracts, right ventricular pressure increases and right ventricular volume decreases. The right atria can fill since right ventricular volume is relatively small. However, at the beginning of diastole, since the volume encompassed by the heart and the pericardial fluid is fixed, very little right atrial filling can occur. This set of events leads to elevated right atrial pressures and a right atrial (or jugular venous) pressure contour that is associated with an *x* descent but no *y* descent, since right atrial filling can only occur during systole.

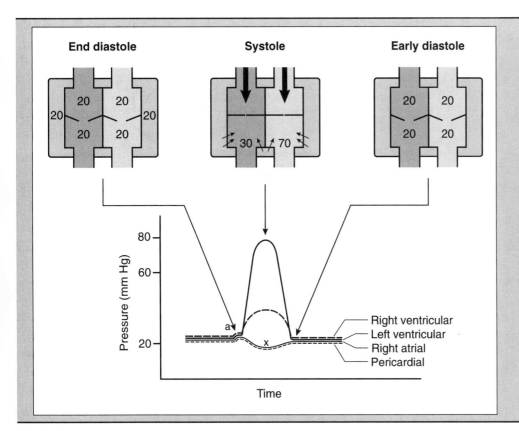

FIG. 5-14
CARDIAC PRESSURE TRACINGS IN A PATIENT WITH PERICARDIAL TAMPONADE. Filling of the atria can occur only during systole (since ventricular contraction allows more room within the pericardial space), which causes the right atrial pressure tracing to show an x descent but no y descent. (*Source:* Adapted with permission from Reddy PS: Hemodynamics of cardiac tamponade in man. In *Pericardial Disease.* Edited by Reddy PS, Leon DF, Shaver JA. New York, NY: Raven Press, 1982, p 161.)

Pericardial Tamponade

1. Elevated right atrial pressure
2. Reduced cardiac output (particularly during inspiration)

Second, increased pericardial fluid causes reduced cardiac output, particularly with inspiration. As pericardial pressure increases and equilibrates with right ventricular diastolic pressure, right ventricular filling is markedly reduced. Reduced right ventricular filling leads to reduced left atrial and left ventricular filling, which reduces cardiac output (Fig. 5-15). In addition, in pericardial tamponade, the reduction in cardiac output is most pronounced during inspiration. Normally, stroke volume decreases by approximately 7%, and arterial blood pressure decreases by 3% during inspiration. Inspiration causes a small decrease in left ventricular volume and an increase in venous return to the right side of the heart by the following mechanism. The more negative intrathoracic pressure associated with inspiration reduces venous return in the pulmonary veins and increases flow in the pulmonary arteries. Reduced preload to the left ventricle results in reduced left ventricular size and reduced arterial blood pressure. In 1873, the German physiologist Kussmaul (remember Kussmaul's sign?) noticed the apparent paradox of the disappearance of the pulse while the heartbeat continued in a patient with pericardial tamponade. His observation of an exaggerated inspiratory decrease in the arterial blood pressure is called *pulsus paradoxus*. Pulsus paradoxus can be seen in patients with severe lung disease, where excessively negative intrathoracic pressure causes an exaggerated reduction in arterial pressure with inspiration. However, pulsus paradoxus is most commonly associated with pericardial tamponade. In pericardial tamponade, during inspiration, more negative intrathoracic pressure results in increased flow into the right atria and ventricles. Since the right-sided chambers now make up a larger percentage of the small, confined space that is due to the presence of pericardial fluid, the left ventricle fills less well (Fig. 5-16). The exaggerated shift means that arterial pressure decreases more than the normal 3% and can be up to 30% in response to inspiration.

FIG. 5-15
As pericardial fluid is increased, pericardial (Peri), right ventricular (RV), and left ventricular (LV) pressures increase, cardiac output (CO) decreases, and the inspiratory fall in arterial pressure increases (pulsus paradoxus). (*Source:* Adapted with permission from Reddy PS, Curtiss EI, Eretsky BF: The spectrum of hemodynamic abnormalities in pericardial effusion. *Am J Cardiol* 66(20):1488, 1990).

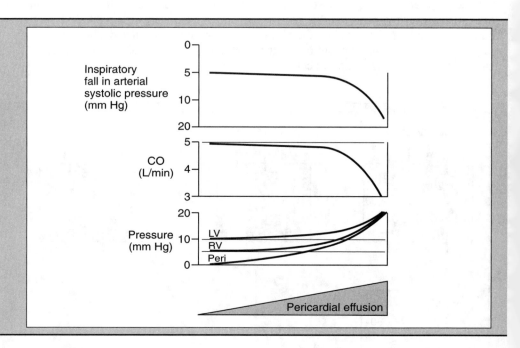

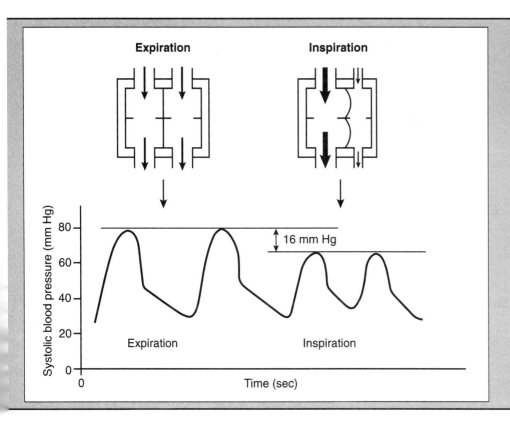

Expiration   Inspiration

FIG. 5-16
**SCHEMATIC SHOWING THE GEN-
ESIS OF PULSUS PARADOXUS
IN PERICARDIAL TAMPONADE.**
With inspiration, negative intrathoracic pressure is transmitted to the heart and leads to a
relative increase in right-sided
blood flow and chamber size.
Since the intrapericardial volume is fixed, reduced venous
return to the left-sided chambers and reduced cardiac output are observed. (*Source:*
Adapted with permission from
Reddy PS: Hemodynamics of
cardiac tamponade in man. In
Reddy PS, Leon DF, Shaver JA
(eds): *Pericardial Disease.* New
York, NY: Raven Press, 1982,
p 161.)

DIFFERENCES BETWEEN CONSTRICTIVE PERICARDITIS AND PERICARDIAL TAMPONADE

The similarities and distinctions between constrictive pericarditis and pericardial tamponade are summarized in Table 5-2. Both constrictive pericarditis and pericardial
tamponade alter ventricular filling (leading to elevated right atrial pressures) and reduce
cardiac output. However, in constrictive pericarditis the heart is not restricted during
early diastole, while in pericardial tamponade, increased pericardial pressure exerts its
effects throughout all of diastole.

PARAMETER	CONSTRICTIVE PERICARDITIS	PERICARDIAL TAMPONADE
Pathophysiology	Thickening of the pericardium, which leads to poor distensibility	Accumulation of fluid in the pericardial space, which compresses the heart
Cardiac output	Reduced	Reduced
Right atrial pressure	Elevated	Elevated
Right atrial venous waveform	Bimodal: sharp *x* and *y* descents	Unimodal: absent or blunted *y* descent
Respiratory variation of right atrial pressure	Decreased intrathoracic pressure resulting from inspiration is *not* transmitted to the pericardial space. Right atrial pressure does not decrease with inspiration. In some cases, right atrial pressure actually increases with inspiration (Kussmaul's sign).	Decreased intrathoracic pressure resulting from inspiration is transmitted to the pericardial space. Right atrial pressure decreases normally with inspiration.
Respiratory variation of cardiac output	Normal inspiratory drop in arterial blood pressure (8–9 mm Hg)	Exaggerated inspiratory drop of systemic blood pressure > 10 mm Hg (pulsus paradoxus)

Table 5-2
Pathophysiologic Similarities and Differences between Constrictive Pericarditis and Pericardial Tamponade

In constrictive pericarditis, the left ventricular pressure tracing shows a "spike-and-plateau" morphology, while in pericardial tamponade the left ventricular pressure is elevated but has a normal pattern. In constrictive pericarditis, right atrial filling occurs in a normal pattern, but there is an exaggerated *y* descent resulting from the sharp decrease in ventricular pressures during early diastole (see Fig. 5-12). In pericardial tamponade, atrial filling occurs only during systole, which leads to an *x* descent but an absent or blunted *y* descent (see Fig. 5-14). In constrictive pericarditis, increased negative transthoracic pressure changes are not transmitted to the heart so that the right atrial pressure does not fall normally with inspiration. In pericardial tamponade, respiratory variability is exaggerated; with inspiration, right atrial pressures decrease normally, and systemic arterial pressures display a supernormal decrease (pulsus paradoxus).

∎ SUMMARY

The pericardium is a double layer of connective tissue (visceral and parietal pericardium) that forms a sac that surrounds the heart. The pericardium is very compliant at low volumes, but as cardiac volume increases it begins to have a constraining effect. Diseases of the pericardium can be due to inflammation of the pericardial tissue (pericarditis) or the accumulation of fluid within the space formed by the visceral and parietal pericardial layers (pericardial effusion). While less common than other cardiac conditions, pericardial diseases may have catastrophic consequences that must be quickly recognized by the physician. Understanding pericardial physiology and pathophysiology is a necessary component for understanding cardiovascular pathophysiology.

KEY POINTS

- The pericardium forms a double-layered sac around the heart. The space between the two layers (the visceral and parietal pericardium) is normally filled with a small amount of fluid.
- The pericardium is elastic at small volumes and inelastic at large volumes. The pericardium prevents acute dilatation of the ventricle.
- Diseases of the pericardium can be due to inflammation of the pericardium (pericarditis) or the accumulation of abnormal amounts of fluid within the pericardial space (pericardial effusion). Pericarditis and pericardial effusion are not mutually exclusive.
- Pericarditis can be either acute or chronic. Acute pericarditis causes sudden onset of chest pain often associated with a rub on physical examination and ST-segment elevation on the ECG. In chronic pericarditis, the symptoms are often more insidious, rubs are frequently not heard, and the ECG shows only nonspecific changes. In some cases of chronic pericarditis, an exuberant inflammatory response can lead to constrictive pericarditis.
- Pericardial effusions are frequently asymptomatic (unless due to acute pericarditis), until the accumulated fluid begins to affect filling of the left ventricle. At this point the patient has pericardial tamponade, which is characterized by hypotension, pulsus paradoxus, and an elevated jugular venous pressure.

Case Study:
Resolution

Mr. Mickelsen developed a large pericardial effusion over the last several days. The accumulation of fluid in the pericardial space led to compression of the heart, poor filling, and pericardial tamponade. A needle was introduced into the pericardial space, and fluid was removed, which significantly alleviated Mr. Mickelsen's symptoms (Fig. 5-17). The original cause for pericarditis was not determined.

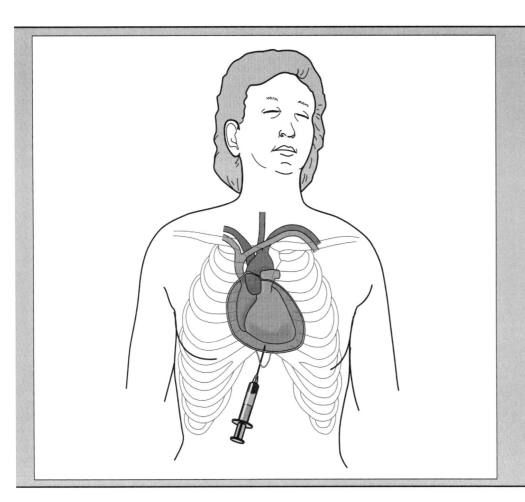

FIG. 5-17
To remove pericardial fluid, a needle is directed toward the left shoulder just under the xyphoid process, and fluid is aspirated. (*Source:* Adapted with permission from Netter FH: *The Ciba Collection of Medical Illustrations: Heart*, vol 5. East Hanover, NJ: Novartis Pharmaceuticals, 1992, p 253.)

▮ REVIEW QUESTIONS

Directions: For each of the following questions, choose the **one best** answer.

1. Which of the following findings is associated with pericardial tamponade?

   (A) Kussmaul's sign
   (B) Increased cardiac output
   (C) Pulsus paradoxus
   (D) ST-segment elevation on the electrocardiogram (ECG)

2. Ms. C. K. has just been involved in a head-on collision. She comes to the emergency room complaining of severe chest pain. Her blood pressure is 70 mm Hg, and during inspiration her blood pressure drops to 50 mm Hg. Which of the following findings would the emergency room physician most likely observe?

   (A) Kussmaul's sign
   (B) A friction rub
   (C) Diffuse ST-segment elevation on the surface electrocardiogram (ECG)
   (D) An enlarged cardiac silhouette on chest radiograph

3. Which of the following statements best describes normal pericardial physiology?

   (A) The pericardial sac is extremely compliant.
   (B) The pericardial sac is extremely noncompliant.
   (C) The pericardial sac is initially very compliant but as it is stretched becomes noncompliant.
   (D) The pericardial sac is initially very noncompliant but as it is stretched becomes compliant.

4. Which of the following statements about chronic pericarditis with constrictive physiology is true?

   (A) Kussmaul's sign (increased jugular venous pressure with inspiration) may be observed.
   (B) Increased cardiac output is often observed.
   (C) Pulsus paradoxus is always observed.
   (D) Decreased right atrial pressure is present.
   (E) A pericardial rub is usually present.

■ ANSWERS AND EXPLANATIONS

1. The answer is C. In pericardial tamponade, abnormal amounts of fluid accumulate in the pericardial space, thus effectively reducing the volume available for the heart itself. This significantly limits the amount of ventricular filling (since filling requires cardiac expansion). Although the pericardial space is fluid filled, changes in intrathoracic pressure are transmitted to the heart, so that jugular venous pressure, while significantly elevated, still decreases with inspiration. In patients with constrictive pericarditis, the pericardium forms a "shell" around the heart that does not transmit changes in intrathoracic pressure so that jugular venous pressure does not decrease and at times increases with inspiration (Kussmaul's sign). In pericardial tamponade, cardiac output is significantly reduced because of poor left ventricular filling. Normally with inspiration, right-sided flows increase as a result of reduced intrathoracic pressure (normal inspiratory fall in jugular venous pressure). However, the right-sided chambers now take up a larger amount of the fixed intrapericardial space so that cardiac output and systemic blood pressure markedly drop during inspiration (pulsus paradoxus). The ECG in pericardial tamponade is not associated with ST-segment elevation (no superficial myocardial inflammation such as in acute pericarditis), rather the pericardial fluid leads to reduced QRS voltages on the ECG.

2. The answer is D. One of the complications of a motor vehicle accident is rupture of the wall of the heart, which can lead to the accumulation of blood in the pericardial space (pericardial tamponade). Since blood accumulates rapidly, patients decompensate very quickly and have profound hypotension and pulsus paradoxus. While acute pericardial inflammation (acute pericarditis) leads to chest pain, diffuse ST-segment elevation on the ECG, and a pericardial rub, diffuse ST-segment elevation and pericardial rubs are frequently not observed with a sudden accumulation of blood in the pericardial space. Kussmaul's sign (inspiratory increase in jugular venous pressure) only occurs if the pericardium is chronically inflamed, and constrictive physiology develops where the pericardium acts as a "hard sac" around the heart. Kussmaul's sign is usually not observed in pericardial tamponade.

3. The answer is C. As pericardial tissue is stretched, it is initially very compliant; however, as pericardial tissue is continually stretched, it reaches a point where compliance is markedly reduced. This characteristic is responsible for the J-shaped curve observed in pressure–volume studies of pericardial tissue.

4. The answer is A. In constrictive pericarditis, increased inspiratory jugular venous pressure (Kussmaul's sign) may be observed. Kussmaul's sign is thought to occur in constrictive pericarditis because of increased inspiratory venous return from abdominal structures, which cannot be accommodated for by the right-sided chambers. Pulsus paradoxus is observed very infrequently in patients with constrictive pericarditis. Since the pericardium forms a hard shell around the heart, ventricular filling is quickly limited during early diastole, leading to high right atrial pressures and a pericardial "knock." However, pericardial rubs are frequently not present. Limited ventricular filling usually is associated with decreased cardiac output.

■ REFERENCES

Lorell BH: Pericardial diseases. In *Heart Disease: A Textbook of Cardiovascular Medicine.* Edited by Braunwald E. Philadelphia, PA: W. B. Saunders, 1996, pp. 1478–1534.

Shabetai R: Diseases of the pericardium. *Cardiol Clin* 8:4, 1990.

Watkins MW, LeWinter MM: Physiologic role of the normal pericardium. *Ann Rev Med* 44:171–180, 1993.

Chapter 6

CONGENITAL HEART DISEASE

Phoebe Ashley, M.D.

■ CHAPTER OUTLINE

Case Study: *Introduction*	*Gale Etherton was a 30-year-old woman who presented to your office with complaints of progressive dyspnea and fatigue over the previous 6 months. On examination her pulse was 75 beats/min, blood pressure was 124/70 mm Hg, and her respiratory rate was 28 breaths/min. Her jugular venous pulse was normal. Her lung examination revealed crackles in both lung bases. On cardiac examination she had a prominent right ventricular impulse, a distinct first heart sound (S_1), a fixed split second heart sound (S_2), and a systolic ejection murmur heard best over the left second intercostal space. What is your diagnosis based upon Ms. Etherton's symptoms and signs? Can you provide the pathophysiologic basis for these clinical findings?*

■ INTRODUCTION

Abnormalities of the heart and great vessels that are present at birth are grouped together under the term *congenital heart disease*. Most congenital cardiac disorders occur as a result of faulty embryogenesis during gestational weeks 3 through 8, when the cardiovascular system is undergoing development. In the fetus, the parallel nature of the pulmonary and systemic circulatory systems allows the fetus to tolerate most congenital cardiac anomalies with the exception of severe regurgitant lesions. After birth, with the elimination of both the maternal circulation and the fetal pathways (ductus arteriosus and foramen ovale), the hemodynamic impact of an anatomic cardiac abnormality in the newborn often becomes apparent. Some children with congenital anomalies do not develop significant hemodynamic problems for many years, which are thus not recognized until they reach adulthood or develop significant cardiovascular compromise.

The incidence of congenital heart disease is generally reported as 8 per 1000 liveborn, full-term births. The incidence is higher in premature infants (~2%), stillborns (2%), and abortuses (10%–25%). Twelve anomalies account for approximately 85% of cases, with frequencies noted in Table 6-1.

Table 6-1
Relative Frequency of Congenital Heart Disease

LESIONS	PERCENTAGE OF ALL LESIONS
Ventricular septal defect[a]	25–30
Atrial septal defect[a]	6–8
Patent ductus arteriosus[a]	6–8
Coarctation of aorta[a]	5–7
Tetralogy of Fallot[a]	5–7
Pulmonary valve stenosis[a]	5–7
Aortic valve stenosis	4–7
Transposition of the great arteries	3–5
Hypoplastic left ventricle	1–3
Hypoplastic right ventricle	1–3
Truncus arteriosus	1–2
Total anomalous pulmonary venous return	1–2
Tricuspid atresia	1–2
Single ventricle	1–2
Double-outlet right ventricle	1–2
Others	5–10

Note. The table excludes patent ductus arteriosus in the preterm neonate, bicuspid aortic valve, peripheral pulmonic stenosis, and mitral valve prolapse.
Source. Adapted from Behrman RE, Kliegman RM, Arvin AM, et al: *Nelson Textbook of Pediatrics*, 15th ed. Philadelphia, PA: W. B. Saunders, 1996, p 1286.
[a] Lesion is described in this chapter.

The etiology of most congenital cardiac defects is unknown. In many cases the cause of a defect is believed to be multifactorial. *Genetic factors* are known to play some role in the development of congenital heart defects, as evidenced by an increased family incidence of cardiac abnormalities. If a woman has one child with a cardiac anomaly, the risk of a second child having heart defects increases to 2%–6%. The risk of a third affected child may reach 20%–30% if two siblings have congenital cardiac defects. Specific chromosomal abnormalities associated with congenital heart disease have been identified, such as trisomies 21, 18, 13, 22, 9 (mosaic), Turner's (XO) syndrome, and +14q−.

Environmental influences have also been associated with cardiac defects. Perhaps the best described external factor contributing to the development of cardiac malformations is maternal rubella in the first trimester of pregnancy. In addition to the development of microcephaly, cataracts, and deafness, fetuses exposed to rubella may develop a number of cardiac anomalies, including patent ductus arteriosus, pulmonary and aortic valvular stenosis, arterial stenosis, tetralogy of Fallot, and ventricular septal defects. Other cardiac teratogens include ethanol, thalidomide, lithium, isotretinoin (Accutane), and anticonvulsant agents. Finally, *comorbid maternal diseases* such as diabetes mellitus, phenylketonuria, and systemic lupus erythematosus may also predispose the fetus to significant abnormalities during cardiac development.

Causes of Congenital Heart Disease
Genetic factors
Environmental factors
Comorbid maternal diseases

This chapter is divided into three sections. First, normal development of the heart is reviewed. Second, the changes from fetal circulation to the newborn circulation are discussed. Finally, the most common congenital cardiovascular defects are discussed individually.

■ EMBRYOLOGY

While the cardiovascular system develops throughout the entire gestational period, the primary structures of the heart develop between weeks 3 and 8. Although the development of the heart through this critical period is presented temporally here because this arrangement provides a convenient outline for our discussion, it is important for the student to remember that there is significant overlap and variability in the development of the cardiovascular system. For example, atrial septation occurs from weeks 4 to 6, but the entire process is discussed here in week 5.

WEEKS 1–3

Early in gestation, the embryo can obtain enough nutrients by diffusion from the surrounding tissues. However, as the embryo grows, this mode of nutrient delivery is insufficient to sustain its metabolic needs, necessitating the development of the cardiovascular system to promote nutrient delivery. The cardiovascular system is derived from angioblastic tissue that arises from the mesenchymal cells derived from the mesoderm.

At day 17 or 18 of embryogenesis, angioblastic cells begin to proliferate and form clusters of cells on either side of the embryo (Fig. 6-1). These cell clusters spread cephalad, canalize, and finally unite to form a crescent-shaped anterior structure and parallel posterior tubes (Fig. 6-2). At the same time, the intraembryonic coelom develops between these two regions. The intraembryonic coelomic cavity becomes the pericardial cavity, which houses the heart (see Chap. 5, Fig. 5-2). The cells from the anterior and posterior structures coalesce and eventually form a complex structure consisting of an anterior upside-down *U* and, in a perpendicular plane, two upside-down *J*s. The two tubes just posterior to the intraembryonic coelom eventually form the heart. As the embryo develops it undergoes cephalocaudal flexion related to rapid longitudinal growth of the central nervous system. Flexion of the embryo brings the two endocardial heart tubes into proximity to one another along the ventral midline. On days 20 to 22, the heart tubes fuse, forming a single straight endocardial tube, which will invaginate into the intraembryonic coelom, which forms the pericardial cavity (Fig. 6-3). At this time the single heart tube has three layers: an outer mantle one to two cell layers thick, a middle layer of amorphous cardiac "jelly," and an inner single layer of endocardial cells. Shortly after fusion of the two endocardial tubes, the heart begins to beat. It is believed that the forces generated by contraction of the heart influence subsequent cardiac development. As the tubular heart elongates, it develops alternating dilatations and constrictions, which correspond to future components of the heart (see Fig. 6-3).

Mesoderm is the primary germ layer of cells between the ectoderm and endoderm. Muscular, skeletal, circulatory, lymphatic, and urogenital tissues are derived from the mesoderm.

Weeks 1–3
A single heart tube is formed.

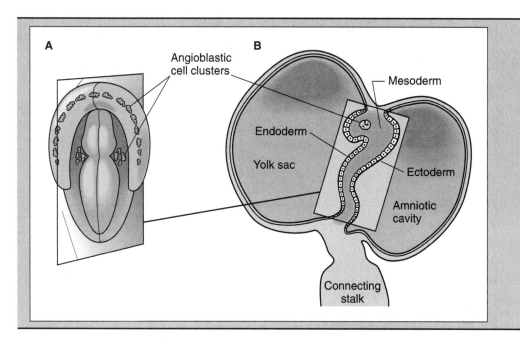

A   B

Angioblastic cell clusters

Mesoderm

Endoderm

Yolk sac

Ectoderm

Amniotic cavity

Connecting stalk

FIG. 6-1
EMBRYO AT DAY 17 OR 18. (A) The figure on the *left* shows a ventral schematic of the embryo. (B) The figure on the *right* shows a sagittal section through the amniotic cavity and the yolk sac. Ectodermal cells of the embryo face the amniotic cavity, and endodermal cells face the yolk sac. The mesodermal layer is formed from ectodermal "buds." Angioblastic cell clusters that will form the circulatory system can be observed in the mesoderm.

WEEK 4

Continued growth of the heart tube within the confines of the pericardial cavity necessitates bending of the heart tube for optimal space conservation. In addition, there appear

Week 4
The heart tube begins to loop.

FIG. 6-2
**DEVELOPING CIRCULATORY SYS-
TEM AND INTRAEMBRYONIC
COELOM.** The developing circulatory system forms a complex
structure shaped like an upside-
down *U* that is associated with
perpendicularly oriented upside-
down *J*s. The intraembryonic
coelom is located above the *U*
and anterior to the *J*s.

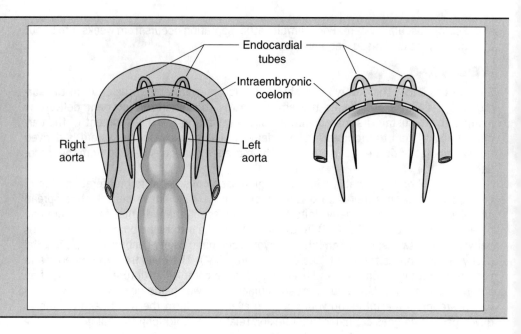

FIG. 6-3
**TWO HEART TUBES FUSE AT
DAY 20 TO 22.** The single heart
tube begins to develop bulges
that will correspond to different
regions of the heart. A cross
section of the heart tube shows
a single layer of endocardial
cells, an outer layer of one or
two cells thick, and an amorphous middle layer of cardiac
"jelly."

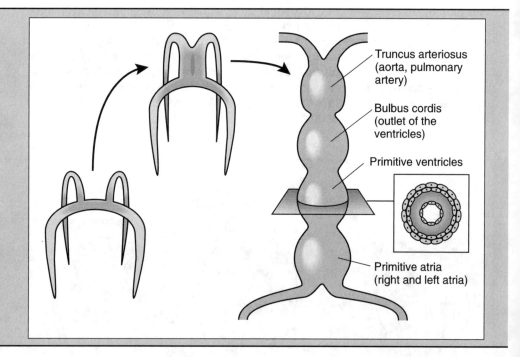

to be intrinsic cellular factors that favor looping of the heart tube. The bulbus cordis and
ventricle grow faster than the other regions of the heart tube. Consequently, the heart
tube bends on itself, forming a *U*-shaped bulboventricular loop. As the heart bends, the
atrium and sinus venosus come to lie behind the bulbus cordis, the truncus arteriosus,
and the ventricle. The bulbus cordis then moves medially within the pericardial sac to
divide the heart into four primitive chambers. At this stage, the area between the
primitive atria and ventricles is termed the atrioventricular (AV) canal. As tubular growth
continues, ventricular growth predominates, and the heart loop takes on an *S*-shaped
configuration with a deep bulboventricular sulcus separating the ventricle from the
bulbus cordis (Fig. 6-4). Abnormalities in cardiac loop formation may lead to malformations associated with ventricular inversion and transposition of the great vessels.

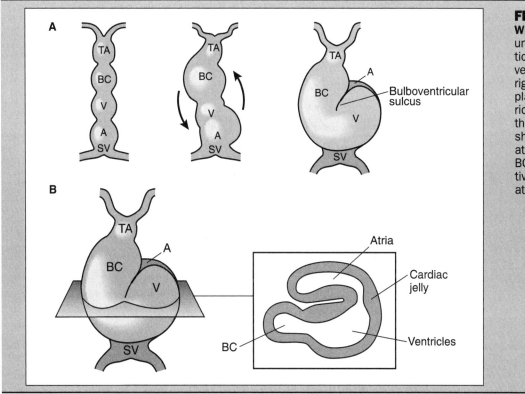

FIG. 6-4
WEEK 4. (A) The cardiac tube undergoes several characteristic bends. The growing bulboventricular loop bends to the right and anteriorly, which places the primitive atria posteriorly. (B) Transverse section of the looped heart tube at week 4 shows the posteriorly located atria. TA = truncus arteriosus; BC = bulbus cordis; V = primitive ventricle; A = primitive atria; SV = sinus venosus.

WEEK 5

During week 5 many of the internal structures of the heart rapidly develop. At this time the AV canal forms, and septation of the atria, ventricles, and great arteries occurs.

AV Canal Formation. During week 4 of development, swellings termed *endocardial cushions* form on the dorsal and ventral walls of the AV canal. During week 5, the endocardial cushions are invaded by mesenchyme cells, move toward one another, and fuse, dividing the AV canal into right and left AV canals (Fig. 6-5).

Atrial Septation. While atrial septal formation begins in week 4, the complex process of atrial septation predominantly occurs during week 5 (Fig. 6-6). The common atrium is divided into right and left atria by the formation and subsequent modification of two septae, the septum primum and septum secundum. The septum primum, a thin membrane of tissue from the roof of the common atrium, begins to grow down into the atrial

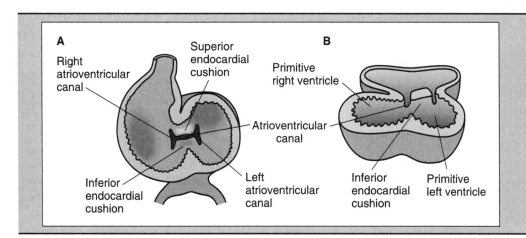

FIG. 6-5
FORMATION OF THE ATRIOVENTRICULAR (AV) CANAL. Endocardial cushions grow superiorly and inferiorly and divide the AV canal into right and left sides. (A) Anterior portion removed. (B) Transverse section.

FIG. 6-6
ATRIAL AND VENTRICULAR SEPTAL FORMATION. (A) Septum primum descends from the roof of the atria. (B) Perforations in the septum primum form the ostium secundum. The septum secundum begins to develop. (C) Septum secundum continues to develop and separates the right and left atria with the exception of a small central region, the fossa ovalis, which is covered by the septum primum. The interventricular septum grows upward from the floor of the ventricle. (*Source:* Reprinted with permission from Moss AS, Adams FH: *Heart Disease in Infants, Children, and Adolescents.* Baltimore, MD: Williams & Wilkins, 1968, p 16.)

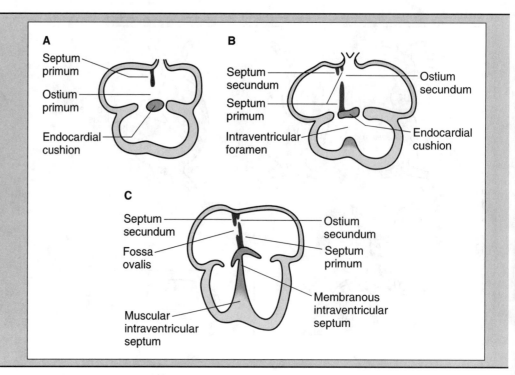

cavity. The area between the descending septum primum and the caudally located endocardial cushions is termed the ostium primum. The ostium primum allows blood to pass from the right to the left atrium. The septum primum and the endocardial cushions grow toward one another, eventually fusing and obliterating the ostium primum. However, before the ostium primum is obliterated, small perforations appear in the septum primum. These perforations coalesce to form a larger opening termed the ostium secundum, which permits continued blood flow from the right to the left atrium. Toward the end of week 5 another membrane of tissue develops, the septum secundum. This thick membrane grows downward from the atrial roof, immediately to the right of the septum primum. As the septum secundum continues to grow, it gradually overlaps the ostium secundum within the septum primum. The septum secundum forms an incomplete partition between the right and left atria, forming an oval opening termed the *foramen ovale*. The cranial portion of the septum primum, attached to the atrial roof, gradually disappears. The remaining portion of the septum primum that is attached to the endocardial cushions forms a flap-like valve over the foramen ovale, termed the *valve of the foramen ovale*. Incomplete growth or excessive resorption of tissue at this stage of development can give rise to interatrial malformations known as atrial septal defects.

Ventricular Septation. While significant changes take place within the atria, the two primitive ventricles begin to dilate. The myocardium on the outside of each ventricle continues to grow while the inner surface of the ventricles thins as a result of the formation of diverticulae and trabeculae. As the ventricles dilate, a muscular ridge of tissue on the floor of the ventricle increases in height (see Fig. 6-6). Subsequently, active proliferation of myoblasts within this ridge of tissue leads to the formation of a thick, muscular interventricular septum. Until the end of week 7 there exists an interventricular foramen between the free edge of the interventricular septum and the fused endocardial cushions. This last region of ventricular septation is called the membranous septum because it is much thinner than the rest of the ventricular septum (see Fig. 6-6C).

Great Artery Septation. During week 5, active proliferation of mesenchymal cells within the walls of the bulbus cordis and truncus arteriosus results in the formation of bulbar and truncal ridges, respectively. The spiral orientation of these ridges results in the formation of a spiral aorticopulmonary (AP) septum when the ridges fuse. Fusion of the truncal ridges divides the bulbus cordis and truncus arteriosus into two channels, the pulmonary and aortic trunk, respectively. As a result of the spiraling of the AP septum, the pulmonary trunk twists around, and anterior to, the ascending aorta. The septum created by fusion of the bulbar ridges connects each ventricle with the appropriate channel (Fig. 6-7). As the AP septum forms, the bulbus cordis is incorporated into the walls of the ventricle. In the right ventricle, the bulbus cordis is represented by the infundibulum, which gives rise to the pulmonary trunk. In the left ventricle, the bulbus cordis forms the walls of the aortic vestibule just inferior to the aortic valve. As the bulbar ridges fuse, the interventricular septum decreases in size. By the end of week 7, the interventricular septum closes, the result of fusion of the right and left bulbar ridges and the endocardial cushions. An extension of tissue from the right side of the fused endocardial cushion merges with the AP septum and the muscular portion of the interventricular septum, forming a thin membranous portion of the interventricular septum that serves to close the interventricular septum. Abnormal development or positioning of the bulbus cordis may give rise to ventricular outflow anomalies as well as interventricular defects.

Week 5
AV canal formation
Atrial septation
Ventricular septation
Separation of the aorta and main
    pulmonary artery

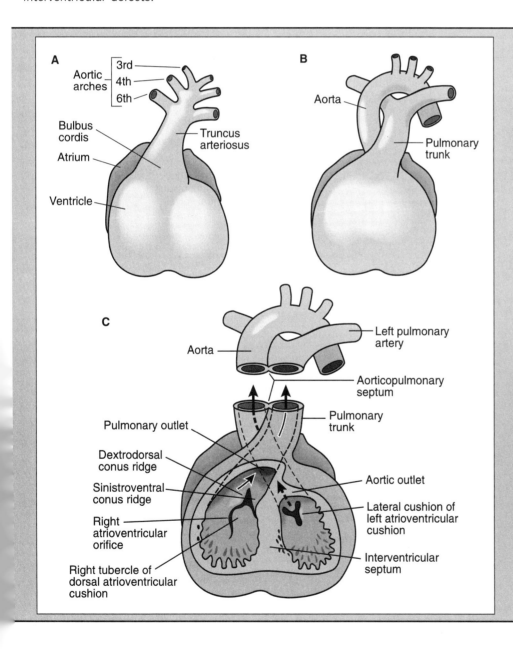

FIG. 6-7
SEPTATION OF AORTA AND MAIN PULMONARY ARTERY. (A) Flow from the right ventricle goes anteriorly into (B) the pulmonary artery. (C) Flow from the left ventricle travels posteriorly and out the aorta.

WEEK 6 AND LATER

During week 6, septation of the atria and ventricles is almost completed. Prior to completion of the AP septum, the semilunar valves begin to develop. This process begins when three valve swellings of subendocardial tissue develop at the orifices of the aortic and pulmonary trunks during week 5. These swellings become hollowed out on their upper surfaces and are reshaped to form the three thin-walled cusps of each mature semilunar valve (the aortic and pulmonary valves). Abnormalities at this stage of development may lead to aortic and pulmonary valve anomalies. Following formation of the right and left AV canals, the subendocardial tissue surrounding the canals begins to proliferate, ultimately forming the two valve cusps of each AV valve. The right and left AV valves are termed the tricuspid and mitral valves, respectively. Subsequent myocardial cell death on the ventricular surface of the AV valves results in string-like muscular strands of tissue connecting the valve cusps to the ventricular wall. Eventually, these strands of tissue degenerate and are replaced by dense connective tissue strands termed *chordae tendinae*. The chordae tendinae are attached to the ventricular wall via muscles termed *papillary muscles* (Fig. 6-8).

FIG. 6-8
DEVELOPMENT OF ATRIOVENTRICULAR VALVES. (A) Formation of the primitive valve cusps. (B) Trabeculation of the ventricular wall. (C) Formation of chordae tendinae and the papillary muscles.

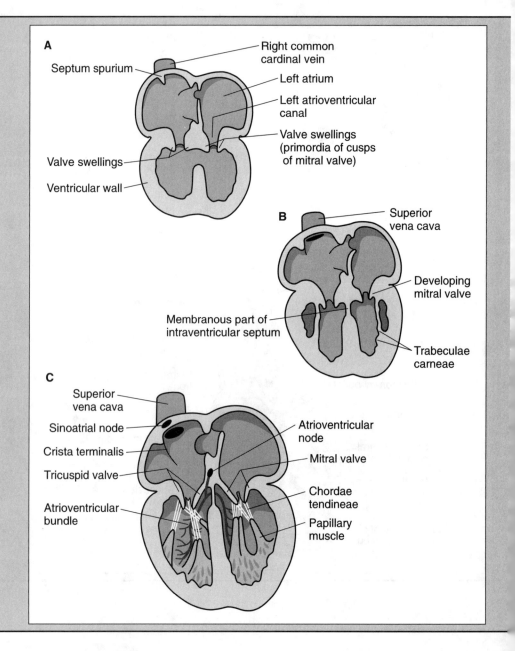

FETAL TO NEWBORN CIRCULATION

As noted previously, the fetus tolerates most cardiac abnormalities, given the parallel nature of the fetal-maternal circulation. The changes in fetal circulation that occur after birth may bring to light embryologic abnormalities. The fetal circulation was eloquently described by Harvey in 1628. In the fetus, approximately one-half of the oxygenated blood from the placenta passes directly into the liver, while the remainder enters the inferior vena cava (IVC) via the ductus venosus, thereby bypassing the liver (Fig. 6-9). From the IVC, blood enters the right atrium and is mixed with deoxygenated blood from the lower portion of the body. Most blood in the right atrium passes into the left atrium via the foramen ovale. A small amount of deoxygenated blood from the lungs also returns to the left atrium.

Unlike the newborn lung, the fetal lung extracts oxygen from the blood.

Placenta means "pancake" in Greek.

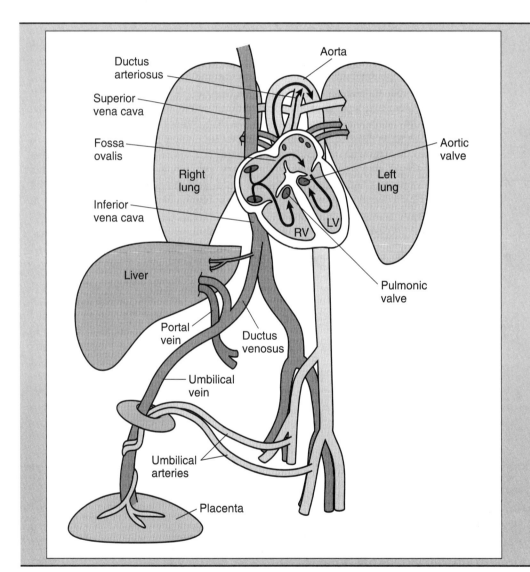

FIG. 6-9
FETAL CIRCULATION. Oxygenated blood flows through the umbilical vein to the fetus. The ductus venosus allows approximately one-half of the oxygenated blood to bypass the fetal liver. Oxygenated blood bypasses the fetal lung via the fossa ovalis and the ductus arteriosus. LV = left ventricle; RV = right ventricle. (*Source:* Reprinted with permission from Moss AS, Adams FH: *Heart Disease in Infants, Children, and Adolescents*, 2nd ed. Baltimore, MD: Williams & Wilkins, 1977, p 12.)

From the left atrium, blood flows across the mitral valve into the left ventricle. From here, the blood leaves the left ventricle through the aortic valve to supply the body with predominantly oxygenated blood. The small amount of blood in the right atrium that did not pass into the left atrium mixes with the deoxygenated blood from the superior vena cava and coronary sinus and crosses the tricuspid valve to enter the right ventricle. The blood then flows across the pulmonic valve into the pulmonary trunk. A small portion of this blood goes to the lungs; however, most blood passes through the ductus arteriosus

Fetal circulation: high pressure pulmonary circulation and low pressure systemic circulation.

Newborn circulation: Low pressure pulmonary circulation and high pressure systemic circulation.

Three Fetal Shunts
Ductus venosus
Ductus arteriosus
Foramen ovale

into the aorta and subsequently to the systemic circulation. Approximately 50% of the blood in the descending aorta returns to the placenta for oxygenation. The remaining 50% supplies the viscera and lower half of the body.

During fetal life the lungs are collapsed, resistance to blood flow through the lungs is high, and the pulmonary arterial pressure is high. In the fetal aorta there is little resistance to blood flow, and the pressure in the aorta is less than the pulmonary artery pressure. Thus, in the fetus, unlike the newborn, the pulmonary system is a high-resistance, high-pressure, low-flow system and the systemic system is a low-resistance, low-pressure, high-flow system. As a result of this pressure gradient, blood tends to bypass the lungs and flow from the pulmonary artery to the aorta via the ductus arteriosus, providing recirculation of blood through the systemic arteries of the fetus.

At birth, the alveoli fill with air, resistance to pulmonary blood flow decreases, and pulmonary artery pressure falls. Also, aortic pressure rises as a result of cessation of placental blood flow. As a consequence of the fall in pulmonary artery pressure and the rise in aortic pressure, forward blood flow through the ductus arteriosus ceases, and the ductus arteriosus occludes within hours to days of birth. During fetal life the blood passing through the ductus arteriosus was venous. After birth, blood flow reverses, and oxygenated blood passes through the ductus arteriosus. The high oxygen content of this blood is believed to lead to constriction of the ductus muscle of the ductus arteriosus. It has long been known that a persistently patent ductus arteriosus (PDA) is more common at higher altitudes. For example, the incidence of a PDA is less than 0.1% of births at sea level but approximately 1% for births at 15,000 feet.

In essence, the three shunts of the fetus—the ductus venosus, the ductus arteriosus, and the foramen ovale—all play an important role in fetal circulation. The ductus venosus supplies blood to the fetus from the placenta, and the ductus arteriosus and the foramen ovale divert blood away from the fetal lungs. Normally all three shunts cease to function after birth. In some conditions these shunts do not close and significantly affect the hemodynamic properties of the infant, child, or adult.

■ CONGENITAL HEART DISEASE

Cardiac defects may be divided into various groups based on the physiologic changes associated with the pathologic defect (Table 6-2). First, congenital cardiac defects can be divided according to the presence or absence of cyanosis. Cyanotic lesions generally include obstruction to pulmonary blood flow as well as a right-to-left shunt that permits venous blood to enter the systemic circulation. One of the most common cyanotic lesions described is tetralogy of Fallot. Second, cardiac lesions may be further subdivided according to the physiologic load placed on the heart (Table 6-3). Cardiac lesions can be associated with *volume overload* (resulting from a shunt or abnormal communication between the pulmonary and systemic circulations), *pressure overload* (resulting from obstruction), or *mixed* lesions.

Table 6-2
Differentiation of Cyanotic and Acyanotic Cardiac Lesions

Cyanotic lesions
Tetralogy of Fallot (with an occluded ductus arteriosus)

Potentially cyanotic lesions
Atrial septal defect (cyanosis appears with Eisenmenger's syndrome)
Ventricular septal defect (cyanosis appears with Eisenmenger's syndrome)
Patent ductus arteriosus (cyanosis appears with Einsenmenger's syndrome)
Pulmonary stenosis (cyanosis appears with elevated right atrial pressure and a patent foramen ovale)
Tetralogy of Fallot (with a patent ductus arteriosus)

Acyanotic lesions
Aortic coarctation
Aortic stenosis

Hemodynamic volume overload occurs primarily in association with cardiac lesions that cause left-to-right shunts: atrial septal defect (ASD), ventricular septal defect (VSD), and PDA. The common pathophysiologic feature of these defects is a circulatory commu-

Table 6-3
Physiologic Categorization of Cardiac Lesions

Pressure overload, or obstructive lesions
Pulmonary stenosis
Aortic stenosis
Aortic coarctation

Volume overload, or shunt lesions
Atrial septal defect
Ventricular septal defect
Patent ductus arteriosus

Combined lesions
Tetralogy of Fallot

Table 6-3
Physiologic Categorization of Cardiac Lesions

nication between the systemic and pulmonary systems, resulting in oxygenated blood being returned to the lungs rather than to the systemic circulation. The determinants of shunt direction and magnitude are the size of the defect and the relative resistances of the pulmonary and systemic vascular circuits. As with most aspects of the cardiovascular system, these factors are dynamic. Eventually, volume overload may lead to ventricular failure and pulmonary hypertension. Increased pulmonary circulation resistance causes flow through the left-to-right shunt to decrease; once pulmonary circulation resistance exceeds systemic circulation resistance, flow eventually reverses, and unoxygenated blood is shunted into the systemic circulation. Reduced arterial oxygen content leads to cyanosis.

Obstruction to the normal flow of blood is the pathophysiologic feature of pressure overload lesions. Lesions producing ventricular outflow obstruction (pulmonary and aortic valvular stenosis and aortic coarctation) are the most common forms of congenital pressure overload. Ventricular hypertrophy, ventricular dilatation, and eventual ventricular failure are the common features associated with ventricular outflow obstructions. In the presence of left heart lesions, ventricular failure is complicated by pulmonary congestion and progressive acidosis. In the presence of right heart lesions, ventricular failure is complicated primarily by venous congestion.

ATRIAL SEPTAL DEFECT (ASD)

An ASD results in a persistent direct flow of blood between the right and left atria after birth. ASDs account for approximately 7% of all congenital heart lesions. They are the most common form of congenital heart disease in adults, with a female predominance of 2:1.

Etiology. ASDs can occur anywhere along the atrial septum (Fig. 6-10). Classically, four different ASDs have been described. A fifth type of ASD, a patent foramen ovale, occurs in up to 25% of people; however, this is not generally considered to be a pathologic occurrence. The four pathologic forms of ASD include secundum ASD, endocardial cushion defect, sinus venosus type, and common atrium. *Secundum ASD* is the most common type of atrial congenital heart defect. Abnormal resorption of the septum primum during the formation of the foramen secundum, inadequate development of the septum secundum, and an abnormally large foramen ovale are all considered possible etiologies for a secundum ASD. An *endocardial cushion defect* with a primum-type ASD occurs when the septum primum does not fuse with the endocardial cushions, resulting in a patent foramen primum. Less commonly, the endocardial cushions fail to fuse, resulting in a large defect in the center of the heart, a common AV canal also known as atrioventricularis communis. This particular lesion occurs in about 20% of persons with Down syndrome; otherwise, it is a relatively uncommon heart defect. Endocardial cushion defects are commonly associated with a cleft mitral valve, which frequently is associated with mitral regurgitation. A *sinus venosus ASD* occurs in the superior portion of the interatrial septum and results from incomplete absorption of the sinus venosus into the right atrium or abnormal development of the septum secundum. The *common atrium* is a rare form of ASD in which the interatrial septum is completely absent. It is the result of failure of the septum primum and septum secundum to develop.

Classification of ASDs
Secundum
Endocardial cushion defect (primum)
Sinus venosus
Common atrium

FIG. 6-10
ANATOMIC LOCATION OF ATRIAL SEPTAL DEFECTS (ASDs).

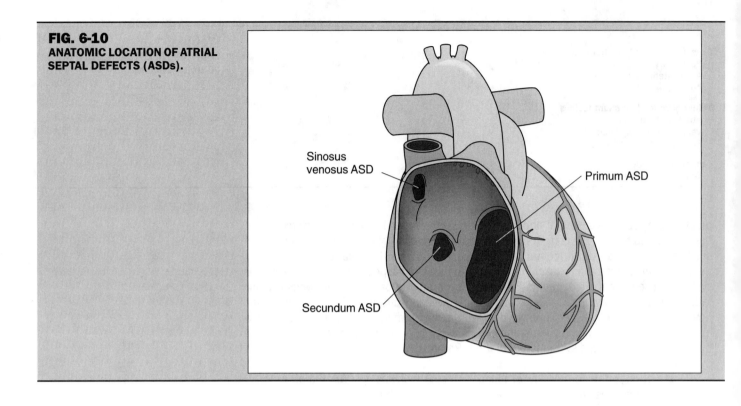

Sinosus venosus ASD

Primum ASD

Secundum ASD

Patients with an ASD remain minimally symptomatic until the following conditions develop:

Left ventricular dysfunction
Atrial arrhythmias
Pulmonary hypertension

Pathophysiology. In essence, there is a communicating hole connecting the two atria. The basic physiology of an ASD is shunting of blood from the left to right atrium (Fig. 6-11). The degree of the shunt is dependent on the size of the defect, the compliance of the right and left ventricles, and the relative resistance of the pulmonary and systemic vascular beds. The course of blood within the heart generally follows the path of least resistance. In the presence of an ASD, blood initially passes more easily from the higher pressure left heart to the more compliant, lower pressure right heart. The shunt occurs during systole and early diastole and produces right atrial and ventricular volume overload and increased pulmonary blood flow. To compensate for this increased volume, both right-sided cardiac chambers hypertrophy and subsequently dilate. In addition, pulmonary blood flow increases, with subsequent enlargement of the pulmonary arteries and veins. Over time, this continued volume overload of the pulmonary vascular beds produces pulmonary vascular disease and pulmonary hypertension. With increased right heart pressures, the shunt of blood from left to right decreases, right ventricular compliance decreases, and eventually the shunt reverses, promoting a predominantly right-to-left shunt and the development of cyanosis (Fig. 6-12). The development of right-to-left shunting and cyanosis is termed Eisenmenger's syndrome. Essentially, three pathophysiologic changes typically lead to the clinical deterioration of patients with ASDs: left ventricular dysfunction, supraventricular arrhythmias, and pulmonary hypertension. Left ventricular dysfunction is often attributable to associated conditions, such as hypertension and coronary artery disease. The supraventricular arrhythmias, particularly atrial fibrillation, atrial flutter, and atrial tachycardia, increase in frequency after the fourth decade and may precipitate or contribute to the development of right ventricular failure. Lastly, pulmonary hypertension secondary to the long-standing left-to-right shunting of blood places further demands upon the right ventricle with both volume and pressure overload.

Clinical History. Patients with an ASD are generally asymptomatic until the third or fourth decade of life. However, on historical review, most patients are likely to have shunned vigorous physical exercise during childhood. In the third and fourth decades patients begin to develop left and right ventricular failure, which leads to a significant increase in symptoms. Patients often complain of dyspnea, fatigue, chest discomfort, effort cyanosis, and hemoptysis.

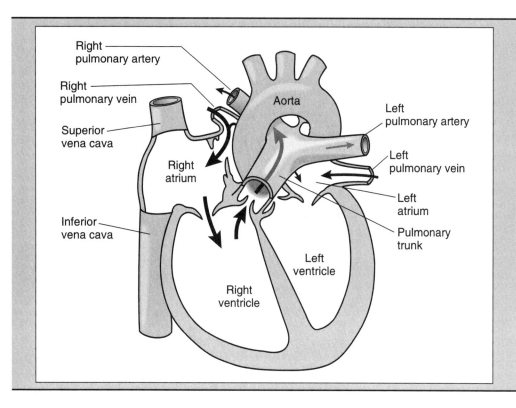

FIG. 6-11
PATHOPHYSIOLOGY OF ATRIAL SEPTAL DEFECTS (ASDS). Blood flows from the left atrium to the right atrium, which leads to increased flow through the pulmonary circulation.

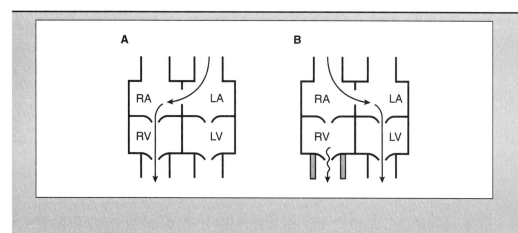

FIG. 6-12
DEVELOPMENT OF CYANOSIS. (A) Persistent increased flow through the atrial septal defect (ASD) causes hypertrophy of the pulmonary vasculature and increased pulmonary pressures. (B) When pulmonary pressure exceeds systemic pressure blood flow, the ASD reverses (right to left) and unoxygenated blood enters the systemic circulation, causing cyanosis. LA = left atrium; LV = left ventricle; RA = right atrium; RV = right ventricle.

Physical Examination. The arterial pulse is normal or diminished. Initially the jugular venous pulse is normal. The hallmark of an ASD is a fixed, widely split S_2 on cardiac auscultation. In the normal heart, during inspiration the S_2 has two components, closure of the aortic valve (A_2), followed by closure of the pulmonic valve (P_2). During inspiration, increased inspiratory venous return and reduced pulmonary vascular impedance cause prolongation of the right ventricular ejection period and delayed P_2; in contrast, during inspiration, reduced pulmonary venous return and reduced left ventricular filling cause A_2 to occur earlier. In expiration, the two valves close simultaneously, and only a single S_2 is audible (Fig. 6-13). With an ASD, the increase in right ventricular stroke volume secondary to left-to-right shunting causes a further delay in P_2, producing a widely split S_2. Since the right and left atria communicate with one another, the stroke volume of each chamber varies in the same way throughout the respiratory cycle, producing a fixed, widely split S_2.

Physical Findings Associated with an ASD
Fixed, widely split S_2
Right ventricular heave
Pulmonic valve ejection murmur resulting from increased flow
Mid-diastolic murmur resulting from increased flow across the tricuspid valve

FIG. 6-13

COMPONENTS OF THE SECOND HEART SOUND (S_2). (A) Normally, with inspiration, increased flow across the pulmonic valve and reduced pulmonary vascular resistance causes the component of S_2 produced by pulmonic valve closure (P_2) to become delayed. (B) In patients with atrial septal defect (ASD), the P_2 becomes delayed as a result of increased flow. In the presence of a large ASD, venous return is similar for the left and right atria, and the relationship between the closure of the aortic valve (A_2) and P_2 becomes constant during the respiratory cycle (fixed splitting) during both inspiration and expiration. (C) In pulmonic stenosis, increased resistance to right ventricular contraction causes a significant prolongation of the right ventricular ejection period. P_2 is delayed, particularly during inspiration (wide physiologic splitting). (D) In aortic stenosis, left ventricular hypertrophy causes delay of the aortic component of S_2 so that splitting is heard during expiration (paradoxic splitting). It is obvious from these examples why Leatham referred to S_2 as the "key to auscultation of the heart."

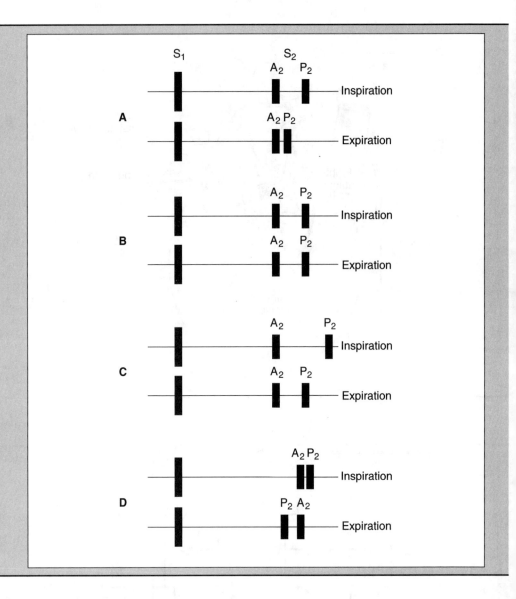

Additional Findings if the Patient Develops Eisenmenger's Syndrome
Right-sided S_4
Pansystolic murmur secondary to tricuspid regurgitation
Early diastolic murmur resulting from pulmonic valve regurgitation
Cyanosis

Often the right ventricular impulse is prominent, with a palpable systolic impulse along the lower left sternal border. Also present is a pulmonic systolic ejection murmur secondary to increased right heart volume with subsequent increased flow through the pulmonic valve. With larger shunts, a mid-diastolic tricuspid murmur may also be audible. An ASD should be suspected whenever a murmur is best heard in the left second intercostal space. Fig. 6-14 summarizes the cardiac auscultatory findings associated with an ASD.

When right heart pressures become greater than left heart pressures, shunt reversal occurs, and patients exhibit central cyanosis, digital clubbing, right ventricular disease, and pulmonary hypertension. Shunt reversal with the above signs represents Eisenmenger's syndrome. On examination, these patients are cyanotic, they have a prominent right ventricular heave; a palpable P_2; a right-sided fourth heart sound (S_4), representing a noncompliant right ventricle; a regurgitant tricuspid murmur; and an early diastolic murmur related to pulmonary regurgitation. The physical examination findings of an ostium primum defect are identical to those of an ostium secundum defect with the addition of a pansystolic murmur at the apex related to mitral valve regurgitation.

Management. A patient with a small ASD and normal heart size should be regularly followed with serial echocardiography. Echocardiography, which uses sound waves to delineate the structure of the heart (see Appendix II), can assess the location and size of

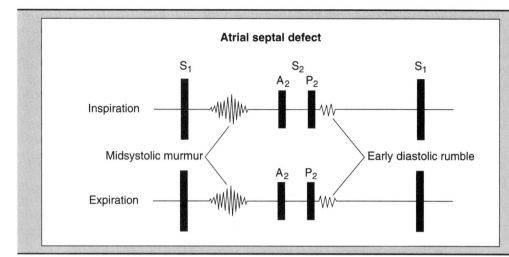

Atrial septal defect

Inspiration

Midsystolic murmur

Early diastolic rumble

Expiration

S_1 S_2 A_2 P_2 S_1 A_2 P_2

FIG. 6-14
CARDIAC AUSCULTATORY FINDINGS WITH ATRIAL SEPTAL DEFECT (ASD). The second heart sound (S_2) is widely split, and the split sound is fixed. Increased flow through the pulmonic valve produces a midsystolic murmur, and increased flow across the tricuspid valve is responsible for a mid-diastolic rumble.

the atrial defect. In addition, echocardiography can be used to determine left and right ventricular function. Patients with moderate to large ASDs in whom pulmonary blood flow exceeds systemic flow should undergo defect repair even if they are asymptomatic. Traditionally, surgical intervention has been the primary mode of repair for ASDs. Transcatheter closure of an ASD is now being investigated as a second form of therapy.

Ms. Etherton was a 30-year-old woman who presented to her internist with complaints of progressive dyspnea and fatigue. Coronary artery disease, congestive heart failure (CHF), dysrhythmia, and congenital heart disease were possible cardiac etiologies for her symptoms. Given her young age, a dysrhythmia or a congenital cardiac defect was the most likely cause for her current decompensated state. Both her history and her physical examination findings were most consistent with the diagnosis of an ASD. The key feature of her case was the presence of a fixed, split S_2. As a result of the existence of an intraatrial communication with left-to-right shunting of blood, there is an increase in the right ventricular stroke volume, which produces a prolonged delay in closure of the pulmonic valve, giving rise to a widely split S_2. In addition, the communication between the two atria creates a symmetry of function between the two chambers throughout the respiratory cycle; thus, the stroke volumes of each chamber are matched, producing a fixed, widely split S_2. The increased volume of blood in the right heart dictates that more blood flows through the pulmonic valve, which produces a systolic ejection murmur heard over the left second intercostal space. Ms. Etherton's complaints of dyspnea and fatigue were most likely related to both pulmonary vascular congestion and left ventricular dysfunction. The cause of her dyspnea may have been twofold: increased pulmonary blood flow related to increased right heart volume and pooling of blood in the lungs secondary to left ventricular dysfunction. In both cases, pulmonary pressures increase and eventually lead to pulmonary vascular congestion.

Case Study:
Continued

VENTRICULAR SEPTAL DEFECT (VSD)

VSDs are the most common congenital cardiac malformation in infants and children, accounting for approximately 25% of all congenital cardiac malformations (see Table 6-1). VSDs are less common in adults because of spontaneous or early surgical closure. By definition, a VSD is a direct communication between the left and right ventricles. Males and females are affected equally.

Etiology. The ventricular septum is usually divided into four components: the membranous septum, the inlet septum, the trabecular septum, and the outlet (infundibular) septum (Fig. 6-15). VSDs are classified by the anatomic portion of the septum that is involved. The most common type of VSD, the perimembranous VSD, occurs in the region

Classification of VSDs
Perimembranous
Muscular
Outlet septal (supracristal)
Inlet septal

of the membranous septum. These defects are described as perimembranous because they usually involve both the membranous septum and a portion of adjacent muscular septum. Perimembranous defects account for 65% of VSDs. The second type of VSD involves only the trabecular or muscular septum. Muscular defects account for 15%–18% of VSDs. Muscular septal defects may appear anywhere in the muscular portion of the interventricular septum (IVS). The defect is probably the result of excessive resorption of the myocardial tissue during the formation of the IVS. The defects may be multiple, giving rise to a Swiss cheese appearance of the muscular septum. The third type of defect is located in the outlet septum and accounts for approximately 8%–10% of VSDs. This type, often called a supracristal VSD (since the defect is above the crista supraventricularis), can be associated with prolapse of the aortic valve (through the defect) and aortic regurgitation. Finally, defects of the inlet septum account for approximately 8%–10% of VSDs.

FIG. 6-15
ANATOMIC COMPONENTS OF THE VENTRICULAR SEPTUM.
The anatomic components of the ventricular septum are the outlet septum (which includes the crista supraventricularis), the trabecular septum, the inlet septum, and the membranous septum. Most ventricular septal defects (VSDs) involve some portion of the membranous septum and are referred to as perimembranous. VSDs are classified by their anatomic location.

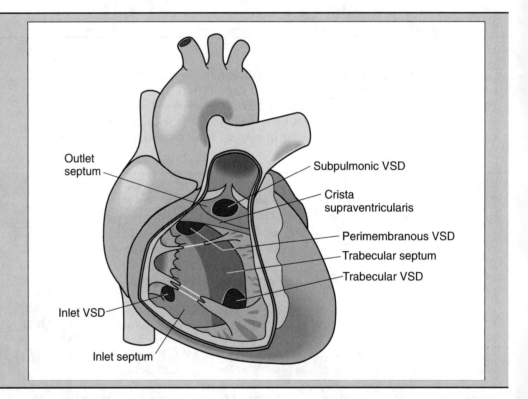

Pathophysiology. Like that of ASDs, the pathophysiology of all VSDs is left-to-right shunting (Fig. 6-16). The degree of shunting is related to the size of the defect and the relative resistances of the pulmonary and systemic circulation. With small defects, there is a significant resistance to flow with a large pressure gradient between the two ventricles. With small defects, right heart pressures are normal and only a small left-to-right shunt exists. In cases of large defects, there is no restriction to flow between the ventricles and equilibration of pressure within the ventricles occurs. Large defects with significant pulmonary vascular resistance result in bidirectional shunting with a predominant right-to-left shunt, which leads to cyanosis.

Clinical History. Patients with a small VSD may be asymptomatic, while those with large shunts may complain of dyspnea and exercise intolerance. Patients with compromise of the aortic valve resulting from defects close to the valve (outlet septum VSDs) often experience aortic cusp prolapse. These patients are more likely to have dyspnea on exertion and exercise intolerance as a result of aortic valve regurgitation. As with ASDs, long-term left-to-right shunting may lead to increased right heart pressures with subsequent shunt reversal, right to left, producing Eisenmenger's syndrome. These patients develop cyanosis, markedly diminished exercise tolerance, severe dyspnea, hemoptysis, angina, and palpitations secondary to atrial and ventricular dysrhythmias.

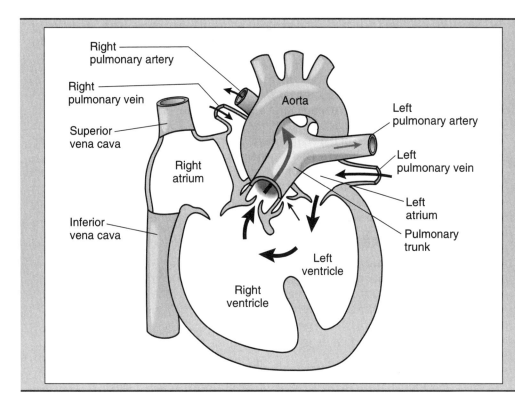

FIG. 6-16
PATHOPHYSIOLOGY OF VENTRIC-ULAR SEPTAL DEFECTS (VSDS). Blood flows through the VSD from left to right, causing an increased volume load on the ventricles.

Physical Examination. On physical examination, the prominent clinical feature in patients with a moderate or large VSD is a pansystolic murmur along the lower left sternal border that is also occasionally audible at the apex. The murmur has a rough quality and is often accompanied by a thrill (vibrations palpable from the chest wall) at the left sternal border. The murmur is the result of blood escaping from one ventricle into an area of lower pressure, that is, from the left ventricle to the right ventricle. It starts simultaneously with the S_1 and may run over into early diastole. With larger shunts, an apical mid-diastolic murmur may be appreciated secondary to increased flow through the mitral valve. An early diastolic murmur of aortic regurgitation may be appreciated in those defects associated with aortic cusp prolapse. In patients with small VSDs, which offer significant restriction to flow between the left and right ventricle, the murmur will be midsystolic, similar in character to the murmur of aortic stenosis (Fig. 6-17).

As with ASDs, patients with long-standing VSDs may subsequently develop Eisenmenger's syndrome and present with central cyanosis, clubbing, and signs of pulmonary hypertension, notably elevated jugular venous pressure, right-ventricular heave, palpable

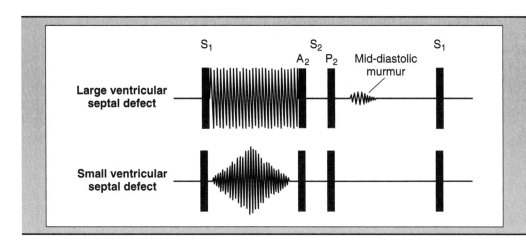

FIG. 6-17
CARDIAC AUSCULTATION FINDINGS WITH VENTRICULAR SEPTAL DEFECTS (VSDS). Larger VSDs are associated with a pansystolic murmur, while smaller VSDs are associated with a mid-systolic murmur.

Physical Findings Associated with a VSD
Systolic murmur (usually pan-systolic, midsystolic if the defect is small)
Systolic thrill
Mid-diastolic rumble

P_2, right-sided S_4, and a loud P_2. Additional murmurs often arise with the development of pulmonary hypertension. These include an early diastolic murmur of pulmonary regurgitation and a second pansystolic murmur related to tricuspid regurgitation.

Management. Some VSDs, small and large, spontaneously decrease in size or close. Spontaneous closure of a VSD occurs in approximately 45% of patients by 3 years of age. Spontaneous closure is more common in smaller defects but has been reported in some patients with very large defects. Optimal management of a VSD depends on an accurate diagnosis and an evaluation of the hemodynamic parameters associated with the defect. Generally, patients with small VSDs are managed medically. Patients with large VSDs often undergo surgical repair early in childhood. Some frail children undergo palliative pulmonary artery banding, with the hope that they will become strong enough to undergo surgical closure of their defect. Operative repair in adults with VSDs is usually undertaken when pulmonary blood flow is more than twice systemic flow.

PATENT DUCTUS ARTERIOSUS (PDA)

The fetal connection between the aorta and pulmonary artery, the ductus arteriosus, normally becomes functionally closed within several hours after birth. In some cases the ductus arteriosus fails to close and remains patent. Maternal rubella in the first trimester is associated with a higher incidence of a PDA.

Etiology. Postnatal closure of the ductus arteriosus is attributed to contraction of the medial smooth muscle within the wall of the ductus. Subsequently the vessel shortens, the wall thickens, and the vessel lumen is obliterated. Over time, necrosis and hemorrhage of the intimal layer of the ductus occurs. Eventually, connective tissue formation begins and fibrosis of the lumen occurs, leaving a residual ligamentum arteriosus. In cases of a PDA, these stages of vessel degeneration do not take place and blood continues to flow between the pulmonary artery and the aorta through the ductus arteriosus (Fig. 6-18).

FIG. 6-18
DUCTUS ARTERIOSUS. Prior to birth, blood flows through the ductus arteriosus from the pulmonary artery to the aorta. After birth, with expansion of the lungs and reduction in pulmonary circulation resistance, flow reverses and oxygenated blood flows from the aorta into the pulmonary artery.

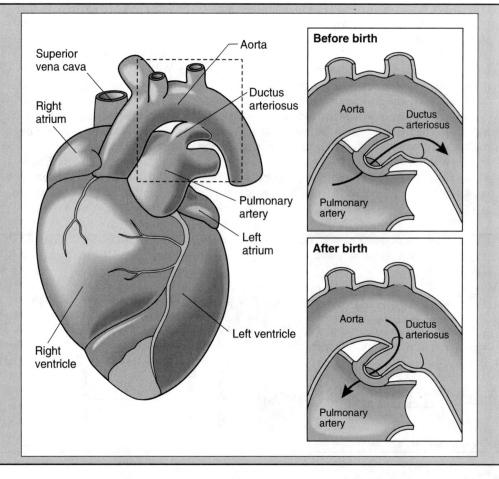

Pathophysiology. Failure of the ductus arteriosus to close results in PDA, which allows blood to flow from the aorta into the lower pressure pulmonary circulation. A PDA does not cause significant problems early in an infant's life. However, over time, the pressure difference between the aorta and the pulmonary artery progressively increases, with a further increase in blood flow from the aorta into the pulmonary artery. In an older child with a PDA, up to two-thirds of the aortic blood flow passes through the ductus arteriosus to the lungs, the left atrium, and on to the left ventricle. This pulmonary-cardiac blood cycle continues for several passes before the blood enters the systemic circulation. There is enhanced oxygenation of the blood reaching the systemic circulation as a result of the additional circulatory passes through the lungs. Also, there is a tremendous increase in left ventricular outflow secondary to the increased accessory blood flow through the lungs and the left side of the heart. As a consequence of the increased pulmonary flow, there is an increase in the pulmonary pressures, which over time leads to pulmonary vascular congestion. Likewise, the increased flow through the left heart increases left ventricular pressures. The left ventricle hypertrophies in an attempt to compensate for this increased flow and pressure. Patients with an uncorrected PDA often die between the ages of 20–40 years as a result of pulmonary hypertension and heart failure.

Clinical History. As with ASDs and VSDs with left-to-right shunting, patients with a PDA may be asymptomatic or complain of effort intolerance. With time and reversal of the shunt to right to left, patients develop symptoms of pulmonary vascular congestion, notably exertional dyspnea and fatigue.

Physical Examination. The classic finding of a PDA is a continuous, harsh murmur heard over the first or second intercostal space along the left sternal border; radiation of the murmur may also be heard in the medial to left midscapular region. The murmur peaks at or near S_2, and the murmur waxes and wanes with each heartbeat, producing a "machinery murmur." The waxing and waning of the PDA blood flow resembles aortic regurgitation. In addition to the murmur, a PDA can be associated with a series of clicks heard during systole. The auscultatory findings with a PDA are summarized in Fig. 6-19.

Physical Findings Associated with PDA
"Machinery-like" murmur
Widened pulse pressure and bounding pulses
Differential cyanosis when pulmonary hypertension develops

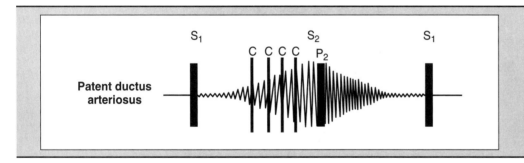

FIG. 6-19
PATENT DUCTUS ARTERIOSUS (PDA). On cardiac auscultation, patients with a PDA have a murmur that spans systole and diastole and peaks at or near the second heart sound (S_2). The murmur is often associated with a series of high-pitched clicks during systole. C = click.

Like patients with aortic regurgitation, patients who have a PDA with large left-to-right shunts have brisk or even bounding carotid pulses and wide pulse pressures. Patients often demonstrate signs of left ventricular overload with a laterally displaced, hyperactive apical impulse. Left ventricular hypertrophy and dilatation occur as a result of the extra work necessary to compensate for the deficit in the systemic circulation.

Over time, with the development of pulmonary hypertension and the eventual development of a right-to-left shunt, the patient's examination reveals cyanosis, clubbing, a right ventricular heave, and an increased P_2. In patients with a PDA associated with pulmonary hypertension, unoxygenated blood flows into the descending aorta. For this reason cyanosis and clubbing are often more prominent in the toes compared to the fingers.

Management. Patients with a PDA require surgical closure. In cases of small PDAs, surgical closure is performed in an attempt to prevent infective endarteritis and embolic events. In patients with moderate-to-large PDAs, closure is performed to prevent the development of CHF and pulmonary vascular disease. Ideally, surgical closure should be performed before cardiomegaly develops.

Shunt Lesions
Atrial septal defect
Ventricular septal defect
Patent ductus arteriosus

PULMONIC VALVE STENOSIS

Pulmonic valve stenosis consists of narrowing or constriction of the orifice of the pulmonary valve. Pulmonic valve stenosis may occur as an isolated cardiac anomaly, or it may be a feature of a more complex cardiac problem.

Etiology. In pulmonic valve stenosis, the pulmonary valve is dysplastic, and the valve cusps are ill formed and thickened, which limits valve movement. Often the valve is a mobile, dome-shaped structure with a very small central orifice.

Pathophysiology. Significant valvular stenosis produces a significant degree of afterload against which the right ventricle must pump (Fig. 6-20). To compensate for this increased pressure, the right ventricle hypertrophies and, in severe cases, subsequently dilates. Dilatation of the right ventricle can stretch the tricuspid valve ring and result in tricuspid regurgitation. Over time, progressive tricuspid regurgitation leads to increased right atrial pressures and subsequent venous engorgement and right heart failure. With severe tricuspid regurgitation, right atrial pressures may be substantial and right-to-left shunting across a stretched foramen ovale may occur.

FIG. 6-20
PATHOPHYSIOLOGY OF PULMONIC VALVE STENOSIS. Increased resistance to flow across the pulmonic valve causes right ventricular enlargement and hypertrophy. Increased right ventricular pressures favor the development of tricuspid regurgitation.

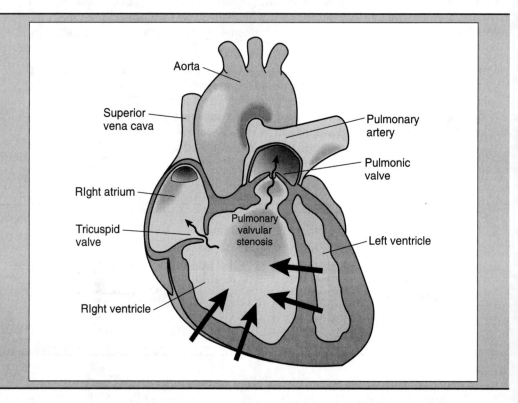

Clinical History. Patients with severe pulmonic valve stenosis are usually recognized and treated in childhood; however, some patients reach adulthood with few symptoms. Symptomatic patients may complain of dyspnea on exertion and fatigue related to inadequate increases in cardiac output during exercise. Occasionally patients experience lightheadedness or syncope.

Physical Examination. A distinctive feature of pulmonic valve stenosis is wide splitting of the S_2 resulting from delayed P_2, producing a delayed interval between A_2 and P_2, the two components of S_2 (see Fig. 6-13). The delay in P_2 is related to the obstruction to right ventricular emptying imposed by the stenotic valve. The murmur associated with pulmonic valve stenosis is best heard over the left second intercostal space and radiates toward the left shoulder. The murmur is loud, harsh, and occupies most of systole. A palpable thrill over the left second intercostal space often accompanies the murmur of

Physical Findings Associated with Pulmonary Valve Stenosis
Wide physiologic splitting of S_2
Midsystolic murmur heard at the left sternal border and left clavicle
Early systolic ejection click

pulmonic valve stenosis. Sudden "checking" of the stenotic pulmonary valve often produces an early systolic ejection click. Fig. 6-21 summarizes the cardiac auscultatory findings with pulmonic valve stenosis.

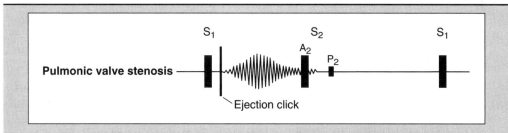

FIG. 6-21
PHYSICAL EXAMINATION FINDINGS WITH PULMONIC VALVE STENOSIS. The second heart sound (S_2) is widely split, a midsystolic murmur produced by turbulent flow across the pulmonic valve can be heard, and there is an early systolic ejection click.

With increasing severity of stenosis, patients develop increased splitting of S_2, and the duration of the systolic murmur increases secondary to prolongation of right ventricular ejection time. With severe stenosis, the duration of the murmur may extend beyond A_2, obliterating the A_2 component of S_2.

Management. Valvotomy is the preferred therapy for pulmonic valve stenosis. Valve replacement is rarely required in cases of isolated pulmonic valve stenosis. Valvotomy is usually considered when the gradient across the pulmonary valve is greater than or equal to 50–60 mm Hg. Today, balloon valvuloplasty has replaced surgical valvotomy. Pulmonary regurgitation may occur but is usually well tolerated.

COARCTATION OF THE AORTA

The term *coarctation* is derived from the Latin word *coarctatus*, meaning "compressed together." A coarctation of the aorta is typically a constriction of tissue located near the aortic attachment of the ductus arteriosus or ligamentum arteriosum (Fig. 6-22). The luminal wall of the aorta is narrowed at the point of constriction while the aorta distal to

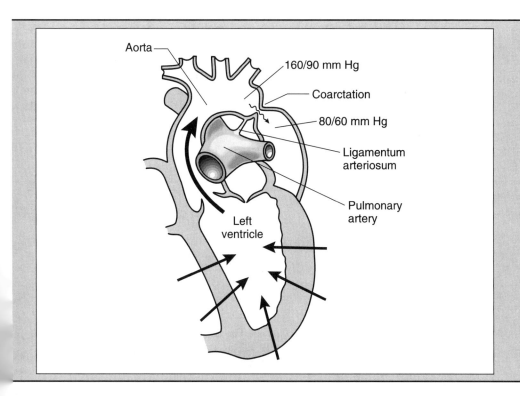

FIG. 6-22
COARCTATION OF THE AORTA. Most commonly, the narrowing is associated with the ligamentum arteriosum. The narrowing places increased afterload on the left ventricle. There is usually a significant pressure gradient between the aortic arch and the descending aorta (160/90 versus 80/60 in the example shown).

the coarctation is usually dilated. Coarctation of the aorta may be a single lesion or may occur in association with other intracardiac abnormalities such as bicuspid aortic valve, VSD, or left ventricular outflow obstruction.

Etiology. In coarctation, the anatomic problem appears to be a sling of ductal tissue producing luminal constriction of the aorta. Another theory of the development of coarctation suggests that hypoplasia of the vessel occurs as a result of diminished flow through the vessel, which contributes to vessel narrowing (which may, in part, explain the relatively common association between aortic stenosis resulting from a bicuspid aortic valve and coarctation).

Pathophysiology. Obstruction of the aorta generally occurs in proximity to the ductus arteriosus. The presence of luminal constriction within the aorta increases the afterload placed on the left ventricle (see Fig. 6-22). As a consequence of this afterload, patients develop elevated upper extremity blood pressures. Beyond the coarctation, blood pressure falls, and the lower extremity pressures are diminished. To compensate for aortic constriction and to maintain adequate blood supply to the lower part of the body, extensive collateral circulation develops. The internal mammary, intercostal, and scapular arteries and others increase in size tremendously to supply the lower part of the body with adequate blood flow. Also, the left ventricle hypertrophies in an attempt to overcome the tremendous load against which it must pump. Eventually, if the coarctation is not treated, left ventricular failure develops.

Clinical History. Most patients with aortic coarctation are asymptomatic. In a hypertensive patient, the lesion may be discovered during the routine investigation of treatable causes of hypertension. Patients may complain of headache, epistaxis, visual changes, and symptoms of left ventricular failure related to the increased pressure proximal to the coarctation. Patients may also complain of lower extremity fatigue or intermittent claudication as a result of diminished perfusion distal to the coarctation.

Physical Examination. Patients with aortic coarctation often have body asymmetry with marked development of the upper body compared to the lower body. Upper extremity blood pressures are much higher than lower extremity blood pressures (just the opposite of normal blood pressure, where lower body pressures exceed upper body pressures by 10–12 mm Hg). The femoral arterial pulse is generally of smaller amplitude than the brachial pulse, and there is a marked radiofemoral delay. In patients with mild coarctation, the apical impulse may be normal; in patients with severe coarctation, the apical impulse may be sustained, reflecting the hypertrophied, power-loaded left ventricle. Upon auscultation, the coarctation produces a systolic murmur in the region between the two scapulae (Fig. 6-23). Since the coarctation is downstream from the left ventricle, the murmur often extends into diastole. If the coarctation causes sufficient narrowing so that a significant gradient exists during diastole (as in Fig. 6-22), the murmur produced by the coarctation can become continuous. A continuous murmur can also be heard in patients with coarctation that is due to turbulent flow through the dilated intercostal collateral vessels. The pulsations of the collateral vessels may be easily seen and palpable.

Physical Findings Associated with Coarctation of the Aorta
Arterial pressure difference between the upper and lower extremities
Systolic murmur resulting from turbulent flow through the coarctation
Continuous murmur if there is a significant gradient during diastole or turbulent flow through collateral vessels

FIG. 6-23
PHYSICAL EXAMINATION FINDINGS WITH COARCTATION OF THE AORTA. Turbulent flow through the coarctation produces a late systolic and early diastolic murmur. If the coarctation is associated with a significant gradient during diastole, a continuous murmur can sometimes be appreciated.

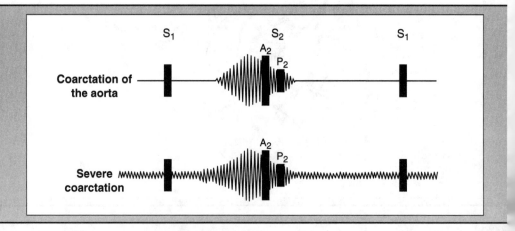

Management. Intervention is usually undertaken when a gradient of 50 mm Hg is identified across the aorta. Surgical repair has produced excellent results. Postoperative survival appears to be best when surgery is performed early in life. Balloon angioplasty is also emerging as a useful method of therapy for aortic coarctation. Hypertension may persist after repair and may be secondary to both changes in vascular compliance and renal renin–angiotensin activity. Additional complications associated with coarctation include accelerated malignant hypertension, dissection of an aortic aneurysm, endocarditis, accelerated coronary atherosclerosis related to long-standing hypertension, and berry aneurysms within the circle of Willis.

AORTIC STENOSIS

Aortic stenosis is fully discussed in Chap. 4. The primary feature of aortic stenosis is left ventricular outflow obstruction.

Etiology. In most cases of aortic stenosis in childhood, the aortic valve is bicuspid or unicuspid, related to fusion of the commissures.

Pathophysiology. The obstruction to left ventricular outflow imposed by the narrowed orifice of the stenotic valve leads to increased systemic pressures to pump blood across the valve and into the aorta. The afterload created by the stenotic valve leads to progressive and concentric left ventricular hypertrophy. Eventually the left ventricle dilates and the symptoms of CHF develop. In addition, the forceful, high-pressure jet of blood that passes through the stenotic valve continuously pounds against the wall of the aorta, eventually causing the dilatation of the proximal aorta.

Clinical History. The clinical picture of aortic stenosis depends on the severity of valvular stenosis. Most children are asymptomatic. When symptoms develop, patients complain of fatigue, exertional dyspnea, angina pectoris, and syncope. With severe aortic stenosis, symptoms of CHF may develop with dyspnea, cough, orthopnea, and paroxysmal nocturnal dyspnea.

Physical Examination. On examination, the patient with aortic stenosis has a slow-rising, delayed pulse, termed *pulsus parvus et tardus*. A narrow pulse pressure is generally noted, with the systolic blood pressure only slightly higher than the diastolic blood pressure. The apical impulse is usually sustained and displaced laterally and inferiorly, related to hypertrophy and dilatation of the left ventricle. A systolic thrill may be palpable with the patient leaning forward with breath held in expiration. S_1 is distinct in aortic stenosis, while S_2 may be obscured by the systolic murmur associated with this condition. Early in the course of disease the normal closure of the aortic valve followed by pulmonic valve closure is maintained, with normal splitting of S_2 into its two components, A_2 followed by P_2. However, with increasing severity of the stenosis and the prolonged excursion of blood from the left ventricle to the aorta, A_2 is delayed, resulting in a single S_2. Over time, the aortic valve may close after the pulmonic valve, producing paradoxic splitting of S_2, with P_2 followed by A_2 (see Fig. 6-13). A systolic ejection click produced by the abrupt "checking" of the aortic valve often can be appreciated. The murmur of aortic stenosis starts early in systole, is loud and rough, and is transmitted into the left ventricular outflow tract and toward the apex.

Management. Severe aortic stenosis in the newborn, if unrecognized, carries a high mortality. In mild cases of aortic stenosis, close follow-up is necessary to determine the appropriate timing of therapeutic interventions. As with pulmonic valve stenosis, valvotomy, either surgical or by balloon valvuloplasty, is the favorable first-line therapy for the seriously ill newborn or child with congenital aortic stenosis. The major complication of valvotomy is aortic regurgitation, which may be mild or severe. For patients in whom palliative valvotomy fails, valve replacement should be undertaken. The timing of replacement is crucial. In children, replacement should be deferred as long as possible because of the complications of growth and anticoagulation in this population. The critical factor in timing valve replacement is left ventricular function. Valve replacement should be performed before significant impairment of left ventricular function develops.

Physical Findings Associated with Aortic Stenosis
Midsystolic murmur
Ejection click
Paradoxic splitting of S_2

Obstructive Lesions
Pulmonary valve stenosis
Coarctation of the aorta
Aortic valve stenosis

TETRALOGY OF FALLOT

In 1888, French physician Etienne Fallot described a group of patients with a combination of congenital cardiac abnormalities. Tetralogy of Fallot is the most common form of cyanotic congenital heart disease that is compatible with life beyond the first few years of infancy. The four cardiac anomalies that constitute the tetralogy include (1) right ventricular outflow obstruction (commonly associated with pulmonic valve stenosis), (2) perimembranous VSD, (3) an overriding aorta, and (4) right ventricular hypertrophy related to right ventricular outflow obstruction (Fig. 6-24).

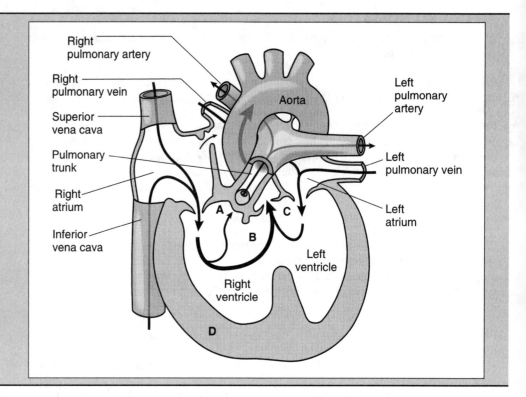

FIG. 6-24
TETRALOGY OF FALLOT. (A) Right ventricular outflow obstruction (muscular thickening or pulmonic valve stenosis). (B) Perimembranous ventricular septal defect. (C) Overriding aorta. (D) Right-ventricular hypertrophy.

Etiology. Tetralogy of Fallot is believed to arise from an abnormal anterosuperior and leftward displacement of the conus septum (see Fig. 6-7) located below the aortopulmonary septum, which results in three anatomic abnormalities: (1) obstruction to the flow of blood exiting from the right ventricle, (2) an overriding aorta that communicates with both ventricles, and (3) a perimembranous VSD.

Pathophysiology. The degree of right ventricular outflow obstruction can predict the clinical picture. In the first hours or days of life, if the ductus arteriosus has not closed, a patient with tetralogy of Fallot may not be cyanotic since the PDA maintains fairly good pulmonary circulation (Fig. 6-25). However, when the ductus closes, blood cannot easily pass from the right ventricle into the lungs because of the stenotic pulmonary valve. As right heart pressures rise, blood from the systemic circulation passes across the VSD and into the aorta without passing through the lungs to become oxygenated. The continued delivery of deoxygenated blood to the systemic circulation produces persistent cyanosis.

Clinical History. In tetralogy of Fallot, exercise-induced hypoxemia and increased carbon dioxide in the blood stimulate ventilation, which is perceived by the patient as dyspnea. A history of squatting to relieve dyspnea is common among children with tetralogy of Fallot. Squatting increases peripheral vascular resistance, thereby augmenting venous return, pulmonary arterial flow, and left ventricular output. These measures subsequently improve systemic arterial oxygenation and relieve the patient's dyspnea. Hypoxic spells are important features of tetralogy of Fallot. The spells are thought to be due to an abrupt

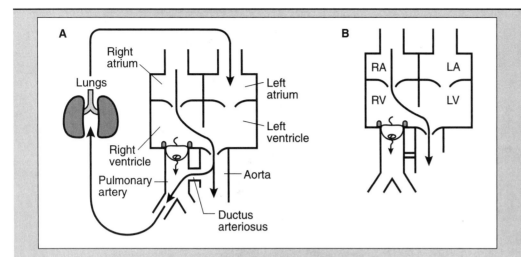

FIG. 6-25
PATHOPHYSIOLOGY OF TETRALOGY OF FALLOT. Diagrams show the four cardiac chambers, the stenotic pulmonic valve, the perimembranous ventricular septal defect, and the overriding aorta. (A) In the presence of a patent ductus arteriosus (PDA), unoxygenated blood can flow through the PDA to the lungs and become oxygenated. (B) However, when the ductus arteriosus closes after birth, unoxygenated blood is transmitted to the systemic circulation and the infant becomes cyanotic.

decrease in pulmonary blood flow and a sudden increase in right-to-left shunting. Children become tachypneic, hypoxic, cyanotic, and may even experience syncope, seizure, stroke, or death. Most infants do not develop cyanosis until days or weeks after birth owing to a PDA. Once the ductus arteriosus closes, cyanosis ensues. Some individuals may not develop cyanosis until they reach adolescence or young adulthood. These cases are related to acyanotic forms of tetralogy of Fallot, and patients complain primarily of exercise intolerance and dyspnea.

Physical Examination. Patients are generally cyanotic and underdeveloped. Clubbing of fingers and toes is also seen. Both the arterial pulse and the jugular venous pressure are normal in tetralogy. A right ventricular impulse may be appreciated in the subxiphoid area or along the left sternal border in the fourth or fifth intercostal space. A systolic thrill may be palpable in the third intercostal space owing to the right ventricular infundibular obstruction. On auscultation, S_1 is normal. S_2 is frequently singular with only an aortic component (A_2) and an inaudible pulmonic component (P_2). The murmur of tetralogy of Fallot relates to the degree of right ventricular outflow obstruction and is located in the left third intercostal space. The cardiovascular auscultatory findings in tetralogy of Fallot are summarized in Fig. 6-26.

Physical Findings Associated with Tetralogy of Fallot
Cyanosis, clubbing
Systolic murmur of turbulent flow across the VSD or through the narrowed right ventricular outflow tract

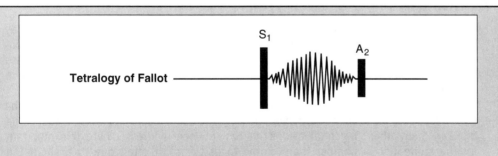

Tetralogy of Fallot

S_1 A_2

FIG. 6-26
CARDIAC AUSCULTATION FINDINGS IN TETRALOGY OF FALLOT. A harsh systolic murmur resulting from turbulent flow through the stenotic pulmonic valve or narrowed right ventricular outflow tract is often heard. Closure of the pulmonic valve is usually not heard, so the second heart sound (S_2) has a single component (A_2).

Management. In the past, palliative surgery was the primary means of managing young patients with tetralogy of Fallot. Various palliative procedures have been created. Two well-recognized palliative procedures are the Blalock-Taussig shunt (subclavian artery to pulmonary artery anastomosis) and the modified Blalock-Taussig (Gore-Tex tube between the subclavian artery and the pulmonary artery [Fig. 6-27]). These procedures increase pulmonary blood flow and alleviate systemic desaturation. Today, most children with tetralogy are diagnosed and undergo corrective surgery in the first few years of life. Surgery is also recommended for adults with tetralogy. Radical surgical repair involves resection of the muscle of the right ventricular outflow tract and closure of the VSD. Adults with small pulmonary arteries that would not permit radical repair can undergo a

FIG. 6-27
MODIFIED BLALOCK-TAUSSIG SHUNT. A Gore-Tex tube between the subclavian artery and the pulmonary artery allows unoxygenated blood to flow to the lungs.

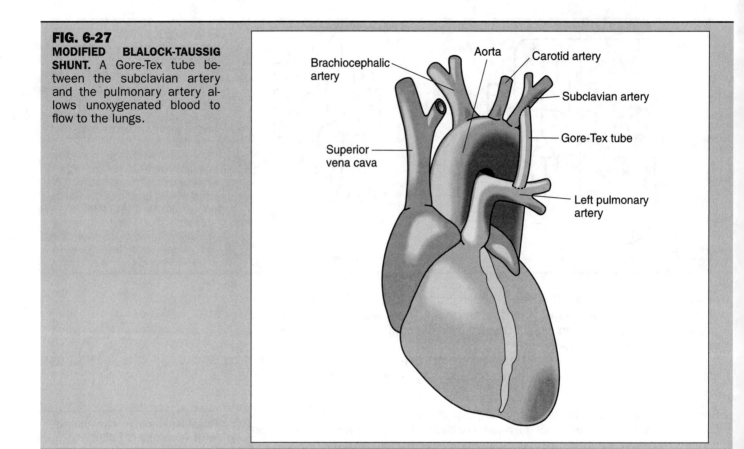

Aorta
Brachiocephalic artery
Carotid artery
Subclavian artery
Gore-Tex tube
Superior vena cava
Left pulmonary artery

palliative procedure. Adults tend to have a greater risk of bleeding compared to children because of compensatory erythrocytosis, prominent collateral circulation, and coagulation defects.

SUMMARY

Congenital heart disease encompasses a wide spectrum of anatomic anomalies that may lead to a variety of hemodynamic and pathophysiologic changes within the cardiovascular system. A general understanding of the pathophysiology of congenital heart disease aids one in understanding and differentiating various cardiac lesions. The ability to recognize such lesions may have significant clinical implications.

In general, congenital abnormalities should be classified pathophysiologically by the type of load they place on the heart: volume loads, pressure loads, and mixed loads. While there are many other congenital lesions that have not been addressed here, it is important for the student to remember that volume loads are most often due to a shunt (an abnormal connection between the systemic and pulmonic circulations), pressure loads are due to some type of obstruction to flow, and finally, mixed loads are usually due to abnormalities that combine both a shunt and an obstruction.

Knowledge of the underlying pathophysiology of cardiac lesions allows the physician to diagnose a congenital abnormality as well as to anticipate complications related to a lesion. Today, many individuals with congenital heart lesions are surviving into adulthood. Consequently, both adult and pediatric physicians must be able to recognize, diagnose, and treat patients with congenital heart disease.

KEY POINTS

- **Embryology.** The main structures of the heart develop between the third and eighth weeks of life. In weeks 1–3 a single vascular tube is formed. In week 4, the major event is the looping of the cardiovascular heart tube. In week 5 a number of complex events continue, including: septation of the atria, septation of the ventricles, and septation of the major arteries. During week 6, septation and valve formation are completed.

- **Fetal-to-newborn circulation.** In the fetus, fetal tissue receives oxygenated blood via the placenta. With the infant's first breath, the lungs expand, and pulmonary resistance decreases, which leads to reduced flow across the foramen ovale and reversed and reduced flow through the ductus arteriosus.
- **Volume overload.** Lesions that cause volume overload are most commonly due to an abnormal communication between the systemic and pulmonary circulations that leads to shunting of blood (ASD, VSD, PDA). Shunting normally occurs from left to right because systemic pressures are normally higher than pulmonary pressures.
- **Pressure overload.** Lesions that cause pressure overload are normally due to some type of obstruction to blood flow (pulmonary valve stenosis, aortic valve stenosis, coarctation of the aorta).
- **Mixed loads.** In mixed lesions, both obstruction to flow and an abnormal communication exist. The classic example is tetralogy of Fallot, where obstruction of flow out of the right ventricle and a VSD lead to right-to-left shunting. Right-to-left shunting causes unoxygenated blood to reach the peripheral tissues, which causes cyanosis.

Case Study: Resolution

Knowing that Ms. Etherton had an ASD, you could anticipate several complications related to this defect. When she presented, she appeared to have evidence of early left ventricular failure with mild pulmonary congestion. If she had remained untreated, the constant volume overload of the pulmonary vascular beds would have produced pulmonary vascular disease and subsequent pulmonary hypertension. The increase in right-heart pressures resulting from the development of pulmonary hypertension would have led to decreased compliance of the right ventricle. Failure of the left ventricle in conjunction with decreased right ventricular compliance would have promoted shunt reversal and the development of cyanosis—Eisenmenger's reaction. Once she developed pulmonary hypertension and cyanosis her clinical course would have deteriorated rapidly.

It is important to treat patients before pulmonary hypertension develops. Ms. Etherton was referred for cardiac surgery, where she received a dacron patch over a large secundum-type ASD. After surgery, she had an uneventful course and resolution of her symptoms.

▪ REVIEW QUESTIONS

Directions: For each of the following questions, choose the **one best** answer.

1. Hayden Reynolds, a 55-year-old man, presents to the physician's office following a syncopal episode this morning. Upon further questioning, the physician discovers that this patient has had stable angina for the past year. He also complains of increasing fatigue over the last 4 months. The physician examines the patient and determines that he has aortic stenosis. Which of the following examination findings would be consistent with this diagnosis?

   (A) Paradoxic splitting of the second heart sound (S_2)
   (B) A collapsing pulse
   (C) A pansystolic murmur best heard over the cardiac apex with radiation to the axilla
   (D) Fixed, widely split S_2
   (E) An early diastolic murmur with a decrescendo character

2. An Eisenmenger's reaction may occur in which of the following cardiac conditions?

   (A) Aortic stenosis
   (B) Pulmonic stenosis
   (C) Atrial septal defect (ASD)
   (D) Coarctation of the aorta
   (E) Aortic regurgitation

3. A 25-year-old cyanotic man presents to the physician's office for evaluation. He reports that he has been told that he has a heart murmur. He notes that his skin has been blue-tinged since approximately the age of 10. Which of the following is a possible etiology of the patient's cyanosis?

   (A) Tetralogy of Fallot with a patent ductus arteriosus (PDA)
   (B) Coarctation of the aorta
   (C) Aortic stenosis
   (D) Mitral regurgitation

4. David Singer is 40 years old. He presents to the physician's office with complaints of dyspnea on exertion, cough, and occasional episodes of blood in his sputum. He denies fever, chills, night sweats, or weight loss. He has smoked two packs of cigarettes a day for the last 10 years. Upon examination, he is afebrile, blood pressure is 137/74 mm Hg, pulse is 90 beats/min, and his respiratory rate is 24 breaths/min. He is in no acute distress. His head, eyes, ears, nose, and throat (HEENT) examination is unremarkable. His lung examination reveals coarse breath sounds bilaterally. His apical impulse is identified in the sixth intercostal space in the midclavicular line. His right ventricular impulse is prominent. His cardiac examination reveals a distinct first heart sound (S_1), a fixed split second heart sound (S_2), and a third heart sound (S_3). A II/VI systolic murmur is identified over the left second intercostal space. The patient has mild hepatomegaly. Evaluation of the extremities reveals 1+ pitting lower extremity edema bilaterally. Which of the following is true?

   (A) The patient has Eisenmenger's syndrome.
   (B) A chest x-ray is necessary to evaluate further for pulmonary vascular congestion, pneumonia, or malignancy.
   (C) The fixed split S_2 is due to increased left ventricular stroke volume and a delay in closure of the aortic valve.
   (D) The electrocardiogram (ECG) for this patient will probably be normal.

5. A 32-year-old man presents to the physician's office with complaints of mild calf pain, decreased exercise tolerance, and fatigue when he plays basketball or when he walks briskly. He denies dyspnea, chest pain, fevers, chills, or sick contacts. He denies tobacco use. He has been active all of his life. His blood pressure is 138/50 mm Hg, pulse is 80 beats/min, and his respiratory rate is 16 breaths/min. He is in no acute distress. His pulses are bounding and symmetric, his apical impulse is identified in the sixth intercostal space in the axillary line, his apical rate is regular, and a harsh continuous murmur is audible over the left second intercostal space. His lung examination is without adventitious sounds. Which of the following statements concerning this patient is true?

   (A) The patient has an aortic coarctation.
   (B) The patient may develop cyanosis.
   (C) The patient's chest x-ray is likely to show notching of the lower rib borders.
   (D) The patient has aortic stenosis.

6. Which of the following findings is associated with tetralogy of Fallot?

   (A) A large R wave in lead V_1 of the surface electrocardiogram (ECG)
   (B) Bounding arterial pulses
   (C) Paradoxic, split second heart sound (S_2)
   (D) A large R wave in lead V_6 of the surface ECG
   (E) Left axis deviation on the surface ECG

7. Which of the following intra-atrial connections can be normally present?

   (A) Secundum atrial septal defect (ASD)
   (B) Endocardial cushion defect
   (C) Sinus-venosus type defect
   (D) Patent foramen ovale
   (E) Common atrium

8. Which one of the following forms of atrial septal defect (ASD) occurs most commonly in patients with Down syndrome?

   (A) Secundum ASD
   (B) Endocardial cushion defect
   (C) Sinus-venosus type defect
   (D) Patent foramen ovale
   (E) Common atrium

■ ANSWERS AND EXPLANATIONS

1. The answer is A. The patient has aortic stenosis. Features of aortic stenosis include the following: a narrow pulse pressure; a slow rising, delayed pulse (pulsus parvus et tardus); a sustained, laterally displaced apical impulse; paradoxic splitting of S_2, and an early systolic murmur identified at the right upper sternal border with transmission into the left ventricular outflow tract and toward the apex. A collapsing pulse is characteristic of aortic insufficiency with a dramatic loss of pulse volume associated with an incompetent, regurgitant valve. An early diastolic decrescendo murmur is also associated with aortic regurgitation. A pansystolic murmur would be heard in a patient with a large ventricular septal defect or mitral regurgitation. A fixed split S_2 is the characteristic physical finding in patients with an atrial septal defect.

2. The answer is C. Eisenmenger's reaction involves right-to-left shunting of blood with the development of cyanosis. In aortic stenosis, pulmonic stenosis, and coarctation of the aorta, blood flow across a narrowed valve or narrowed aorta is limited, but generally no reversal of flow or cyanosis occurs. If the aortic valve is regurgitant, blood may flow back into the left ventricle only to be thrust out through the valve again; no complete reversal of blood flow occurs. The pressure within the left ventricle is greater than the systemic pressure as a result of the increased force of contraction generated in an attempt to push blood through the narrowed aortic valve; thus, blood flows from the left ventricle into the left ventricular outflow tract. Also, the blood in the left ventricle has already passed through the lungs and become oxygenated; hence, central cyanosis does not develop. The only listed lesion that is associated with Eisenmenger's syndrome is a long-standing ASD. Continued increased flow through the pulmonary artery may cause an increase in pulmonary vascular resistance which, if pulmonary vascular resistance increases enough, will lead to right-to-left shunting.

Over time, right-to-left shunting of blood (reversal of the normal flow of blood) can occur across a defective intra-atrial septum, as in the case of an ASD, across a defective intraventricular septum as in the case of a ventricular septal defect, in tetralogy of Fallot, or across a patent ductus arteriosus in which case deoxygenated blood flows from the pulmonary artery into the aorta.

3. The answer is A. The question necessitates that the reader recognize the potential complications of long-standing congenital heart disease. Generally, tetralogy of Fallot with a PDA does not produce cyanosis; however, shunt reversal through the ventricular septal defect (VSD) or the PDA may develop over time and lead to the development of cyanosis. The presence of the PDA maintains blood oxygenation; however, the increased pulmonary flow through the lungs and the left heart eventually leads to pulmonary vascular congestion and left ventricular hypertrophy, respectively. With the subsequent development of pulmonary hypertension and left ventricular failure, the shunt through the VSD or the PDA reverses right to left as the pulmonic pressures exceed systemic pressures and cyanosis develops.

Aortic stenosis and coarctation of the aorta cause an increased pressure overload on the left ventricle and may lead to shortness of breath, if the patient develops left ventricular failure. Mitral regurgitation places an abnormal volume load on the left ventricle and may lead to shortness of breath if the left ventricle fails. However, none of these three lesions would be associated with cyanosis in the absence of other lesions.

4. The answer is B. The patient has an atrial septal defect (ASD) with evidence of left heart failure and increased right heart volume. Left ventricular failure is demonstrated by the presence of S_3 and coarse bilateral breath sounds, which suggests pulmonary congestion. Additionally, there are findings suggestive of right heart failure with hepatomegaly and bilateral lower extremity edema. He does not have evidence of right-to-left shunting from Eisenmenger's syndrome (no cyanosis).

The patient's tobacco use history in conjunction with his report of hemoptysis mandates that a chest x-ray be performed to rule out the possibility of malignancy. There are several possible etiologies for hemoptysis including the following: bronchitis, pneumonia, malignancy, tuberculosis, congestive heart failure, and mitral stenosis. A chest x-ray may quickly limit the differential diagnosis and, in conjunction with the history and physical examination, may provide a diagnosis.

The hallmark of an ASD is a fixed, widely split S_2. With an ASD, the increase in right ventricular stroke volume as a result of left-to-right shunting further delays the normal closure of the *pulmonic* valve producing the widely split S_2. Since the two atria are in direct communication with one another, the stroke volume of each chamber varies similarly throughout the respiratory cycle producing a fixed, widely split S_2. Additional features associated with an ASD include a prominent right ventricular impulse along the left sternal border and a pulmonic systolic ejection murmur. Both of these findings are related to increased blood volume in the right heart secondary to a left-to-right shunt.

The ECG of an ostium secundum ASD depicts right axis deviation and a right bundle branch block (RBBB) related to hypertrophy of the right ventricle and a delay in right ventricular activation, respectively. In the case of an ostium primum or endocardial cushion defect, the ECG reveals left axis deviation and a RBBB related to an aberrant anatomic position of the conduction system rather than left ventricular enlargement. The ECG aids in the differentiation of the two forms of ASD and is rarely normal.

5. The answer is B. The patient's clinical history and physical examination findings are consistent with the presence of a patent ductus arteriosus (PDA). The hallmark of a PDA is a continuous, harsh, blowing murmur heard over the first or second intercostal space along the left sternal border. The murmur waxes and wanes with each heartbeat producing a "machinery-like murmur" that is more prominent during systole. Additionally, patients have bounding pulses, a wide pulse pressure, and lateral displacement of the apical impulse. Over time, excessive blood flow through the lungs leads to the development of pulmonary hypertension. With the onset of pulmonary hypertension, the flow of blood through the PDA reverses, producing a right-to-left shunt from the pulmonary artery into the aorta rather than from the aorta into the pulmonary artery. Subsequently, patients develop cyanosis as deoxygenated blood passes into the systemic circulation.

Coarctation of the aorta may produce lower extremity fatigue or intermittent claudication as a result of diminished perfusion distal to the coarctation. Patients may be hypertensive and may have obvious upper-lower body asymmetry. The apical impulse may be sustained reflecting an increased load placed upon the left ventricle. A continuous murmur may be heard over both scapulae as a result of turbulent flow through the intercostal collateral vessels. Unlike the murmur of a PDA, there is no alteration in the character of the murmur associated with a coarctation. A chest x-ray may be pathognomonic for coarctation with notching of the lower rib borders. The murmur of aortic stenosis is not continuous but occurs only in midsystole since the aortic valve is normally closed during diastole.

6. The answer is A. Patients with tetralogy of Fallot develop significant right ventricular hypertrophy related to the degree of right ventricular outflow obstruction. Right ventricular hypertrophy is identified on an ECG by the presence of a large R wave in lead V_1, since the right ventricle is anatomically the most anterior chamber. Conversely, since the left ventricle is located posteriorly, left ventricular hypertrophy is associated with a prominent R wave in lead V_6. Left ventricular hypertrophy is not associated with tetralogy of Fallot. In general, enlargement of the ventricle distorts the vector of myocardial depolarization toward the hypertrophied side of the heart. Left ventricular hypertrophy is associated with left axis deviation, and right ventricular hypertrophy is associated with right axis deviation. A fixed, split S_2 would be associated with an atrial septal defect, rather than tetralogy of Fallot, producing right axis deviation. Finally, although tetralogy of Fallot is associated with right-to-left shunting of blood, bounding arterial pulses would not be expected.

7. The answer is E. There are five forms of ASD; however, only four forms are considered pathologic. The four pathologic forms of ASD include the following: secundum ASD, endocardial cushion defect, sinus-venosus type, and a common atrium. A patent foramen ovale exists in up to 25% of people and is not generally considered to be a pathologic occurrence.

8. The answer is B. Endocardial cushion defects occur in approximately 20% of persons with Down syndrome, otherwise the lesion is relatively uncommon. The defect occurs when the endocardial cushions fail to fuse, resulting in a large defect in the center of the heart.

■ REFERENCES

Bashore TM, Lieberman EB: Aortic/mitral obstruction and coarctation of the aorta. *Cardiol Clin* 11:617–641, 1993.

Behrman RE, Kliegman RM, Arvin AM, et al: *Nelson's Textbook of Pediatrics*, 15th ed. Philadelphia, PA: W. B. Saunders, 1996.

Driscoll DJ: Evaluation of the cyanotic newborn. *Pediatr Clin North Am* 34:1–23, 1990.

Haworth S, Bull C: Physiology of congenital heart disease. *Arch Dis Child* 68:707–711, 1993.

Mahoney LT: Acyanotic congenital heart disease, atrial and ventricular septal defects, atrioventricular canal, patent ductus arteriosus, pulmonic stenosis. *Cardiol Clin* 11:603–616, 1993.

Moore KL: *The Developing Human: Clinically Oriented Embryology*, 4th ed. Philadelphia, PA: W. B. Saunders, 1988.

Perloff JK: *The Clinical Recognition of Congenital Heart Disease*, 4th ed. Philadelphia, PA: W. B. Saunders, 1994.

Warnes CA: Tetralogy of Fallot and pulmonary atresia/ventricular septal defect. *Cardiol Clin* 11:643–650, 1993.

Chapter 7

VASCULAR ABNORMALITIES

Fred M. Kusumoto, M.D.

▮ CHAPTER OUTLINE

Case Study: *Introduction*	*Ms. Maud Kelly was a 35-year-old healthy woman who had no history of medical problems. She had had a recent history of worsening headaches and episodic blurred vision. The most important finding on her physical examination was a blood pressure of 226/108 mm Hg. The remainder of Ms. Kelly's physical examination was notable for two findings. Auscultation of her heart revealed a loud fourth heart sound (S_4). In addition, auscultation of the left side of her abdomen revealed a harsh, rasping sound that occurred simultaneously with her cardiac apical impulse. Was Ms. Kelly's blood pressure normal for her age? What are the possible causes for her physical examination findings?*

▮ INTRODUCTION

Abnormalities of the arterial system are a commonly encountered problem. High arterial blood pressure is present in over 15% of adults in the United States. High arterial blood pressures are associated with a variety of medical conditions, including catastrophic situations involving the largest vessel of the body, the aorta. In this chapter the pathophysiology of high arterial blood pressure (hypertension), aortic diseases (which are frequently associated with hypertension), and profound low arterial blood pressure (hypotension, commonly referred to as "shock") are discussed.

▮ HYPERTENSION

Blood travels through the arteries of the body propelled by the force of cardiac contraction. Blood pressure was first measured by Jean Poiseuille in the 1820s, and the modern sphygmomanometer was developed in the 1880s by Samuel von Basch. Today, an auscultatory method, first described by the Russian physician Korotkoff in 1905, that indirectly measures brachial artery pressure is commonly employed (Fig. 7-1). An inflatable cuff is wrapped around the upper arm at the level of the heart. The cuff is inflated to pressures higher than the systolic pressure, completely occluding blood flow in the brachial artery. As the pressure in the cuff is lowered below the level of systolic pressure, pulsating turbulent blood flows through the brachial artery and repetitive, faint, but crisp sounds can be heard using a stethoscope (Korotkoff's sounds). As the pressure in the cuff is further reduced, blood flow in the brachial artery becomes continuous but is still relatively turbulent, and the Korotkoff's sounds become muffled. Muffled Korotkoff's sounds are usually heard when the cuff pressure is approximately 5–10 mm Hg greater than the diastolic pressure. Once the pressure in the cuff drops below the diastolic pressure, continuous normal flow returns to the brachial artery, and the Korotkoff's sounds disappear. In conditions associated with increased flow (e.g., exercise), intra-arterial turbulence can be heard at cuff pressures well below the actual diastolic pressure, so that the point at which the Korotkoff's sounds become muffled actually becomes a better approximation of the diastolic pressure.

FIG. 7-1
When cuff pressure is greater than the systolic pressure (> 120 mm Hg in this example), the brachial artery is occluded, and no blood flow occurs. As the cuff pressure is lowered below systolic pressure, pulsatile turbulent flow occurs in the brachial artery and can be heard by auscultation (Korotkoff's sounds). As cuff pressure is further reduced, the brachial arterial flow becomes continuous but remains turbulent and the Korotkoff's sounds become muffled (60–50 mm Hg in the example). When the cuff pressure is reduced below diastolic pressure (50 mm Hg), laminar blood flow returns to the brachial artery and the Korotkoff's sounds disappear.

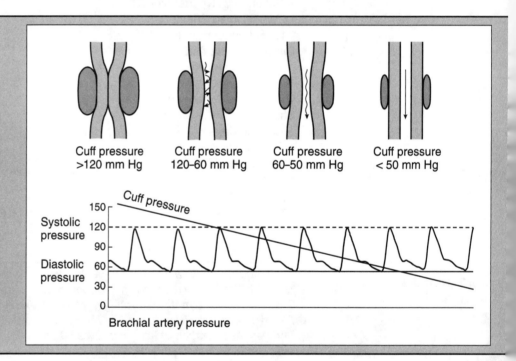

Normal blood pressure is usually defined as systolic pressures less than 140 mm Hg and diastolic pressures less than 90 mm Hg. In general, blood pressure is lower at night, and some data suggest that reduction in the circadian variation of blood pressure is associated with a worse prognosis. Blood pressures are normally lower in children. For example, systolic blood pressures greater than 120 mm Hg and diastolic blood pressures greater than 80 mm Hg should be considered inappropriately high in children under 10 years of age.

The pressure in the vascular bed relates to cardiac output and peripheral resistance in the following manner:

$$\text{Blood pressure} = \text{cardiac output} \times \text{total peripheral resistance}$$

In simplistic terms, abnormally elevated blood pressure is due to increased cardiac output, increased peripheral vascular resistance, or a combination of increased cardiac output and peripheral vascular resistance (Fig. 7-2). Since cardiac output is the product of stroke volume and heart rate, both increased heart rate and increased left ventricular contractility can lead to elevated blood pressure. Increased peripheral vascular re-

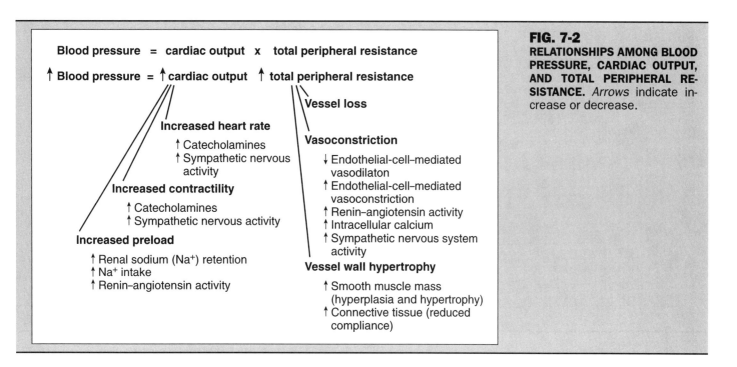

Blood pressure = cardiac output x   total peripheral resistance

↑ Blood pressure = ↑cardiac output ↑ total peripheral resistance

Vessel loss

Increased heart rate
   ↑ Catecholamines
   ↑ Sympathetic nervous
      activity

Increased contractility
   ↑ Catecholamines
   ↑ Sympathetic nervous activity

Increased preload
   ↑ Renal sodium (Na⁺) retention
   ↑ Na⁺ intake
   ↑ Renin–angiotensin activity

Vasoconstriction
   ↓ Endothelial-cell–mediated
      vasodilaton
   ↑ Endothelial-cell–mediated
      vasoconstriction
   ↑ Renin–angiotensin activity
   ↑ Intracellular calcium
   ↑ Sympathetic nervous system
      activity

Vessel wall hypertrophy
   ↑ Smooth muscle mass
      (hyperplasia and hypertrophy)
   ↑ Connective tissue (reduced
      compliance)

FIG. 7-2
RELATIONSHIPS AMONG BLOOD PRESSURE, CARDIAC OUTPUT, AND TOTAL PERIPHERAL RESISTANCE. *Arrows* indicate increase or decrease.

sistance can be due to arterial vasoconstriction, any process that reduces vessel compliance (arterial wall hypertrophy), or actual loss of capillaries. Clinically, hypertension is classified as primary or secondary, depending on whether a separate definitive cause of high blood pressure can be identified.

PRIMARY HYPERTENSION

Most commonly, no specific cause for high blood pressure can be identified, so that the hypertension is called *primary* (primary hypertension is also termed *essential hypertension*). Primary hypertension accounts for more than 90% of cases of high arterial pressure. Primary hypertension is a multifactorial process that can result from a variety of interrelated mechanisms that cause increased cardiac output or increased peripheral vascular resistance (see Fig. 7-2).

Renal Retention of Excess Sodium (Na⁺). Renal retention of excess Na⁺ can lead to increased intravascular fluid volume, increased preload, and by the Starling relationship (see Chap. 1), increased cardiac output. Several possible mechanisms for renal retention of Na⁺ have been suggested. First, several investigators have suggested that patients with primary hypertension have a decreased number of functional nephrons, which reduces the total available glomerular filtration surface area. Normally, people under 30 years of age have approximately 800,000 nephrons per kidney. Some investigators have suggested that up to 40% of young adults have fewer than this number; it is possible that these patients are predisposed to hypertension, but no causal link between reduced nephron number and the development of hypertension has been firmly established. Second, resetting of the normal pressure–natriuresis relationship could be the mechanism for primary hypertension in some patients. Normally, when blood pressure rises, renal excretion of Na⁺ and water increases (Fig. 7-3). Rightward shifting of the pressure–natriuresis curve (so that higher blood pressures are required to maintain a given amount of Na⁺ excretion) can be caused by a number of mechanisms, including abnormalities of the renin–angiotensin system (see below) or a blunted response to atrial natriuretic hormone.

Increased Peripheral Vascular Resistance. Another mechanism for primary hypertension is increased peripheral vascular resistance resulting from sympathetic nervous system hyperactivity or deficiencies in other vasodilatory systems. Young patients with hypertension have been found to have increased circulating catecholamines and increased vascular responsiveness to circulating catecholamines. Sympathetic nervous

FIG. 7-3
Rightward resetting of the pressure–natriuresis curve means that higher arterial pressures are necessary to maintain a specific amount of renal Na+ excretion.

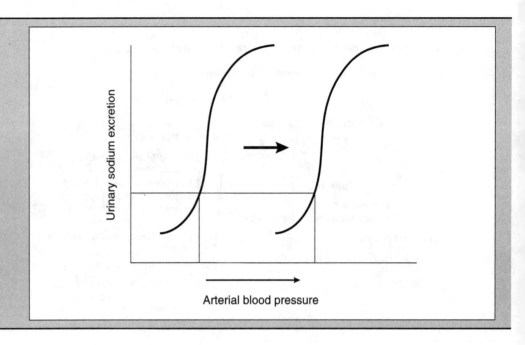

Possible Membrane Protein Defects in Primary Hypertension
(increase intracellular Ca2+ concentrations)
Na+–K+-ATPase inhibition
Na+–H+-exchanger activation
Ca2+-ATPase inhibition

activity can increase cardiac output by increasing the basal heart rate and increasing the cardiac inotropic state or by increasing peripheral vascular resistance by promoting arteriolar vasoconstriction. Kallikrein is a protease that converts kininogen to bradykinin, which is a potent vasodilator. Some investigators have reported that decreased production of renal kallikrein may be a mechanism for hypertension in some patients. Similarly, other investigators have reported decreased production of several vasodilatory prostaglandins in patients with hypertension.

Recent research suggests that hypertension is associated with abnormal function in several important membrane proteins, which could potentially cause an increase in peripheral vascular resistance. First, several investigators have identified endogenous *ouabain-like factors* in the blood of patients with hypertension. Ouabain inhibits sodium–potassium-adenosine triphosphatase (Na+–K+-ATPase). Remember that the Na+–K+-ATPase is important for extruding Na+ from the intracellular space (see Chap. 2). Inhibition of Na+–K+-ATPase could lead to intracellular Na+ accumulation, which could favor increased intracellular calcium ions (Ca2+) through the Na+–Ca2+-exchanger. Increased intracellular Ca2+ could lead to enhanced smooth muscle cell vasoconstriction (see Chap. 3) and a generalized increase in peripheral vascular resistance (Fig. 7-4). Similarly, enhanced Na+–hydrogen (H+)-exchanger activity has been described in cells from hypertensive patients. Enhanced Na+–H+ exchange increases intracellular Na+, which can cause increased smooth muscle cell vasoconstriction as described above. Finally, intracellular Ca2+ concentrations can be directly increased if cytoplasmic Ca2+-ATPase activity is inhibited.

Another potential cause of increased peripheral vascular resistance is a decrease in capillary number. Some investigators have suggested that hypertension is associated with loss in capillary density. It is not clear how important this mechanism is in the pathogenesis of hypertension.

Renin–Angiotensin System. A third possible mechanism for primary hypertension could be an alteration in the renin–angiotensin system. Renin was originally isolated from rabbit kidneys at the turn of the 19th century. Since then we have learned that the renin–angiotensin system is an intricate and complex system that controls blood pressure and cardiovascular function. Normally, increased blood pressure inhibits release of renin from the renal juxtaglomerular cells, which leads to decreased production of angiotensin I and a consequent decrease in angiotensin II (Fig. 7-5). Since angiotensin II is a potent vasoconstrictor and a stimulator of aldosterone (which causes Na+ retention), inappropriately elevated angiotensin II levels could cause hypertension. Large population

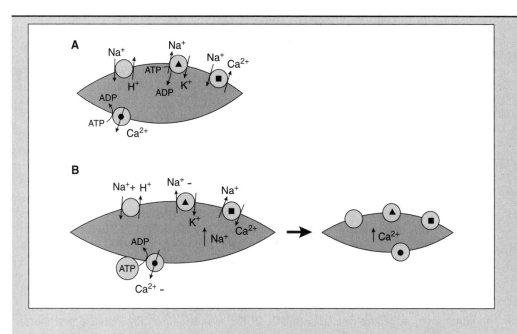

FIG. 7-4
MEMBRANE PROTEIN DEFECTS ASSOCIATED WITH HYPERTENSION. (A) A smooth muscle cell is shown with a schematic representation of three membrane proteins important for ion transport: Na^+–K^+-ATPase ▲, Na^+–H^+-exchanger ○, the Na^+–Ca^{2+}-exchanger ■, and the Ca^{2+}-ATPase ●. (B) Both activation of the Na^+–H^+-exchanger and inhibition of the Na^+–K^+-ATPase lead to increased intracellular Na^+ concentrations. Increased intracellular Na^+ favors accumulation of intracellular Ca^{2+}. Increased intracellular Ca^{2+} increases smooth muscle vasoconstriction. Intracellular Ca^{2+} can also be directly increased by inhibition of the Ca^{2+}-ATPase. ADP = adenosine diphosphate; ATP = adenosine triphosphate; Ca^{2+} = calcium ion; H^+ = hydrogen ion; K^+ = potassium ion; Na^+ = sodium ion.

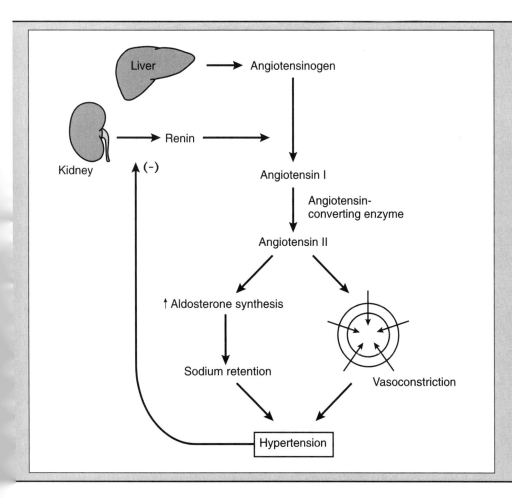

FIG. 7-5
FEEDBACK LOOP FOR THE RENIN–ANGIOTENSIN SYSTEM. The liver produces angiotensinogen. Renin, which is produced by juxtaglomerular cells in the kidney, cleaves a leucine–leucine bond in angiotensinogen to produce angiotensin I.

Increased Peripheral Vascular Resistance in Primary Hypertension
Sympathetic system overactivity
Reduced production of systemic vasodilators or increased production of systemic vasoconstrictors
Increased smooth muscle cell intracellular Ca^{2+} resulting from protein defects
Global loss of capillary density
Endothelial-cell–mediated imbalance of local vasoconstrictors and vasodilators
Endothelial-cell production of growth factors

Primary hypertension is probably multifactorial.

studies of patients have found that 60% of patients with primary hypertension have normal renin levels, and 15% of patients have elevated levels of plasma renin activity.

Insulin Resistance. A fourth possible mechanism for essential hypertension involves insulin resistance. Normally, insulin causes sympathetic activation and vasodilation, which tend to cancel each other and yield no net effect on blood pressure. In some patients with hypertension, the vasodilatory effect of insulin is attenuated as a result of failure to synthesize the potent vasodilator, nitric oxide (NO), which leads to a net hypertensive effect because of unopposed sympathetic activation.

Primary Endothelial Dysfunction. Primary endothelial dysfunction may be the pathophysiologic mechanism of hypertension in some patients (Fig. 7-6). It has been reported that some hypertensive patients have a blunted vasodilatory response to acetylcholine (ACh). In the presence of an intact endothelium, ACh causes vasodilation that appears to be mediated by the release of the potent vasodilator NO (see Chap. 3). Reduced production or reduced sensitivity to vasodilator molecules (such as NO) may be important in the pathogenesis of hypertension. In addition, several investigators have found that patients with hypertension have increased production of endothelial-cell–derived vasoconstrictors. Finally, it is possible that increased production of endothelial-cell–derived growth factors could lead to smooth muscle hypertrophy in the arteries and cause hypertension. To summarize, a generalized abnormality of the endothelium may increase peripheral vascular resistance through a variety of mechanisms and may be the pathophysiologic mechanism for hypertension in some patients.

Primary hypertension is most likely a heterogeneous condition with any of the abovementioned mechanisms having a varying role in each individual patient. It is important to remember that usually the kidneys can handle large volume loads without a consequent increase in blood pressure, which suggests that some abnormality in renal function is present in all types of primary hypertension. Regardless of etiologic mechanism, prolonged periods of hypertension can lead to profound organ damage as outlined below.

FIG. 7-6
ENDOTHELIAL CELL DYSFUNCTION IN HYPERTENSION. (A) Normally, endothelial cells form a thin layer that lines the arteries. Endothelial cells produce nitric oxide (NO) and prostacyclin (PGI_2), which cause smooth muscle vasodilatation. The vasoconstrictor endothelin I is produced in small amounts. In hypertensive patients, the balance is shifted to favor secretion of factors that cause vasoconstriction. Morphologically, the endothelial cells become rounder. Smooth muscle cells become larger (hypertrophy) and proliferate (hyperplasia).

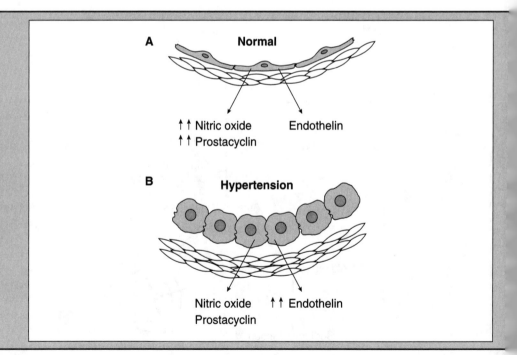

SECONDARY HYPERTENSION

When high blood pressure is a consequence of another well-defined abnormality, it is termed secondary hypertension. Several well-recognized causes of secondary hypertension are listed in Table 7-1 and Fig. 7-7.

Table 7-1
Causes of Secondary Hypertension

CAUSE	PATHOPHYSIOLOGY
Oral contraceptives	Estrogen component stimulates angiotensinogen production.
Renal disease	Almost any form of renal disease can cause hypertension.
Renovascular disease	Narrowing of the renal arteries can cause hypertension. Relatively decreased glomerular perfusion leads to increased renin production. Increased renin ultimately causes increased angiotensin I and angiotensin II production.
Adrenal disease	*Adrenal cortex:* Any condition associated with increased cortisol production can be associated with hypertension (Cushing's syndrome, Cushing's disease).
	Adrenal medulla: Pheochromocytoma can be associated with hypertension.
Coarctation of the aorta	Focal narrowing of the aorta just after the takeoff of the left subclavian artery results in hypertension in the upper extremities and decreased blood pressure to abdominal organs and the lower extremities.
Pregnancy	Pregnancy is sometimes associated with hypertension due to prostaglandin release.

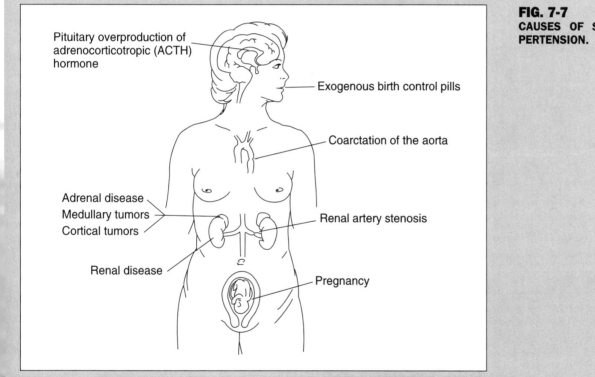

FIG. 7-7
CAUSES OF SECONDARY HYPERTENSION.

Oral Contraceptive and Postmenopausal Estrogen Use. Oral contraceptives tend to increase blood pressure. The estrogen component of birth control pills tends to stimulate production of angiotensinogen in the liver. In addition, estrogen and synthetic progestogens may induce fluid retention in some individuals. Finally, plasma insulin levels may be increased in women taking oral contraceptives, which suggests that some type of peripheral insulin resistance is present. Overall, the incidence of oral contraceptive–mediated hypertension is low, probably less than 5% of all women who use oral contraceptives.

Renal Disease. As discussed earlier, the kidney has a central role in maintaining Na+ homeostasis and normal blood pressure. Almost any form of kidney disease (glomerulonephritis, interstitial nephritis, polycystic kidney disease) can be associated with hypertension. Kidney disease can be both a cause and effect of hypertension, thus setting up a positive feedback loop. Hypertension is frequently associated with both acute and chronic renal insufficiency. Approximately 80%–90% of patients with end-stage renal disease have accompanying hypertension.

Renovascular Disease. Obstruction of a renal artery can cause reduced blood flow to the kidney and cause the release of renin from the abnormally perfused kidney. Obstruction of the renal arteries can be due to atherosclerosis or fibromuscular dysplasia. Atherosclerosis of the renal artery is most common in older men, while fibromuscular dysplasia is most commonly observed in younger women. As discussed earlier, increased renin leads ultimately to increased angiotensin II production, which causes both vasoconstriction and Na+ retention resulting from increased aldosterone synthesis. The possibility of renovascular hypertension should be considered in any patient with hypertension but particularly in those patients with elevated serum creatinine levels (which suggest renal dysfunction) or sudden onset of refractory hypertension.

Chromaffin cells are neuroectodermal cells that stain black when exposed to chromium salts.

Adrenal Disease. Diseases of the adrenal medulla and the adrenal cortex can be associated with hypertension. Tumors of the adrenal medulla (pheochromocytomas) consist of chromaffin cells that secrete norepinephrine and other catecholamines. Increased circulatory catecholamines cause arterial vasoconstriction and elevated blood pressures. Adrenocortical tumors that produce excess aldosterone or cortisol can also be associated with hypertension. Similarly, excess production of corticotropin (adrenocorticotropic hormone, ACTH) from pituitary adenomas or from nonpituitary sources (oat cell carcinoma) can be associated with hypertension. Excess cortisol from any mechanism causes hypertension by stimulating the synthesis of renin substrate and expression of angiotensin receptors and partial activation of renal mineralocorticoid receptors (which leads to Na+ retention).

Coarctation of the Aorta. In coarctation of the aorta, there is a discrete narrowing in the aortic arch, just after the origin of the left subclavian artery. The obstruction causes left ventricular hypertrophy, relative hypertension in the upper extremities, and relative hypotension to the abdominal organs and lower extremities. Generalized vasoconstriction resulting from an increase in the renin–angiotensin system (the result of reduced renal blood flow) and increased sympathetic nervous activity contribute to the pathophysiology of hypertension.

Pregnancy. Hypertension can appear in up to 10% of pregnant, previously normotensive women during the last trimester or immediately after delivery (gestational hypertension). This response is most common in young women during their first pregnancy. It appears that the key mechanism for gestational hypertension is failure of the placenta to invade fully the maternal uterine arteries, which leads to relative placental ischemia. As a compensatory response, the placenta releases prostacyclins and endothelins, which cause increased vascular volume and increased arterial blood pressure. Some data suggest that the primary reason for the failure of placental invasion is a maternal immunologic response to placental antigens.

TARGET ORGAN EFFECTS

Hypertension from any cause can be associated with profound effects on several target organs, including the eye, brain, heart, and kidneys (Fig. 7-8).

Retinal microinfarcts are often called "cotton wool spots." In severe cases of hypertension, the optic nerve disk becomes edematous and swollen (papilledema).

Retina. The effects of hypertension on the retinal arteries can be directly observed by ophthalmoscopic examination and were first described by Keith in 1939. Since intraocular pressure determines the capillary flow and intraocular pressure does not increase with arterial hypertension, the retinal arteries are particularly vulnerable to the effects of systemic hypertension. Characteristic changes of the retina actually allow the examiner to evaluate the severity and duration of hypertension (Fig. 7-9). The retinal arteries constrict and hypertrophy in response to systemic hypertension. On ophthalmoscopic examination, the arteries reflect more light and take a "copper-wire" appearance. Where arteries and veins cross, the thickened arteries compress the vein and arteriovenous "nicking" is observed. With elevated arterial pressure for long duration, the retinal vessels may leak fluid onto the retinal surface. The aqueous portion of this fluid is rapidly cleared, often leaving an accumulation of hard lipid exudates. Hard exudates can also be associated with diabetes mellitus. If arterial pressure increases rapidly, the vessel wall can burst, causing hemorrhages and microinfarcts to be observed on the retina.

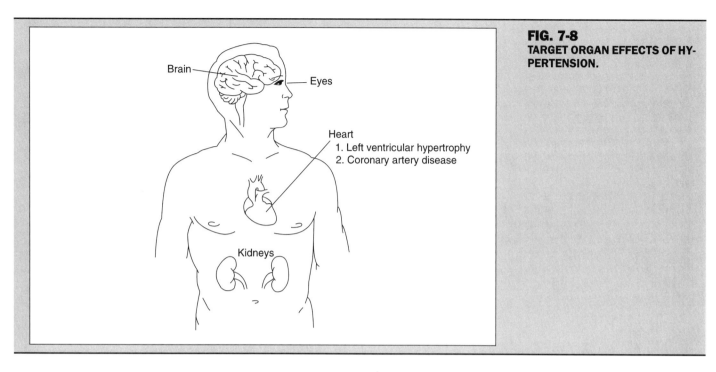

FIG. 7-8
TARGET ORGAN EFFECTS OF HYPERTENSION.

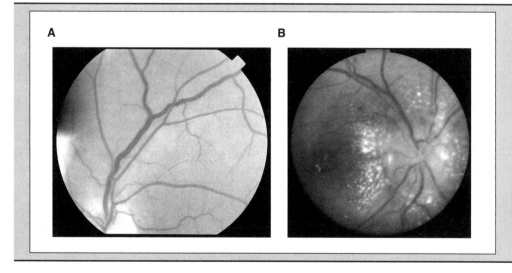

FIG. 7-9
RETINAS IN HYPERTENSION. (A) Arteriovenous (A/V) nicking changes along the superotemporal vascular arcade of a left eye in early hypertensive retinopathy (15-degree field fundus photo). (B) Grade 4 hypertensive retinopathy with optic nerve head swelling, yellow lipid deposition from leaking exudate, and retinal swelling in a right eye (15-degree field fundus photo). (*Source:* Courtesy of Gregory S. H. Ogawa, M.D., University of New Mexico, Albuquerque, New Mexico.)

Central Nervous System. Severe hypertension can cause a generalized encephalopathy. Hypertension is a significant risk factor for stroke, usually resulting from atherosclerosis and thrombosis of the large arteries that supply the brain (vertebrobasilar and carotid arteries) or the cerebral arteries themselves. In addition, hypertension is associated with thrombosis of the small penetrating cerebral arteries, which can cause small (2 mm–5 mm) strokes (lacunae). Hypertension can also cause aneurysmal dilatation of small cerebral arteries (Charcot-Bouchard aneurysms), which can burst and cause intracerebral hemorrhage.

Heart. Hypertension causes increased afterload on the heart (Fig. 7-10). In response to the increased afterload, the left ventricular wall thickness increases. As discussed in Chap. 1, left ventricular hypertrophy can cause abnormal filling of the left ventricle, producing congestive heart failure. In addition, hypertension is an important risk factor for the development of atherosclerotic coronary artery disease (see Chap. 3).

Left ventricular hypertrophy resulting from hypertension causes several distinctive findings on physical examination. First, left ventricular hypertrophy reduces left ventricular compliance. Ventricular filling becomes more dependent on atrial contraction and a

FIG. 7-10
(A) Hypertension causes increased afterload on the heart, since ventricular pressure must now be higher than the elevated systemic pressure (*curve 1*). Increased afterload initially reduces the stroke volume (SV) of the ventricle. To maintain SV, the heart begins operating on the steeper portion of the diastolic pressure volume curve (*curve 2*). (B) Over time the left ventricle thickens, which shifts the diastolic pressure curve upward and the isovolumic systolic pressure curve to the left.

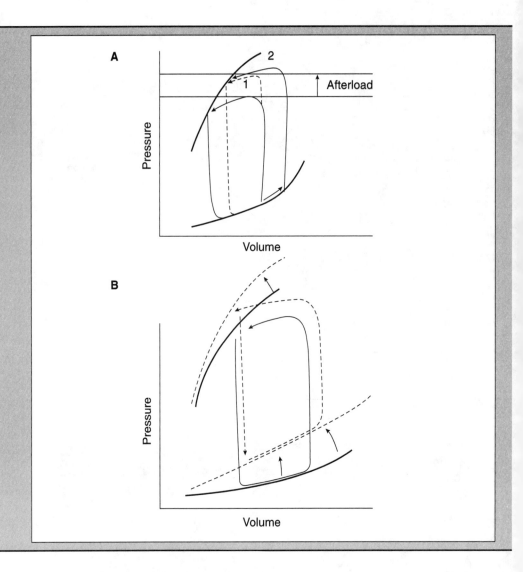

presystolic fourth heart sound (S_4) can sometimes be appreciated. Second, the apical impulse can become more prominent and sustained. Normally, the point of maximal impulse (PMI) is felt before the carotid upstroke. If the PMI can be felt simultaneously with the carotid impulse, the PMI is sustained and left ventricular hypertrophy should be suspected. Finally, the portion of the second heart sound (S_2) produced by aortic valve closure (A_2) becomes accentuated.

Increased left ventricular wall thickness causes several changes to be observed on the surface electrocardiogram (ECG), which are summarized in Fig. 7-11. First, since ventricular mass is larger, the QRS complex (which represents ventricular depolarization) has a larger magnitude. In addition, left ventricular hypertrophy causes abnormal ventricular repolarization, which is associated with ST-segment depression and T-wave inversion.

Kidneys. Hypertension can also cause atherosclerotic lesions in the afferent and efferent arterioles and capillaries of renal glomeruli. Structural damage to the nephrons can lead to microalbuminuria and progressive renal insufficiency.

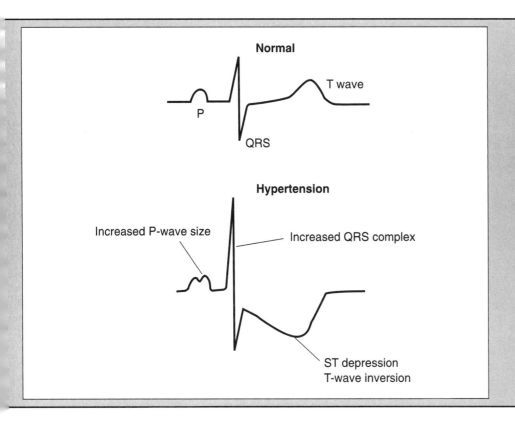

FIG. 7-11
Several characteristic electrocardiogram findings are associated with left ventricular hypertrophy. When the left ventricle hypertrophies, the QRS magnitude increases, and repolarization (ST segment and T wave) becomes abnormal. The atria also hypertrophy in response to the increased end-diastolic ventricular pressure, which leads to P-wave enlargement. Since the left atrium is activated later than the right atrium, left ventricular hypertrophy is associated with lengthening of the P-wave duration.

Ms. Kelly had renal artery stenosis (as a result of fibromuscular dysplasia) which was responsible for her elevated blood pressure and the auscultatory findings in her abdomen. Turbulent flow across the stenotic renal artery caused the harsh, rasping abdominal sound, which is called a bruit. The fourth heart sound (S_4) was due to left ventricular hypertrophy.

Ms. Kelly was scheduled for an elective balloon dilatation of her renal artery when she suddenly developed severe substernal chest pain one evening. The pain radiated to her back. She was brought to the emergency room. Radial artery and femoral artery pulses were difficult to palpate.

Case Study:
Continued

◀ DISEASES OF THE AORTA

Blood is ejected from the heart into the aorta, which then provides branches to the head and extremities. In addition to serving as a conduit, the aorta has an important role for forward propagation of blood. When the heart contracts, the aorta distends, thus converting kinetic energy from the contracting ventricle to potential energy stored in the vessel wall. As illustrated in Fig. 7-12, when the aorta recoils, the potential energy stored in the vessel wall is converted back into kinetic energy, and blood is propelled forward (since the aortic valve is closed). Like other arteries, the wall of the aorta has three layers, the intima, the media, and the adventitia (see Chap. 3). However, the medial layer of the aorta contains relatively little smooth muscle and large amounts of spirally arranged elastic tissue that are responsible for the aorta's important compliance properties.

Since the aorta is the main artery of the body, diseases of the aorta can have catastrophic consequences. In general, aortic diseases can be divided into (1) *aortic aneurysm*, in which the aorta responds to increased stress by abnormal expansion and (2) *aortic dissection*, in which a tear in the intimal layer results in separation of tissue within the medial layer of the aorta.

FIG. 7-12
(A) During systole, left ventricular contraction causes distention of the aorta. At this time the mitral valve (MV) is closed, and the aortic valve (AV) is open. (B) During diastole, the MV opens, and the AV is closed; however, recoil of the aorta leads to continued forward motion of blood. (*Source:* Berne RM, Levy MN: *Cardiovascular Pathophysiology*, 7th ed. St. Louis, Mo: Mosby–Year Book, 1997, p 136.)

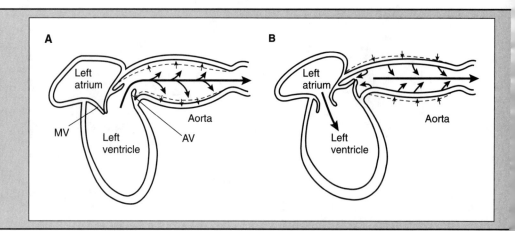

The word *aneurysm* is derived from the Greek word *aneurysma*, which means "widening."

Pseudoaneuryms are associated with vessel wall dissection.

AORTIC ANEURYSM

Normally the aorta is approximately 3 cm in diameter at its aortic valve origin, decreases to 2.5 cm in the descending thoracic aorta, and gradually tapers to 1.8–2 cm in the abdomen. An aneurysm is an abnormal dilatation of a vessel; traditionally, any localized dilatation greater than 1.5 times the expected diameter has been considered abnormal. While aneurysms can be observed in any blood vessel, aneurysms of the aorta can have catastrophic consequences. The first accurate description of an aortic aneurysm was made by Galen in the second century. In 1542, Fernelius recognized that aneurysms arose from localized thinning of the arterial wall. A true aneurysm involves all three layers of the vessel wall, whereas in a pseudoaneurysm, the intima and media layers are disrupted, and the dilated region is lined only by the adventitial layer (Fig. 7-13).

Aortic aneurysms are generally classified by location and shape. While aneurysmal

FIG. 7-13
In a true aneurysm, the vessel lumen dilates, and increased vessel size involves all three layers of the artery. In a false aneurysm, a tear in the intimal layer leads to bleeding into the medial layer (dissection). If the amount of bleeding is large, a false aneurysm, in which a portion of the dilated vessel is subtended by the media and adventitia, can occur.

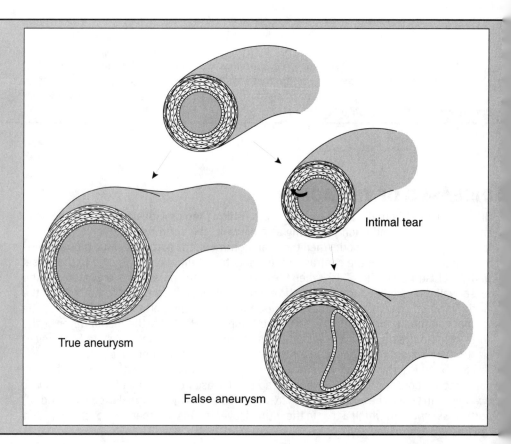

dilatation can be observed in any portion of the aorta, the intra-abdominal aorta is by far the most common site for aortic aneurysms (Fig. 7-14). Aortic aneurysms can be classified as *fusiform* if there is circumferential dilatation of the aorta or *saccular* if a balloon-like dilatation with a relatively small neck is observed. Regardless of their location or shape, the main threat of aortic aneuryms is the possibility of rupture, which is a medical emergency associated with very high mortality.

Aneurysms isolated to the ascending aorta are usually associated with cystic degeneration of the media layer of the aorta (cystic medial necrosis). In this condition, small cysts filled with basophilic material replace the smooth muscle cells of the media. Usually, patients with cystic medial necrosis have a normal body habitus, but some patients have a peculiar body habitus (tall stature, arachnodactyly) referred to as Marfan's syndrome. Other rare causes of cystic medial necrosis include Ehlers-Danlos syndrome type IV and pregnancy. Very rarely, syphilis can be associated with ascending aortic aneurysm because small stellate scars form in the media of the ascending aorta. Aneurysms of the descending aorta and abdominal aorta are usually due to atherosclerosis. However, familial clustering of some cases suggests that a hereditary mo-

Vasa vasorum are the small arteries present in the larger arteries and veins that supply blood and nutrients to the adventitial and outer medial layers.

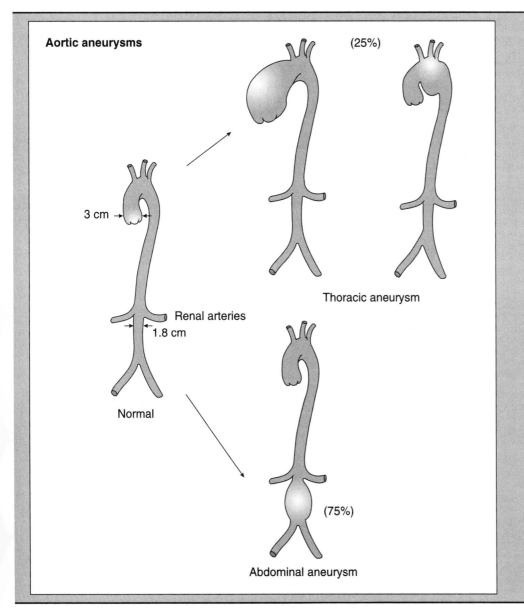

Aortic aneurysms

(25%)

3 cm

Renal arteries

1.8 cm

Normal

Thoracic aneurysm

(75%)

Abdominal aneurysm

FIG. 7-14
Aortic aneurysms can be found in any portion of the aorta, but most commonly they involve the abdominal aorta just below the renal arteries.

lecular defect of the media may also have an important pathogenetic role. Abdominal aortic aneurysms are usually fusiform and localized to the abdominal aorta distal to the renal arteries. Some researchers have postulated that since the intrarenal abdominal aorta does not have a vasa vasorum, atherosclerotic lesions in this region cause relative ischemia and increased injury to the inner wall of the media. Abdominal aortic aneuryms are more common in older people; it has been estimated that approximately 3% of people older than 50 years old have an abdominal aortic aneurysm.

While aortic aneurysms in any location can be associated with pain as they compress adjacent structures, in general they are asymptomatic until they rupture, which has catastrophic consequences. In general, the risk of rupture is related to size. For abdominal aortic aneurysms less than 4 cm in diameter, the risk for rupture has been estimated to be 0%–2% per year, while those greater than 5 cm in diameter have a 22% risk of rupture within 2 years. Less is known about thoracic aneurysms, but several small studies have suggested that the risk of rupture is higher when the aortic diameter increases to greater than 5 cm.

AORTIC DISSECTION

Dissection of the aorta is a catastophic event in which circulating blood causes separation of the media (see Fig. 7-13). Contrary to popular belief, aortic dissection is not commonly associated with aortic aneurysm; the term *dissecting aortic aneurysm* should be reserved for the small minority of cases in which patients survive the acute phase of aortic dissection and have aneurysmal dilatation of the false lumen. There are several reports of dissection of the aorta including Nicholl's autopsy of King George II in 1761. The first report of surgical repair of aortic dissection was made by Cooley in 1957.

Aortic dissection can occur in any portion of the aorta: ascending thoracic, descending thoracic, or abdominal aorta. While there are several classification schemes, aortic dissections can be simply classified as type A and type B (Fig. 7-15). In the more common type A dissection, the ascending thoracic aorta is involved. In type B dissections, the ascending thoracic aorta is not involved.

The two important factors for aortic dissection appear to be hypertension and degeneration of the media layer of the aorta. In general, hypertension is the most important factor, since elevated blood pressure is associated with approximately 80% of cases, and primary defects of the media can only be found in a small percentage of cases. However, conditions associated with a defect in the media layer (Marfan's syndrome, cystic medial necrosis) are often associated with an abnormally high incidence of aortic dissection. Aortic dissection can complicate any process that causes arterial inflamma-

FIG. 7-15
CLASSIFICATION OF AORTIC DISSECTION. Type A involves the ascending aorta (with or without involvement of the descending aorta), and type B involves the descending aorta only. (*Source:* Barre AE (ed): *Glenn's Thoracic and Cardiovascular Surgery*, 5th ed, vol 2. Norwalk, CT: Appleton & Lange, 1991, p 1957.)

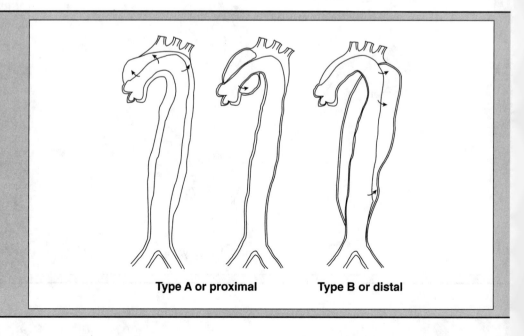

Type A or proximal   **Type B or distal**

tion such as giant cell arteritis. In addition, aortic dissection is associated with pregnancy, usually in the third trimester or in the immediate postpartum period. Table 7-2 summarizes the causes of aortic dissection.

Aortic dissection usually begins with an intimal tear that exposes the medial layer to intraluminal blood. The force of intraluminal blood (generated by ventricular contraction) causes separation of the medial layers. The separation of tissue progresses rapidly along the length of the aorta, within the media. The blood-filled space between the medial layers is called the false lumen. As the false lumen becomes distended with blood, secondary tears on the inner surface can be observed. In some cases, an intimal tear is not observed. It has been suggested that in this small minority of cases, rupture of a vessel in the vasa vasorum is the source of intramedial blood.

Table 7-2
Causes of Aortic Dissection

CAUSE	COMMENTS
Hypertension	The incidence of hypertension in patients with aortic dissection is approximately 75%. There is no solid link between hypertension and the initiation of the process of dissection; however, it is a major factor for progression.
Connective tissue disorders	
Marfan's syndrome	Approximately 4%–12% of patients with acute dissection have Marfan's syndrome.
Giant cell arteritis	
Polyarteritis nodosa	
Trauma	Aortic dissection may occur secondary to cardiac catheterization or surgical trauma.
Pregnancy	About 50% of aortic dissections in women under 40 occur during pregnancy, but the overall incidence is very low.

Aortic dissection is associated with sudden onset of severe chest or back pain. The site of pain will sometimes migrate, often following the path of the dissection itself. On physical examination both hypertension and hypotension can be observed. Absent pulses in the extremities can be observed if the dissection flap occludes the subclavian or femoral arteries. The dissection can rupture into the pleural, peritoneal, or pericardial spaces. Pericardial bleeding inevitably leads to pericardial tamponade physiology and extreme hypotension.

Case Study:
Continued

A transesophageal echocardiogram of Ms. Kelly is shown in Fig. 7-16. In transesophageal echocardiography, a probe is placed through the mouth and esophagus. A small transducer at the tip of the probe is capable of transmitting and receiving multiple ultrasound waves. The signals can be integrated by computer to form an image of the heart that can be observed on a video monitor. Since the esophagus and the aorta are anatomically very close to one another, detailed images of the ascending and descending aorta can be obtained. Notice the linear echogenic structure within the ascending thoracic aorta. Ms. Kelly had a type A aortic dissection (since the ascending thoracic aorta was involved). Suddenly Ms. Kelly's blood pressure precipitously dropped to unmeasurable levels, and she became unresponsive.

FIG. 7-16
TRANSESOPHAGEAL ECHOCAR-DIOGRAM OF MS. KELLY. (A) Schematic of a transesophageal echocardiogram. An ultrasonic transducer on the tip of the probe sends and receives signals that can be integrated into a planar image. (B) Actual image showing the dissection flap in the ascending aorta. (*Source:* Feigbaum H: *Echocardiography*, 5th ed. Philadelphia, PA: Lea & Febiger, 1994, p 110.)

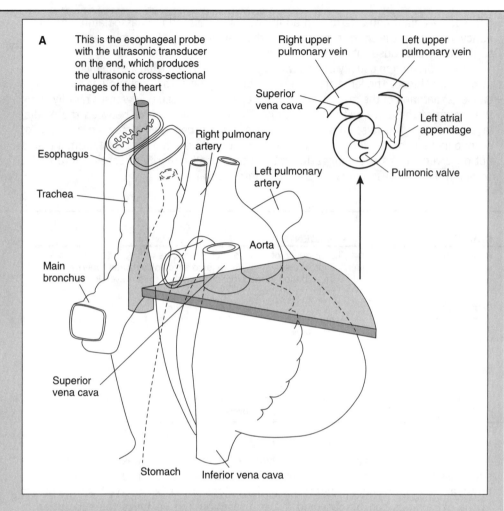

A This is the esophageal probe with the ultrasonic transducer on the end, which produces the ultrasonic cross-sectional images of the heart

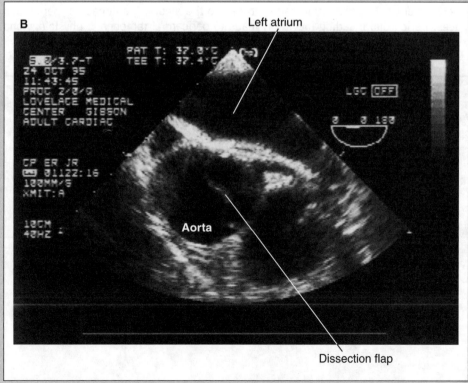

SHOCK

The essential function of the cardiovascular system is to supply adequate blood to tissues and organs to ensure adequate supply of oxygen and other nutrients and to allow removal of metabolic waste products. The word "shock" has been used medically to describe any abnormality that prevents the cardiovascular system from performing this basic function. Shock is normally manifested by low arterial blood pressure (hypotension) and can be broadly classified according to cardiac causes and noncardiac causes (Table 7-3).

TYPE	CAUSE
Cardiac	Electrical problems (bradycardia, tachycardia)
	Mechanical problems (muscle loss, valvular, pericardial tamponade)
Noncardiac	Extracardiac obstruction (pulmonary embolus, tension pneumothorax)
	Volume loss (bleeding, severe burn)
	Volume maldistribution (allergic reaction, sepsis)

Table 7-3
Classification of Shock

CARDIAC CAUSES

Cardiac causes of shock can be further subdivided into electrical and mechanical abnormalities. Shock resulting from an *electrical abnormality* is defined as any heart rhythm that does not allow adequate perfusion of the end-organs. As described in Chap. 2, abnormal heart rhythms can be due to heart rates that are too slow (bradycardia) or too fast (tachycardia). For example, when the heart rhythm is ventricular fibrillation, no measurable forward arterial blood flow occurs (Fig. 7-17). Rapid abnormal rhythms such as ventricular tachycardia can in some rare instances be associated with normal blood pressures, but usually this tachycardia is also associated with profound hypotension.

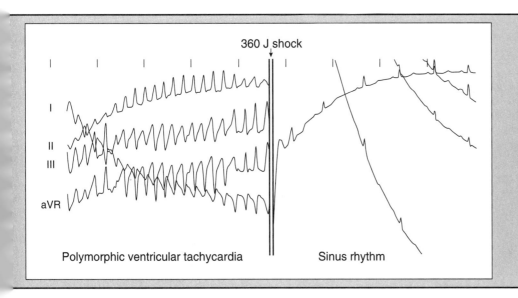

FIG. 7-17
Polymorphic ventricular tachycardia that does not allow adequate perfusion of blood is treated with a 360 J shock applied through the chest wall via special pads. After the shock, the patient returns to sinus rhythm with normal blood pressure.

Mechanical abnormalities of heart dysfunction include loss of systolic function from direct muscle injury (the presence of a large myocardial infarction), valvular abnormalities (severe stenosis or regurgitation of any of the heart valves), or from compression resulting from excess fluid in the pericardial space (pericardial tamponade).

NONCARDIAC CAUSES

Noncardiac shock can be due to acute *extracardiac obstruction* of blood flow. This usually occurs in the pulmonary circulation as the result of a massive pulmonary embolus or a tension pneumothorax that leads to "kinking" of the large pulmonary vessels. More commonly, noncardiac shock is due to profound *volume loss*, which causes reduced preload and reduced cardiac output. Hypovolemia can be due to any cause of acute blood loss or a severe burn, which leads to a large amount of plasma volume loss. The last noncardiac cause of shock has been termed *volume maldistribution*, in which peripheral resistance markedly decreases. One example of such shock is an allergic reaction, which results in release of a large amount of the potent vasodilator histamine. Profound vasodilation leads to profound hypotension despite normal cardiac function.

EVALUATION OF SHOCK

When one is confronted with a patient with shock, the first step is evaluation to see whether any arrhythmias are present (Fig. 7-18). If the patient has an abnormal tachycardia, prompt cardioversion is required to restore normal heart rhythms. This is done by applying large surface electrodes to the body and delivering large amounts of electrical energy (200–360 J). An example of a successful defibrillation is shown in Fig. 7-17. If the patient has profound bradycardia, large electrode patches can use lower energy to capture and depolarize the myocardium (temporary pacing). Temporary pacing in a patient with high-grade artioventricular (AV) block and no intrinsic escape pacemaker (such as the AV node) is shown in Fig. 7-19.

If the patient has a heart rhythm that should be associated with adequate perfusion and arterial pressures, evaluation for mechanical cardiac abnormalities and noncardiac causes should be sought. Physical examination is very important in this situation;

FIG. 7-18
FLOW DIAGRAM OF SHOCK. (*Source:* Kusumoto F: Cardiovascular disorders. In *Pathophysiology of Disease.* Edited by McPhee SJ, et al. Stamford, CT: Appleton & Lange, 1995, p 210.)

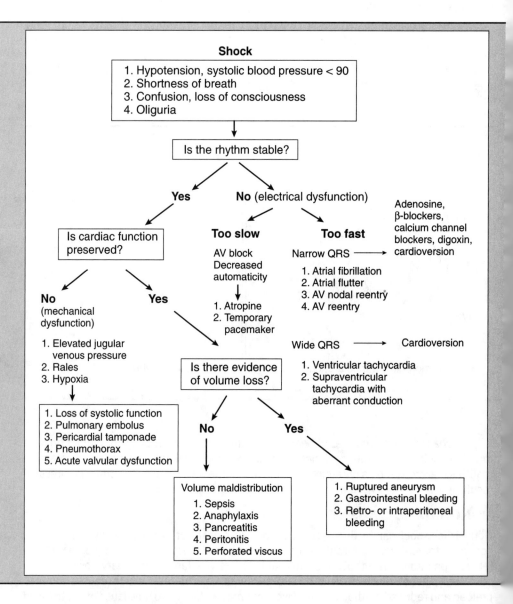

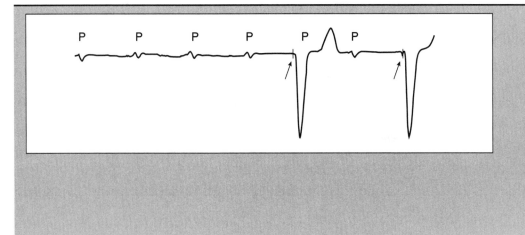

elevated jugular venous pressure and muffled heart sounds suggest pericardial tamponade; absent breath sounds in one lung field suggest a pneumothorax; a pulsating abdominal mass suggests an aortic aneurysm; fever suggests sepsis; and a skin rash could be the result of an allergic reaction. Additional tests such as a complete blood count (CBC), ECG, echocardiogram, and chest radiograph may also be useful in evaluating the patient with profound hypotension.

■ SUMMARY

Hypertension is often classified as primary, when no recognizable cause can be identified, and secondary if a separate cause of hypertension is present. While this classification schema is useful clinically, it reveals our ignorance of the pathophysiology of hypertension. As we learn more about the different etiologic mechanisms of primary hypertension our ability to treat this disease will become more effective. Hypertension causes significant damage to multiple organs: the eyes, kidneys, brain, and heart. Hypertension is an important risk factor for the development of atherosclerotic heart disease as discussed in Chap. 3. Hypertension is also the major cause of diseases of the aorta: aortic aneurysm and aortic dissection. The treatment of significant hypotension (shock) is a medical emergency. Shock can be due to both cardiac and noncardiac causes. Cardiac causes can be subdivided further into mechanical abnormalities and electrical abnormalities. Understanding the pathophysiology of both hypertension and hypotension is a necessary and fundamental part of medical education.

KEY POINTS

- Hypertension can be due to increased peripheral vascular resistance, increased cardiac output, or increases in both parameters.
- Hypertension can be classified as primary or secondary, depending on whether a separate defined cause can be identified. Primary hypertension is probably multifactorial.
- Hypertension causes significant damage to target organs (retina, central nervous system, heart, kidneys).
- Hypertension can lead to aortic aneurysm (dilatation of the aorta) or aortic dissection (bleeding into the medial space of the aorta).
- Shock or profound low blood pressure can be due to cardiac and noncardiac causes.

Case Study:
Resolution

Ms. Kelly's aorta dissected, and she now developed profound shock. Shock in association with an aortic dissection suggests that the ascending thoracic aorta is involved; it can be due to a number of causes. First, hypotension can be due to aortic rupture and exsanguination of blood into the pleural or peritoneal spaces. Second, if the aortic dissection involves the annulus of the aortic valve, severe acute aortic regurgitation can result in hemodynamic compromise. Third, the aortic dissection can extend into the pericardial space, leading to pericardial tamponade. Finally, in rare cases, the dissection can extend into the right coronary artery and cause a myocardial infarction, which can be associated with pump failure and arrhythmias. In Ms. Kelly's case, she was taken to the operating room, where a large type A aortic dissection that was bleeding into the pleural space was confirmed. The dissection was repaired, and Ms. Kelly had an uneventful postoperative course.

■ REVIEW QUESTIONS

1. Hypertension may be associated with

    (A) decreased cardiac output
    (B) increased peripheral vascular resistance
    (C) complete atrioventricular (AV) block
    (D) sepsis
    (E) tension pneumothorax

2. A possible secondary cause of hypertension is

    (A) coarctation of the aorta
    (B) blunted endothelial response to acetylcholine (ACh)
    (C) coronary artery disease
    (D) aortic aneurysm
    (E) aortic dissection

3. An aortic dissection is defined as

    (A) an abnormally narrowed aorta
    (B) a dilated portion of the aorta
    (C) separation of the aortic wall between the endothelium and muscular layers of the aorta
    (D) separation of the aortic wall between the adventitia and the media

4. Severe cardiac shock is characterized by

    (A) increased blood pressure
    (B) cold and clammy skin
    (C) warm skin
    (D) normal blood levels of lactic acid
    (E) increased urinary output

ANSWERS AND EXPLANATIONS

1. The answer is B. Hypertension may be caused by any condition associated with increased cardiac output or increased peripheral vascular resistance. Complete AV block would cause a reduced heart rate and may be associated with hypotension. Sepsis and tension pneumothorax are both noncardiac causes of shock (profound hypotension).

2. The answer is A. Coarctation of the aorta is a congenital abnormality that is characterized by a discrete narrowing in the aortic arch just after the origin of the left subclavian vein. This abnormality reduces blood flow to the renal arteries, which causes activation of the renin–angiotensin system and hypertension, particularly in the upper extremities. Aortic dissection is not a secondary cause of hypertension. As in the case study, hypertension predisposes patients to the development of aortic dissection. Aortic dissection is sometimes associated with profound hypotension (low blood pressure) and shock. Similarly hypertension predisposes patients to develop coronary artery disease or an aortic aneurysm. Blunted endothelial responses to ACh are possible mechanisms for primary hypertension.

3. The answer is C. Aortic dissection is normally characterized by separation of the intimal and medial layers of the aorta. An abnormal dilation of the aorta is termed an aortic aneurysm.

4. The answer is B. Shock can occur as a result of both cardiac and noncardiac causes. Skin color is dependent on the type of shock. When the shock is caused by severely reduced cardiac output, the arterioles and capillaries vasoconstrict in an effort to maintain systemic blood pressure. In shock resulting from endotoxemia, profound vasodilatation of the arterioles leads to warm skin. Shock is associated with low blood pressure and reduced urine output (reduced perfusion of the kidneys). In shock, lactic acid levels are usually elevated (the definition of shock is inadequate tissue perfusion).

REFERENCES

Kaplan N: *Clinical Hypertension*, 6th ed. Baltimore, MD: Williams & Wilkins, 1994.

Appendix I
PHYSICAL EXAMINATION AND ELECTROCARDIOGRAPHIC ABNORMALITIES

Fred M. Kusumoto, M.D.

■ CHAPTER OUTLINE

■ INTRODUCTION

The purpose of this appendix is to integrate some of the concepts that have been discussed in this text. *Cardiovascular Pathophysiology* was organized anatomically. We sequentially discussed overall chamber function, the specialized conduction system, the coronary arteries, the heart valves, the pericardium and the vascular system. However, in medicine, the physician is normally confronted with an abnormal clinical finding for which he or she must construct a differential diagnosis.

In this section the differential diagnosis of selected abnormal *physical examination* and *electrocardiographic findings* are discussed. It is hoped that the student will thus be helped to integrate different aspects of cardiovascular pathophysiology that have been reviewed in this book. Furthermore, it is very important for the student to become comfortable with physical examination skills, particularly cardiac auscultation.

■ PHYSICAL EXAMINATION

HEART SOUNDS

Since the invention of the stethoscope in the 1820s by Laënnec, physicians have carefully and methodically analyzed the sounds produced by the heart. Auscultation of the heart by an experienced examiner often identifies many cardiac disease states. Unfortunately, as technology has advanced and the field of medicine has substantially broadened, the time allotted to teaching auscultatory skills has decreased. However, auscultation of the heart is vitally important for integrating the pathophysiologic processes that we have described in this book.

Heart sounds are relatively short sounds heard by stethoscope. In contrast, heart murmurs, which are due to turbulent blood flow, are characterized by a *prolonged* series of vibrations that can be heard by stethoscope. In general, there are two types of heart sounds: high-frequency sounds made by sudden closing or opening of heart valves and low-frequency sounds that are due to ventricular filling. The first and second heart sounds (S_1 and S_2) are examples of high-frequency sounds associated with abrupt valve closure. While investigators have identified several components to the S_1, the S_1 is primarily due to closure of the mitral and tricuspid valves at the end of diastole. The second heart sound (S_2) is due to closure of the aortic valve (A_2) and pulmonic valve (P_2). Evaluation of the relationship between the A_2 and P_2 is reviewed in Chaps. 4 and 6 and is not discussed further here.

Two Types of Heart Sounds
High-frequency sounds of valve closure (S_1 and S_2)
Low-frequency sounds of ventricular filling (S_3 and S_4)

S_3 is a sound heard during early diastole.

In some conditions, low-frequency heart sounds in early diastole (third heart sound or S_3) and late diastole (fourth heart sound or S_4) can be appreciated (Fig. AI-1). The pathophysiologic causes of S_3 and S_4 are explored below.

FIG. AI-1
THE THIRD (S_3) AND FOURTH (S_4) HEART SOUNDS. In late diastole, just before S_1 and simultaneous with the P wave, a low-frequency S_4 can sometimes be heard. In early diastole, after the T wave, a low-frequency S_3 can sometimes be heard.

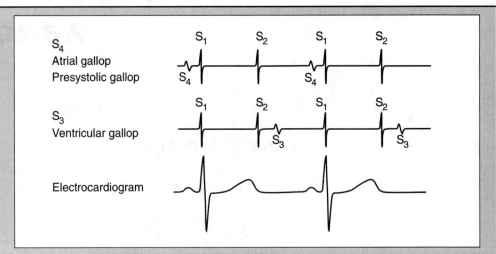

The S_3 can sometimes be heard after the S_2 (Fig. AI-1). The S_3 can be heard in a variety of conditions (Table AI-1); it is thought to be due to any condition associated with rapid early filling of the ventricle. For this reason, a *physiologic* S_3 can often be heard in children, adolescents, and young adults. However after age 40, an S_3 should be considered suspicious.

Table AI-1
Causes of a Third Heart Sound

Physiologic S_3
  Heard in children and young adults

Pathologic S_3
  Very rapid early diastolic ventricular filling
    Anemia
    Hyperthyroidism
    Mitral or tricuspid regurgitation
    "Left-to-right" shunts

  Ventricular dysfunction
    Ischemia
    Valvular abnormalities
    Congenital heart disease

  Restrictive or constrictive filling of the ventricle
    Pericardial constriction (pericardial knock)
    Ventricular hypertrophy

Pathologic S_3
Rapid, early ventricular filling
Ventricular dysfunction
Restricted ventricular filling

The S_3 is thought to arise from sudden deceleration of a column of blood filling the left ventricle when the elastic limit of the left ventricle is reached (Fig. AI-2). The sudden deceleration causes vibration, which can be appreciated as the low-frequency S_3. More recent investigation has suggested that the S_3 heard by cardiac auscultation is due to the actual impact of the left ventricle against the chest wall.

A *pathologic* S_3 can be heard in conditions associated with *rapid early diastolic filling, ventricular dysfunction*, and *restriction of ventricular filling* (Fig. AI-3). An S_3 produced by abnormally rapid early diastolic filling can be heard in anemia, hyperthyroidism, and severe mitral or tricuspid regurgitation. In ventricular dysfunction, the S_3 is due to ventricular enlargement to a point near the elastic limit of the left ventricle. Filling of the enlarged ventricle at elevated pressures leads to a forceful impact of the heart against the chest wall and an S_3. Finally, in conditions associated with restricted filling of the left ventricle, such as severe hypertrophy or pericardial thickening associated with constrictive physiology, an S_3 can be heard. When the sound is due to constrictive pericarditis, it is usually called a "pericardial knock." As mentioned in Chap. 5, the "pericardial knock" usually occurs earlier and is higher pitched than the S_3 resulting from ventricular dysfunction. However, the pathophysiologic genesis of the extra heart sound in both conditions is probably similar.

    S_4 occurs in late diastole and is probably due to vibrations that arise from atrial contraction (Fig. AI-4). For this reason, an S_4 is not heard when the patient does not have coordinated atrial contraction (atrial fibrillation). Like the S_3, the actual reason for an audible S_4 is due to either sudden deceleration of blood during atrial contraction or actual impact of the left ventricle against the chest wall.

S_4 is a sound heard during late diastole.

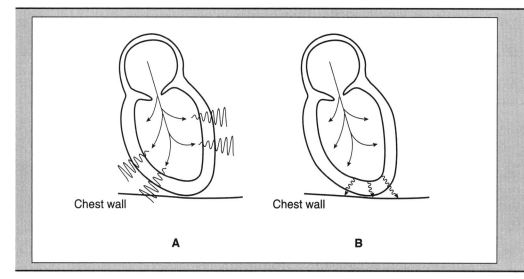

FIG. AI-2
GENESIS OF THE THIRD HEART SOUND (S_3). The genesis of the S_3 is thought to be due to sudden deceleration of the column of blood in the left ventricle (A), or the actual impact of the left ventricular apex against the chest wall (B).

    A soft physiologic S_4 can occasionally be heard in children (Table AI-2). In general, any S_4 should be considered suspicious. A pathologic S_4 is heard in two conditions. First, any condition that *decreases ventricular compliance* can make the vibrations from atrial filling audible. Ventricular hypertrophy and ventricular ischemia are the most common causes for reduced ventricular compliance. Less commonly, *atrial contraction associated with very rapid filling of the ventricle* can produce an audible S_4. Examples of this mechanism include anemia and thyrotoxicosis.

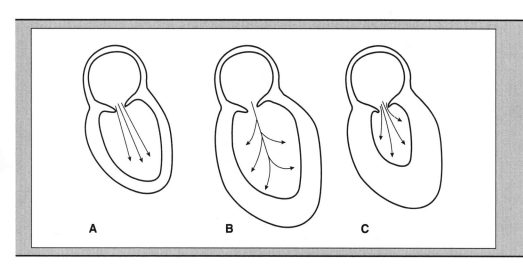

FIG. AI-3
THREE CONDITIONS ASSOCIATED WITH THE THIRD HEART SOUND S_3. Increased flow through the mitral valve (A), sudden cessation of flow into a dilated left ventricle (B), and sudden cessation of flow into a thickened hypertrophied ventricle (C).

FIG. AI-4
GENESIS OF THE FOURTH HEART SOUND (S$_4$). Atrial contraction causes increased flow across the mitral valve. If the ventricle is relatively noncompliant, sudden cessation of blood flow or actual impact of the thickened ventricle against the chest wall produces the S$_4$.

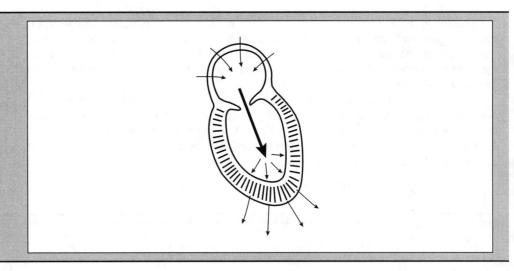

Table AI-2
Causes of a Fourth Heart Sound

Physiologic S$_4$
  Rarely heard in children

Pathologic S$_4$
  Very rapid late diastolic ventricular filling
    Anemia
    Hyperthyroidism
    Mitral or tricuspid regurgitation

  Decreased ventricular compliance
    Ischemia
    Ventricular hypertrophy

HEART MURMURS

The word *murmur* is derived from Latin and originally meant "rumbling or growling." Heart murmurs are prolonged sounds that arise from turbulent blood flow from one of four causes: (1) high rates of flow through normal valves, (2) forward flow through a narrowed or irregularly shaped valve, (3) backward flow through a leaking heart valve, or (4) flow through an abnormal cardiac or extracardiac connection. In general, murmurs are classified by whether they occur during systole (ventricular contraction) or diastole (ventricular filling).

Classification and Description of Murmurs
Timing (systolic versus diastolic)
Loudness (grades I–VI)
Pitch (high versus low frequency)
Radiation (neck, axilla, back)

Murmurs are further characterized by loudness and pitch. Traditionally, the loudness of murmurs is classified by a scheme developed in the early 1930s by Freeman and Levine (Table AI-3). Some murmurs are associated with enough turbulent flow that the vibrations can be palpated from the chest wall. This palpable vibration is called a *thrill*. The pitch of the heart murmur depends directly on the velocity of the turbulent flow. For example, in aortic regurgitation, blood flows from the high-pressure aorta into the low-pressure ventricle. The velocity of the regurgitant flow can be 4–5 m/sec and leads to a high-pitched early diastolic murmur. In contrast, mitral stenosis also causes turbulent flow during diastole, but the velocity is approximately 2 m/sec (since there is a smaller gradient between the two chambers and the orifice causing the turbulent flow is larger). Mitral stenosis is associated with a low-frequency murmur, frequently referred to as a "rumble." Careful attention to the pitch allows differentiation between these two types of diastolic murmurs.

Systolic murmurs are midsystolic or holosystolic.

Systolic Murmur. Systolic murmurs are classified by the portion of systole in which they are heard (Fig. AI-5). Midsystolic murmurs (also called *ejection murmurs*) are characterized by a distinct sound, often with a crescendo-decrescendo character that is separate from S$_1$ and S$_2$. The typical midsystolic murmur is due to turbulent flow in the left ventricular or right ventricular outflow tract or turbulent flow through the aortic or pulmonic valves. Mitral valve closure causes S$_1$; during isovolumic contraction no

Loudness
Grade I—very faint, difficult to hear
Grade II—faint, but easily heard
Grade III—moderately loud
Grade IV—very loud
Grade V—very loud, can be heard with the edge of the stethoscope to the skin
Grade VI—extremely loud, can be heard with the stethoscope off the skin

Pitch
High frequency—heard best with the diaphragm
Low frequency—heard best with the bell

Timing
Systolic
Diastolic
Continuous

Radiation
Neck
Axilla
Back

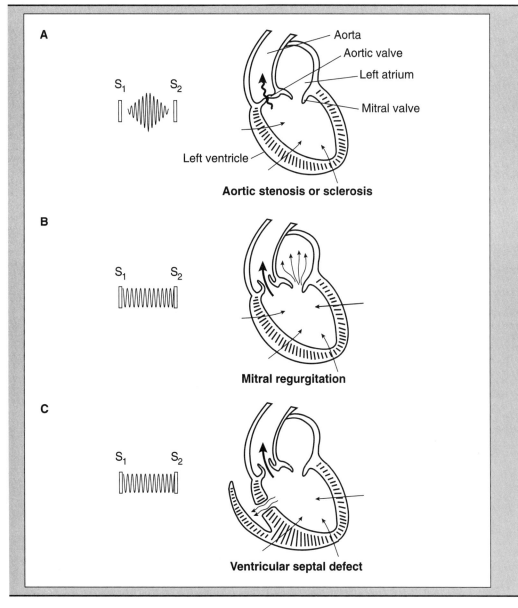

FIG. AI-5
SYSTOLIC MURMURS. (A) Turbulent flow across the aortic valve (stenotic or sclerotic) causes a midsystolic "ejection" murmur. (B) Turbulent flow produced by regurgitation of blood into the left atrium as a result of an incompetent mitral valve produces a holosystolic murmur. (C) Turbulent flow across a moderate ventricular septal defect also produces a holosystolic murmur.

murmur is heard. The ventricles contract, and flow out of the heart causes the murmur. As flow decreases in the latter parts of systole, the murmur decreases in intensity. Mid-systolic murmurs can be due to thickening (sclerosis) of the aortic or pulmonic valve with or without functional stenosis. In addition, left ventricular hypertrophy can sometimes be associated with a gradient in the left ventricular outflow tract and cause a systolic murmur.

The second type of systolic murmur is called holosystolic. Holosystolic murmurs begin with S_1 and end with S_2. Commonly, holosystolic murmurs obscure S_1 and S_2. Holosystolic murmurs occur when there is flow throughout systole from one chamber with higher pressure into another chamber with lower pressure. For example, a holosystolic murmur is heard when the mitral valve leaks and abnormal flow occurs from the left ventricle into the lower pressure left atrium. In addition, a moderate ventricular septal defect can be associated with a holosystolic murmur if flow occurs from the left ventricle into the lower pressure right ventricle.

Diastolic Murmurs. A diastolic murmur suggests that turbulent flow is occurring simultaneously with ventricular filling. Diastolic murmurs are classified by onset into *early*, *mid-*, and *late* diastolic murmurs (Fig. AI-6).

Holos means "entire" in Greek.

FIG. AI-6
DIASTOLIC MURMURS. (A) Turbulent flow produced by regurgitation of blood into the left ventricle as a result of an incompetent aortic valve produces an early diastolic murmur. (B) Turbulent flow across a stenotic mitral valve produces a low-frequency mid-diastolic rumble. The murmur begins after the second heart sound. (C) Turbulent flow across a stenotic mitral valve during atrial contraction produces a late diastolic murmur.

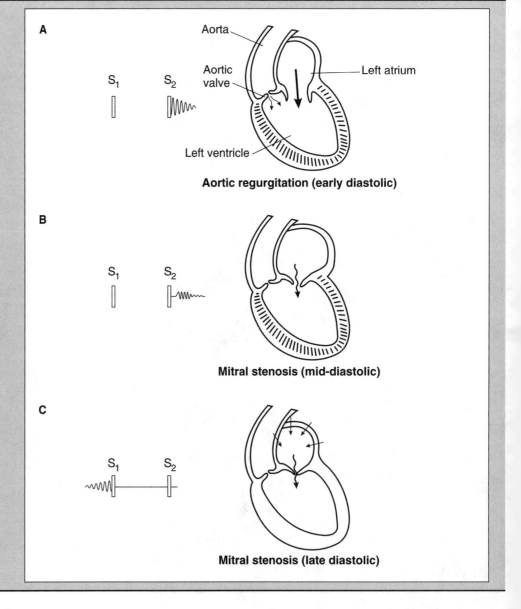

Early diastolic murmurs begin with S_2. The most common cause of an early diastolic murmur is aortic regurgitation. In aortic regurgitation, as left ventricular pressure falls below aortic pressure, blood leaks into the left ventricle through an abnormal aortic valve. In chronic aortic regurgitation, the murmur has a very high frequency; the duration of the murmur depends on the severity of the aortic regurgitation. In moderately severe chronic aortic regurgitation, the murmur can extend throughout diastole. In severe chronic aortic regurgitation, the diastolic murmur has more of a decrescendo character as the difference between aortic and ventricular pressures becomes smaller. In acute severe aortic regurgitation, the murmur is quite short and has a much lower frequency. Another cause of an early diastolic murmur is pulmonary valve regurgitation (normally produced by elevated pulmonary artery pressures), which is called a Graham Steell's murmur.

In a mid-diastolic murmur, the murmur is heard distinctly after S_2. The prototypic cause of mid-diastolic murmurs is tricuspid valve or mitral valve stenosis. Both of these valvular abnormalities produce a low-frequency "rumble." The murmur of tricuspid stenosis increases with inspiration as a result of increased right-sided blood flow.

A late diastolic murmur is heard just before the S_1. Tricuspid valve and mitral valve stenosis both can be associated with a late diastolic murmur as a result of increased flow across these valves during atrial contraction. Another cause of a late diastolic murmur is severe chronic aortic regurgitation. As Austin Flint eloquently described in the mid 1800s, aortic regurgitation can cause partial closure of the mitral valve, which then causes turbulent flow through the mitral valve when the left atrium contracts (see Chap. 4).

ELEVATED JUGULAR VENOUS PRESSURE

Jugular venous pressure is a reflection of right atrial pressure. Any cause of elevated right atrial pressure results in elevated jugular venous pressure. The causes of elevated jugular venous pressure are summarized in Table AI-4.

Table AI-4
Causes of Elevated Jugular Venous Pressure

Pericardial disease
   Constrictive pericarditis
   Pericardial tamponade

Right ventricular failure
   Right ventricular myocardial ischemia and infarction
   Pulmonary hypertension
   Left ventricular failure

Valvular abnormalities
   Pulmonic valve stenosis or regurgitation
   Tricuspid valve stenosis or regurgitation

ELECTROCARDIOGRAPHIC ABNORMALITIES

Like the physical examination, the electrocardiogram (ECG) offers several excellent opportunities for integrating concepts in cardiovascular pathophysiology.

ST-SEGMENT ELEVATION

Causes of ST-Segment Elevation
Early repolarization
Myocardial infarction
Printzmetals's angina
Pericarditis

Normally the ST segment on the ECG is isoelectric. At this time in the cardiac cycle, normally the ventricles are depolarized, and the individual ventricular myocytes are at the plateau phase. For this reason, no large voltage gradients can be measured from the surface ECG. However, several abnormalities can cause a relative voltage gradient to be measured during this period, and it can manifest as ST-segment elevation on the surface ECG.

First, ST-segment elevation can be observed as a normal finding in young people. This condition is commonly referred to as early repolarization (Fig. AI-7). Some experimental data suggest that patients with early repolarization have relatively heterogeneous repolarization. Certain myocytes have a large population of the transient outward current (I_{to}) [see Chap. 2], which causes voltage gradients to exist during the normally isoelectric ST segment.

FIG. AI-7
**A NORMAL 12-LEAD ELECTRO-
CARDIOGRAM SHOWING EARLY
REPOLARIZATION.**

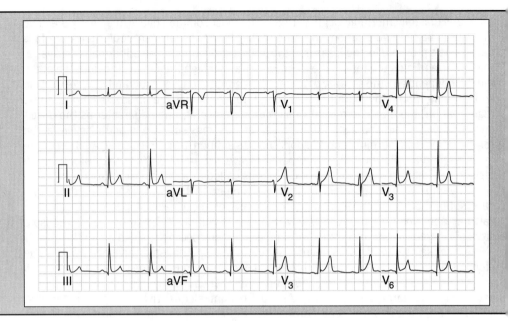

Second, ST-segment elevation can be observed in myocardial infarction. As discussed in Chap. 3, occlusion of blood causes ST-segment elevation to be observed on the ECG if the positive electrode is directly over the injured area. The ST-segment elevation can be due to either systolic or diastolic effects. The ECG is useful for the diagnosis and localization of myocardial injury resulting from coronary artery occlusion. Morphologically, the ST segment often has a domed appearance ("concave down"), but any type of ST-segment elevation in the setting of symptoms suggestive of coronary ischemia should be regarded with suspicion.

ST-segment elevation can also be seen in Printzmetal's angina. Remember that some patients can develop chest pain from myocardial ischemia resulting from spasm of the coronary arteries. In this case, the large epicardial coronary arteries suddenly constrict and cause transmural ischemia to the myocardium supplied by that vessel. For this reason, transient ST-segment elevation can be observed on the ECG.

Finally, ST-segment elevation can be observed in pericarditis. The mechanism for ST-segment elevation in pericarditis is not completely worked out, but it appears to be due to superficial epicardial cell "injury" that is just underneath the inflamed pericardium. This leads to diffuse ST-segment elevation in all leads except for lead aVR (see Chap. 5, Fig. 5-1). The ST-segment elevation in pericarditis often has a "concave up" appearance. In addition to diffuse ST-segment elevation, since inflamed pericardium also covers the atria, diffuse PR-segment depression, particularly in the inferior leads (II, III, aVF), and isolated PR-segment elevation in lead aVR can be observed.

CHANGES IN QRS VOLTAGE AND P-WAVE SIZE

Increased and decreased QRS voltages can be observed in a variety of settings. Increased QRS voltage is due to either increased muscle mass or reduced soft tissue between the heart and the surface electrodes. Decreased QRS voltage can be observed in conditions that increase the distance between the heart and the surface recording electrodes, such as pericardial effusion and chronic obstructive pulmonary disease. Decreased QRS voltages can also be seen in conditions associated with infiltration of normal myocardium with abnormal tissues, such as amyloidosis.

The size of the P wave most commonly reflects the size of the atria. In general, large atria are associated with large P waves. For example, patients with mitral stenosis frequently have very large P waves because of hypertrophy and increased size of the left atrium, which must contract against a narrowed mitral valve orifice.

Lead aVR is the only lead where the positive electrode is located directly "over" the atria.

In **amyloidosis**, abnormal twisted β-pleated sheet proteins are deposited in various organs.

■ REVIEW QUESTIONS

Directions: For each of the following questions, choose the **one best** answer.

1. Tyler Gross is a 48-year-old man with no significant medical history. He was in his usual state of health when he suddenly passed out 5 days ago while running. On physical examination, Mr. Gross is noted to have a systolic murmur on cardiac auscultation, and his carotid upstrokes are delayed. What other physical examination findings would you expect to find?

    (A) The systolic murmur obscures the first (S_1) and second (S_2) heart sounds (holosystolic).
    (B) The diastolic blood pressure is extremely low (48 mm Hg).
    (C) The systolic murmur has a crescendo-decrescendo quality.
    (D) A loud mid-diastolic rumble can be appreciated.

2. Ashley Henderscheid is a 42-year-old woman who is noted to have a holosystolic murmur. What is the valvular abnormality that is the most likely cause of her cardiac auscultatory findings?

    (A) Aortic stenosis
    (B) Pulmonic stenosis
    (C) Mitral regurgitation
    (D) Patent ductus arteriosus

3. Sarah Figueredo is a 33-year-old woman with a history of rheumatic fever as a child. She has had progressive exertional shortness of breath for the past 2 months. On physical examination, her heart rate (HR) is regular (74 beats/min), and she is noted to have a mid-diastolic murmur. What other finding would you expect to note?

    (A) Holosystolic murmur
    (B) Late diastolic murmur
    (C) Increased QRS size on the electrocardiogram (ECG)
    (D) Decreased P wave on the ECG

(*Questions continue*)

4. Hannah Reynolds is a 32-year-old woman who has experienced 2 days of severe chest pain that is worse with inspiration. Her electrocardiogram (ECG) is shown below. What is the likely cause of her symptoms?

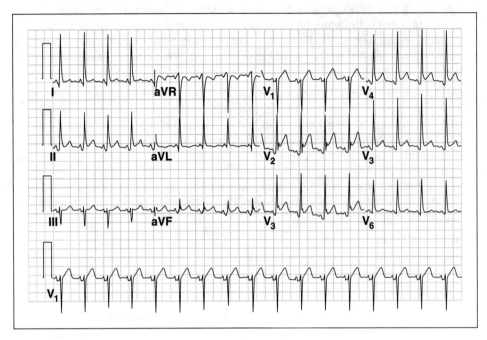

(A) Aortic stenosis
(B) Myocardial infarction
(C) Printzmetal's angina
(D) Pericarditis
(E) Pericardial tamponade

■ ANSWERS AND EXPLANATIONS

1. The answer is C. Systolic murmurs suggest turbulent flow during ventricular contraction. Stenosis of the pulmonic or aortic valves, regurgitation of the mitral or tricuspid valves, or a ventricular septal defect can cause systolic murmurs. The additional physical examination finding of a decreased carotid upstroke makes aortic stenosis the most likely cause for this patient's symptoms. Passing out, or syncope, is a manifestation of aortic stenosis. With exertion, peripheral circulation dilates, but the cardiac output is relatively fixed (since only a small amount of blood can be ejected through the stenotic aortic valve), which leads to decreased perfusion to the brain and syncope. The murmur of aortic stenosis has a crescendo-decrescendo quality. A holosystolic murmur is characteristic of mitral regurgitation; a low diastolic pressure suggests aortic regurgitation; and a mid-diastolic rumble is most commonly associated with mitral stenosis.

2. The answer is C. A holosystolic murmur is usually associated with mitral regurgitation. Aortic stenosis and pulmonic stenosis cause crescendo-decrescendo midsystolic murmurs. A patent ductus arteriosus is usually associated with a continuous murmur heard through both systole and diastole.

3. The answer is B. Ms. Figueredo has mitral stenosis resulting from rheumatic heart disease. In addition, since her HR is regular, she is probably in sinus rhythm. In mitral stenosis the left ventricle is "protected" from abnormal pressure and volume loads (see Chap. 4), and an increase in the size of the QRS complex (which would suggest left ventricular hypertrophy) is uncommon. Similarly, since the left atrium must contract against a gradient, the P wave is normally larger rather than smaller because of left atrial hypertrophy. Atrial contraction against the stenotic mitral valve causes the late diastolic murmur associated with mitral stenosis. Finally, while it is possible that Ms. Figueredo has "mixed" valvular disease (both mitral stenosis and mitral regurgitation), a holosystolic murmur (resulting from mitral regurgitation) is not an expected finding.

4. The answer is D. Ms. Reynold's ECG is characterized by diffuse ST-segment elevation consistent with pericarditis. ST-segment elevation resulting from myocardial infarction or Printzmetal's angina is generally more localized (since occlusion occurs in one coronary artery). Aortic stenosis can be associated with left ventricular hypertrophy and a larger QRS complex but not with ST-segment elevation. Similarly, pericardial tamponade does not characteristically cause ST-segment elevation, but rather the QRS complex is smaller.

In addition to the diffuse ST-segment elevation, notice that there is PR-segment depression in all leads except for aVR, where PR-segment elevation is observed. Diffuse PR-segment changes are fairly specific for pericarditis.

Appendix II

DIAGNOSTIC TESTS

Fred M. Kusumoto, M.D.

■ CHAPTER OUTLINE

Echocardiography
Stress Testing
Cardiac Catheterization

In this appendix a brief description of each of the various diagnostic tests available to the cardiologist is given. It is important for the student to keep in mind that history, physical examination, and (to some extent) the electrocardiogram (ECG) are the most useful tools available to the cardiologist. Technology has complemented these basic skills, not replaced them. Potentially useful diagnostic tests for various pathophysiologic conditions are summarized in Table AII-1.

Table AII-1
Commonly Used Diagnostic Tests for Particular Cardiovascular Conditions

Heart failure
  Echocardiography

Valvular disease
  Echocardiography
  Transesophageal echocardiography
  Cardiac catheterization

Coronary artery disease
  Stress testing (electrocardiography, echocardiography, nuclear imaging)
  Cardiac catheterization

Pericardial disease
  Echocardiography

Congenital heart disease
  Echocardiography
  Transesophageal echocardiography
  Cardiac catheterization

■ ECHOCARDIOGRAPHY

Echocardiography is arguably the most important diagnostic test that has been developed in cardiology. A transducer emits short bursts of high-frequency signals (> 20 kHz) of low intensity. Signal reflection delineates boundaries between cardiac structures. For example, blood is not very echogenic, while the cardiac valves are very echogenic, and myocardial tissue has an intermediate value.

Although there are several different types of echocardiography, this discussion focuses only on two-dimensional echocardiography. In two-dimensional echocardiography, multiple ultrasound beams are directed along an arc (Fig. AII-1). The returning signals are integrated into an image that can be produced on video. Several standardized positions for "slicing" the heart have been developed. Two positions are commonly used: the left parasternal area and the apex (Fig. AII-2). In both of these two positions the plane of the arc can be positioned at right angles, either vertically or horizontally. From the apical position when the plane is oriented horizontally, all four chambers of the heart and the mitral and tricuspid valves can be observed (Fig. AII-3).

The transducer is normally located on a hand-held probe that accesses the heart from the surface. The transducer can also be mounted on a probe that can be placed within the esophagus (Fig. AII-4). The esophagus is located just behind the left atrium and provides an excellent view of the heart.

FIG. AII-1
SCHEMATIC SHOWING THE PROCESS OF TWO-DIMENSIONAL ECHOCARDIOGRAPHY. Low-energy sound waves are continuously emitted from a transducer. Two echogenic structures reflect the sound waves. The returning signals are integrated by a computer and visualized on a video screen.

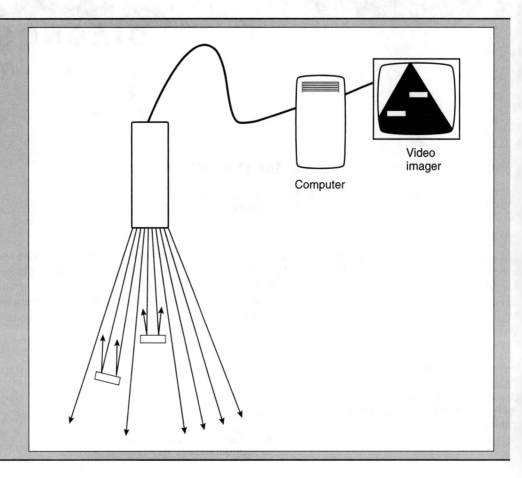

FIG. AII-2
The transducer is placed in the left parasternal area or near the cardiac apex.

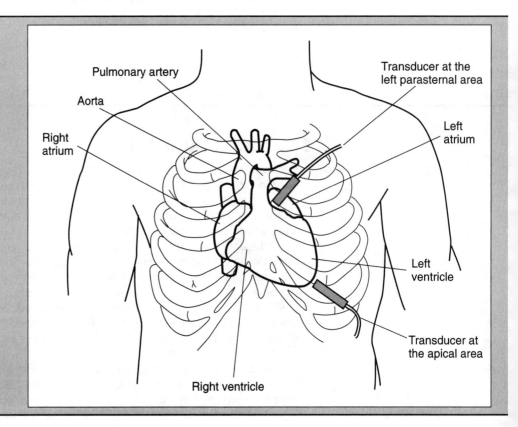

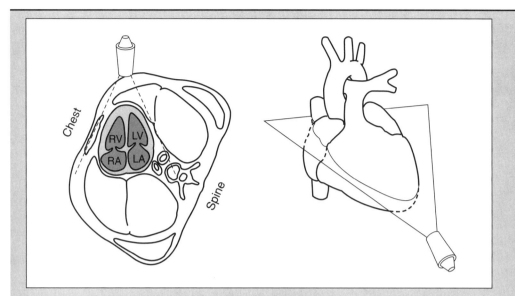

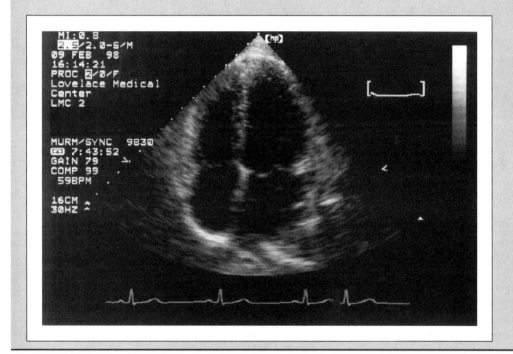

FIG. AII-3
TWO-DIMENSIONAL ECHOCAR-DIOGRAPHIC IMAGE OBTAINED FROM THE APEX WITH THE IMAGING PLANE ORIENTED HORIZONTALLY. In this view the ventricles, the atria, and the mitral and tricuspid valves can be imaged. Transducer position relative to the heart is shown in the *upper left*. A schematic of the chamber anatomy in this plane is in the *upper right*. The *bottom panel* shows the actual echocardiographic image. LA = left atrium; LV = left ventricle; RA = right atrium; RV = right ventricle. (*Source:* Courtesy of Maggie Nielsen, Lovelace Medical Center, Albuquerque, New Mexico.)

FIG. AII-4
THE ULTRASOUND TRANSDUCER CAN ALSO BE MOUNTED ON AN ESOPHAGEAL PROBE. The esophagus is located just behind the left atrium. This anatomic relationship allows transesophageal echocardiography to provide very clear views of the heart. (*Source:* Adapted with permission from Feigenbaum H: *Echocardiography,* 5th ed. Philadelphia, PA: Lea & Febiger, 1994, p 110.)

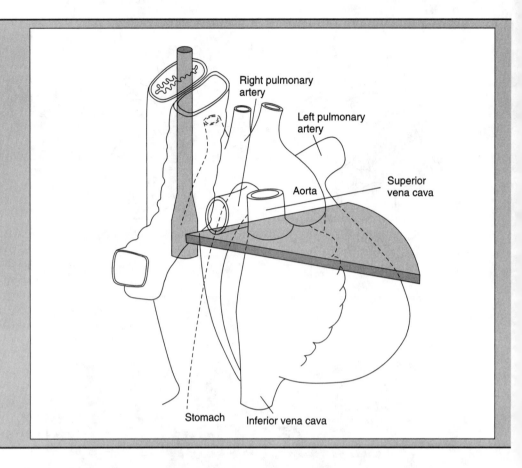

Right pulmonary artery

Left pulmonary artery

Superior vena cava

Aorta

Stomach   Inferior vena cava

■ STRESS TESTING

Coronary artery disease is one of the most commonly encountered cardiology problems. To evaluate for the presence or absence of coronary artery disease, stress testing is commonly used. There are many different types of stress testing, but all involve some sort of physiologic stress (chemical, exercise) and some way of monitoring the heart (ECG, echocardiography, nuclear imaging) both at rest and during stress. Fig. AII-5 shows an ECG in a patient at rest and during peak exercise. The patient has a narrowing of the right coronary artery, which caused myocardial ischemia. Myocardial ischemia, in turn, caused ST-segment depression to be observed on the surface ECG in lead II. Remember from Chap. 3 that ischemia is a common cause of ST-segment depression.

Stress testing is an important tool that provides a noninvasive method for evaluating for the presence or absence of significant narrowing of the coronary arteries. However, it is important to remember that some ischemic syndromes, such as unstable angina and

FIG. AII-5
Electrocardiographic lead II in a patient with a significant narrowing in the right coronary artery both at rest (A) and after 8 minutes of exercise (B). Notice that after exercise, there is significant ST-segment depression (*arrow*), which suggests that the exercise induced myocardial ischemia. (*Source:* Courtesy of Margaret Abeyta, Lovelace Medical Center, Albuquerque, New Mexico.)

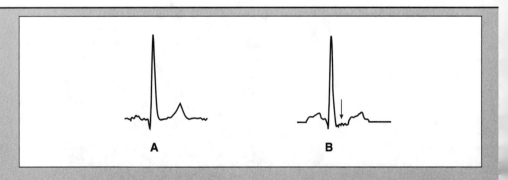

A   B

myocardial infarction, are most commonly due to ulceration of an unstable plaque that leads to intravascular thrombosis. Stress testing can evaluate only for the presence or absence of fixed lesions. Unfortunately there is no test available that evaluates the "stability" of atherosclerotic plaques.

■ CARDIAC CATHETERIZATION

In the period from the 1920s to the 1950s, several intrepid investigators showed the feasibility of placing catheters directly in the heart. In 1929, Werner Forssman inserted a catheter through his own antecubital vein and, using fluoroscopy and a mirror, managed to direct the catheter into his right atrium. He then walked down to the radiology department so that he could obtain a confirmatory roentgenogram (x-ray). After this, Cournand, Richards, and other investigators used direct catheterization of the cardiac chambers (in patients) to evaluate the hemodynamic function of the heart. Direct placement of catheters within the chambers of the heart and the coronary arteries (cardiac catheterization) has become an important and commonly used tool that is currently the "gold standard" test of cardiology.

Measurement of Pressures and Delineation of Cardiac Chambers. Catheters (small tubes) can be placed directly in any of the cardiac chambers to measure pressures (Fig. AII-6). In the example, a patient with aortic stenosis has pressures measured simultaneously in the left ventricle and the aorta to determine the severity of the gradient.

In addition to measurement of pressures, injection of radiopaque dye through the catheters can delineate the internal structure of the heart. This is a way to measure the systolic function of the heart.

Evaluation of the Coronary Anatomy. In 1958, Sones developed a method that allowed selective cannulation of the left and right coronary arteries via a small tube inserted into an antecubital vein. In the mid 1960s, Judkins and Amplatz developed preformed catheters that can be inserted through the femoral artery and reliably cannulate the coronary arteries (Fig. AII-7). After the coronary artery is cannulated, dye can be injected into the artery, and the presence or absence of flow-limiting atherosclerotic lesions can be determined. Once the number and severity of lesions are defined, the appropriate treatment can be chosen.

Cardiac Catheterization
Catheters are placed into the cardiac chambers to measure intracardiac pressures and, using radiopaque dye, determine structure and function of each cardiac chamber. Commonly, only the function of the left ventricle is so tested.

Catheters are placed into the coronary artery orifices. Injected dye delineates coronary anatomy.

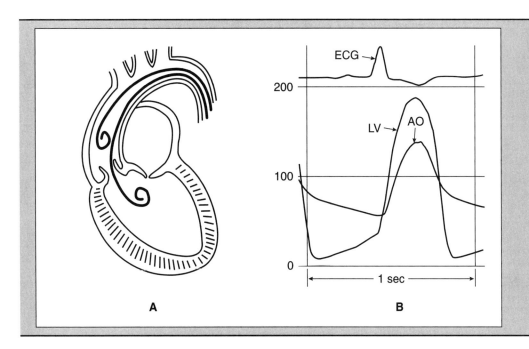

A   **B**

FIG. AII-6
(A) Catheters (this particular type of catheter is called a *pigtail*) are placed in the left ventricle and the aorta of a patient with aortic stenosis. (B) Simultaneous measurement of pressures provides information on the severity of the aortic stenosis. AO = aorta; ECG = electrocardiogram; LV = left ventricle.

FIG. AII-7
A specially shaped catheter is placed in the right femoral artery and maneuvered to the orifice of the coronary artery. Dye is injected through a syringe which delineates the coronary artery anatomy.

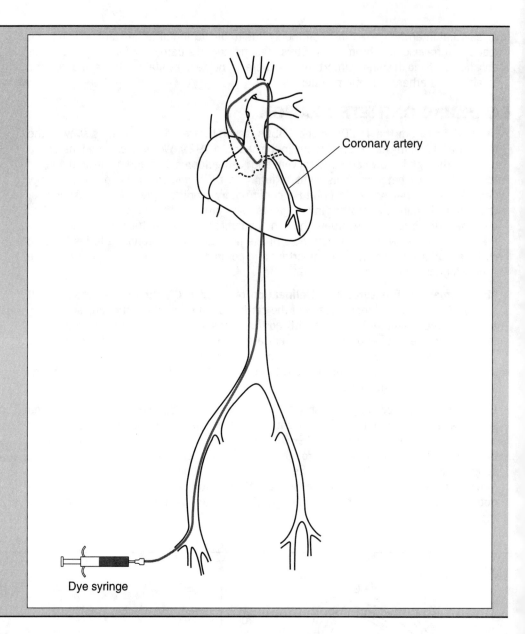

Coronary artery

Dye syringe

■ REFERENCES

Baim DS, Grossman W: *Cardiac Catheterization, Angiography, and Intervention.* Baltimore, MD: Williams & Wilkins, 1996.

Feigenbaum H: *Echocardiography*, 5th ed. Philadelphia, PA: Lea & Febiger, 1994.

Roberts SO, Robergs RA, Hanson P (eds): *Clinical Exercise Testing and Prescription: Theory and Application.* Boca Raton, FL: CRC Press, 1997.

INDEX

NOTE: An "f" after a page number denotes a figure; a "t" after a page number denotes a table.

normal, 224
relationship of to CO and peripheral resistance, 224, 225f
and renal retention of Na+, 224–225, 224f
Borrelia burgdorferi, 27
Bradycardias, 67–70
as cause of shock, 239t
causes and mechanistic sites of, 69f
Bradykinin, 97f, 226
Breathlessness. *See* Dyspnea
Bulbus cordis, 194, 194f, 195f, 197, 197f
Bundle branch block, 68–70, 69f
Bundle branches, 54f

C

CABG. *See* Coronary artery bypass graft surgery
Calcium (Ca2+)
accumulation of in cytoplasm with ischemia, 25
Ca2+-ATPase, 6, 6f, 40, 97, 98f
pump, 6, 6f, 40, 43f, 46
Ca2+–calmodulin complex, 94, 96f
channel(s)
blockers, 120, 240f
general structure of, 43–44, 45f
Ca2+-L, 43t, 51–52
Ca2+-release, 6
α-subunit of, 44, 45f, 51
Ca2+-T, 43f
concentration, intracellular
versus extracellular, 46f, 47f
increased
with hypertension, 226, 227f
with myocardial infarction, 121
with triggered tachycardia, 70
conductance (gCa2+), 46, 50f
current, long-lasting (I_{Ca-L}), 43t, 49f, 55, 58
deposition of in atherosclerotic lesions, 107
and inotropic state of myocyte, 13f, 15, 15f, 16, 16f
inward flow of during action potential, 51
movement of in myocyte during cardiac cycle, 6f, 29, 40
Na+–Ca2+ exchanger, 43f, 121
regulation of intracellular concentration of, 5–7, 6f, 7f
and relaxation of myocyte, 5, 5f, 6f
in smooth muscle
contraction (vasoconstriction), 94–95, 96f, 98–99, 99f
relaxation (vasodilation), 97, 98f
Calmodulin, 94–95, 96f
cAMP. *See* Cyclic adenosine monophosphate
Candida, 178t
Carcinoid syndrome, 167
Cardiac
action potentials. *See* Membrane, action potentials of
cells, classification of, 84
cycle, analysis of. *See* Pressure-time analysis and Pressure-volume analysis
myocytes
cellular architecture of, 2–4, 2f
contractile properties of isolated fiber of, 13–15, 13f–15f
oxygen demand of, 118
output
decreased by
aortic stenosis, 147
pericardial tamponade, 184, 184f
definition of, 11–13, 38
factors affecting, 18
normal, 12t
relationship of to CO and peripheral resistance, 224–225, 225f
physiology
normal, 2–18
right and left, compared, 10–11, 11f
Cardiomyopathy, 1–2, 27–30

alcoholic, 27
congestive, 28
dilated, 28
hypertrophic, 29–33
anatomic classification of, 31t
heart murmurs with, 32f
pressure-volume relationship with, 32f
idiopathic, 27
infiltrative, 30
ischemic, 26
Catecholamines, 6, 13, 225–226, 225f
Catheterization, cardiac, 261–262, 261f, 262f
Cellular
architecture, 2–4
membrane. *See* Membrane
physiology, normal, 2–7
Central nervous system, in hypertension, 231
Chagas' disease, 24t
Channels. *See* Ion channels
Charcot-Bouchard aneurysm, 231
Chemotactic agents, 100–101, 108f
Chest pain. *See* Angina
CHF. *See* Congestive heart failure
Chlamydia, 101
Cholesterol, 103–105
serum levels of, and coronary artery disease rates, 104f
Chordae tendineae, 7, 158f, 161t, 198, 198f
Chromaffin cells, 230
Chylomicrons, 103–105, 104f
Cigarette smoking, 101, 113–114
Circulation, fetal to newborn, 199–200, 199f
CK. *See* Creatine kinase
Clubbing, 207, 209, 215
CO. *See* Cardiac output
Coagulation system activation, 111–112, 113f
Coarctation of aorta. *See* Aorta, coarctation of
Cobalt, 27
Cocaine, 27
Coccidiomycosis, 178t
Cocksackie B virus, 24t, 26, 178t
Coelom, intraembryonic, 193, 193f, 194f
Collagen fibers
degradation of, as initiating cause of plaque disruption, 120
in pericardium, 175, 176f
platelet adherence to, 111, 112f
Collateral flow, 121
Comorbid maternal disease, 192
Compact AV node, 56
Compliance
definition of, 10
measurement of by diastolic pressure curve, 143–144
of ventricle, 17, 28, 40, 143–144, 147
Complicated lesion, atherosclerotic, 105, 106f
Conduction velocities in various tissues, 58t
Congenital heart disease. *See* Heart disease, congenital
Congestive
cardiomyopathy, 28
heart failure (CHF), 148, 165
Connecting stalk, 193, 193f
Connexins, 56, 57f
Contraceptives (oral) and hypertension, 229, 229t
Contractile state. *See* Inotropic state
Contractility
increased
by higher Ca2+ concentrations, 15, 15f, 18
relationship of to CO, blood pressure, and peripheral resistance, 225f
reduced
effect of on volume-pressure curve, 19, 19f, 22, 22f
by myocardial ischemia, 24, 121–122
Contraction
of cardiac myocyte, 4–6, 5f, 6f, 13–15, 13f–15f
isometric, 12, 14, 14f
isotonic, 15